Drugs for Mental Illness

A Series of Books in Psychology

Editors:
Richard C. Atkinson
Gardner Lindzey
Richard F. Thompson

Drugs for Mental Illness

A Revolution in Psychiatry

Marvin E. Lickey
Barbara Gordon

Department of Psychology and Institute of Neuroscience
University of Oregon

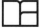

W. H. Freeman and Company
New York

Project Editor: Larry Olson

Copy Editor: Diane Silver

Designer: Gary Head

Production Coordinator: Bill Murdock

Compositor: Graphic Typesetting Service

Printer and Binder: The Maple-Vail Book Manufacturing Group

Library of Congress Cataloging in Publication Data

Lickey, Marvin E., 1937—
   Drugs for mental illness.

   (A Series of books in psychology)
   Includes bibliographies and index.
   1. Psychopharmacology—Popular works. 2. Schizophre-
nia—Chemotherapy. 3. Depression, Mental—Chemotherapy.
I. Gordon, Barbara, 1942–   . II. Title. III. Series.
[DNLM: 1. Mental disorders—Drug therapy. WM 402
L711d]
RC483.L47 1983   616.89'18   83-1569
ISBN 0–7167–1457–4
ISBN 0–7167–1458–2 (pbk.)

Printed in the United States of America.

6 7 8 9 10   VB   5 4 3 2 1 0 8 9 8

Contents

Preface

This book is for everyone who is interested in learning about drug treatments in modern psychiatry. It is a summary and an explanation of some important medical research on schizophrenia, mania, depression, and anxiety. It describes diagnostic procedures, the evidence that drugs are effective, the risks of drug treatment, and how the drugs affect the brain. It begins and ends with a discussion of frequently voiced philosophical and ethical concerns about drug treatments for mental illness.

This book is also for people who are close to mental illness as patients or as family and friends of patients. Most people are uncertain about when psychiatric treatment is needed, how to choose a psychiatrist, or how to evaluate the treatment. We aim to demystify psychiatry. By learning something about psychiatry, you may become less fearful and more capable of responding constructively when mental illness strikes nearby.

This is not a self-help book. It may help you to converse with a psychiatrist or help you to get the most that psychiatry has to offer, but it does not propose do-it-yourself treatments. The disorders we discuss are serious, and people with serious mental illnesses need the professional expertise of psychiatrists. Psychiatry is no longer an inchoate specialty where ignorance is disguised as theory. Biological psychiatry can even be called a fast-moving field. By the time you read this book, some of the treatments we describe may have been replaced by better ones.

Although this book is about drug treatments, we do not want to leave the impression that there is a drug for every mental health problem. There are many conditions for which drug treatment is ill advised or harmful. Psychotherapy is not in danger of being displaced by chemicals. Clinical psychology is also a fast-moving field and, like psychiatry, is becoming more effective as knowledge accumulates through research.

We owe special thanks to our undergraduate students. Without their stimulation we would not have recognized the need for such a book. We also thank Dr. Philip A. Berger of the Stanford University Medical Center and Dr. John M. Davis of the Illinois Mental Health Institutes for their conscientious and penetrating reviews of the manuscript. We thank Mary Ross for typing early drafts of the manuscript and Jeffrey Moran for introducing us to word processing with microcomputers. Finally, we thank our children, Sarah, David, Ingrid, Abe, and Rachel. They gave us time by foregoing automobile rides and riding their bicycles, even in the rain. They gave up vacations and weekends at the coast, did extra chores at home, and tolerated our preoccupations. Most of all we thank them for their encouragement.

January 1983   Marvin E. Lickey
                                                  Barbara Gordon

For Beverly Rogers

Drugs for Mental Illness

1

Drugs Enter Psychiatry

During the decade of the 1950s, the introduction of several new drugs revolutionized psychiatry. Suddenly, psychiatrists were able to treat a variety of serious mental illnesses that had been essentially untreatable before. Hundreds of millions of mental patients throughout the world have received these new treatments. People who would otherwise have been doomed to life in a psychiatric hospital have become able to care for themselves, and some of the most debilitating symptoms of mental illness have become rare. The afflicted and their families have been spared incalculable anguish and have saved hundreds of billions of dollars that would have been spent on incarceration and custodial care. Many psychiatrists believe these drugs are one of the great medical advances of the twentieth century, comparable in their impact to the antibiotics and vaccines.

Our ambition to write about the use of drugs in treating mental illness was kindled by two experiences we had several years ago. The first experience was connected with our work. We are university professors in the Institute of Neuroscience and the Psychology Department at the University of Oregon. Until becoming interested in psychiatric drugs, we had pursued research and teaching without paying much attention to the practical or medical applications of our research. We had thoughtlessly supposed that psychiatry was an unscientific, not really medical, profession whose responsibility was to look after helpless people who were not really ill.

These attitudes were first challenged in the early 1970s, when our undergraduate students began demanding that we demonstrate how our scholarship and research were relevant to people outside of academe. The students' demands were most insistent when we lectured about experiments on the actions of various chemicals on brain cells. The students were intensely interested in this subject. The youth drug culture was then in full flower. Many of the students were taking psychoactive drugs recreationally, and they were curious about what scientists might have to say about one of their favorite activities. Psychopharmacology thus became part of our course syllabus. To provide a balanced treatment, we began to teach about psychiatric drugs as well as recreational drugs. This made us learn more about psychiatry, a subject we had not been familiar with previously.

As we talked with our students and friends about psychiatric drugs, we began to realize that the recent drug revolution in psychiatry is not widely appreciated. Most of our acquaintances believed, as we did before we started studying the subject, that a psychiatrist's only legitimate tool is his words. Most were skeptical or disapproving of the use of drugs to treat mental illness. As we talked and lectured, and as our appreciation of contemporary psychiatric treatment grew, we became convinced that everyone should understand how psychiatry has changed since Freud.

The second event that motivated us to write this book was more personal. A few years ago, a colleague and friend at another university suffered a severe episode of mental illness that seriously disrupted his career and personal life. After long training at several famous universities, and after establishing himself as a competent researcher in neurophysiology, he experienced recurrent outbreaks of anger mixed with hopelessness and despair that brought his work to a halt. His abilities to think and concentrate were displaced by mental turmoil. His relationships with his wife and children began to deteriorate. After nearly two years of floundering with ineffective psychotherapy, misdiagnosis, and inappropriate drugs, our friend finally consulted a psychiatrist who gave the correct diagnosis, an effective drug treatment, and effective psychotherapy. The recovery that ensued was so dramatic that in an earlier age it would have been called a miracle. The recovery, of course, was not magical. Our friend recovered when he received drugs and psychotherapy that constructively changed the activity of his brain cells.

The Drug Revolution in Psychiatry

The drug revolution in psychiatry began in 1949 when the Australian psychiatrist John F. J. Cade reported some of his experiments with lithium. He found that lithium could produce tameness in otherwise wild and fearful guinea pigs. In a great leap of overconfidence that would leave most medical researchers aghast (and would be illegal under present U.S. regulations governing the development of new drug therapies), Cade gave lithium to ten hospitalized manic and agitated psychiatric patients. Lithium worked. The patients assumed emotional tones much closer to the normal range. One of these patients had been hospitalized for five years in an almost continual state of manic agitation. After four weeks on lithium, he became so much calmer that he was capable of leaving the hospital and resuming his old job. A few years later, the French psychiatrists Jean Delay and Pierre Deniker successfully tested the drug chlorpromazine (brand name, Thorazine) for calming psychotic agitation. Later in the 1950s, drugs for the effective treatment of depression became available.[1]

The new drugs were revolutionary because they worked. Previously, effective treatments for severe mental illness had been virtually unknown. Psychiatrists had been searching for treatments since early in the nineteenth century, but, with the exception of electroconvulsive shock treatment for depression, few treatments were successful. Psychiatric patients were given physical treatments such as insulin shock and hydrotherapy. They were also given a variety of psychological therapies, including psychoanalysis. But convincing evidence that these treatments worked was always scarce. By contrast, the new drugs were demonstrably effective. Since the beginning of the drug revolution, new (nonpsychoanalytic) methods of psychotherapy also have been developed that have proved to be effective in the treatment of depression and in the prevention of relapse in patients who suffer from schizophrenia.

The new treatments were also revolutionary because they made psychiatry more accessible to all the people who needed it. Psychotherapy based on Freudian principles is clearly only for the rich. For others it is financially devastating as it requires therapeutic sessions at least once a week for several years. By comparison, drug treatments and the newer forms of psychotherapy are inexpensive. Drug treatments do not require weekly visits to the psychiatrist. The new psychotherapies can often be given to several patients at once in a weekly meeting with the therapist, and they are effective after only a few weeks or months.

The effectiveness of the new drugs can be illustrated by examining the number of patients in United States mental hospitals between 1900 and 1975. During the first half of the twentieth century, the number of patients in mental hospitals steadily increased from 150,000 to about 500,000. In the period just following World War II, mental hospitals were so crowded that it became a common joke that the sane and the insane soon would have to exchange housing. In 1956, the year that the new drugs were first widely used in the United States, the upward trend in the hospitalized population reversed, and by 1975 the number of patients in mental hospitals had declined to 200,000. The downward trend has continued to the present.[2] However, the decline in the number of hospitalized patients has not resulted from a decrease in the rate of new hospital admissions. Rather, the new drugs have made it possible for patients to leave the hospital after a much briefer stay. Before 1956, patients often spent their entire lives in the hospital.

Modern treatment for severe mental illness typically consists of an initial hospital stay lasting from two to eight weeks. While in the hospital, the patient is medically and psychologically evaluated. If drug therapy is warranted and if the patient has no medical problems that would make drugs too risky, an initial drug trial is carried out under close medical supervision. If the treatment is successful, the patient is released after a few weeks, and drug therapy may continue on an outpatient basis. Psychotherapy may be used in conjunction with drugs, depending on the particular illness.

Psychiatric drugs have vastly improved the quality of life inside mental hospitals. Before 1956, the hospital environment was dismal. Typically, the quarters were overcrowded. Hallucinating patients talked to their "voices." Stuperous catatonic patients sat in one place, in one posture, for days, developing pressure sores. Withdrawn patients did not speak to anyone. Manic patients paced the floor purposelessly for days until exhausted, and those who were violent had to be physically restrained. The physicians and other personnel, unable to find more effective ways to relieve the symptoms, desperately used such procedures as insulin shock, warm baths, and strapping patients in wet sheets to calm psychotic agitation. Therapeutic success was usually only temporary, and the physician became mainly a supervisor of custodial care. Often, patients had to be put in straightjackets, isolated in padded rooms or given debilitating sedative drugs. The use of the new drugs has transformed the hospital environment into one in which many patients can enjoy sports, handicrafts, music, entertainment, and even gainful employment.[3]

Reactions to the Drug Revolution

Although nearly everyone agrees that the new drugs have benefited psychiatric patients, the pharmacological approach has encountered several types of resistance. This resistance has been based on four main issues: the issue of whether mental illness is primarily biological or psychological; the issue of whether psychotherapy or drug therapy is the preferred treatment; the issue of whether drug treatment violates patients' legal rights; and the issue of whether negative side effects outweigh the benefits of drug treatment. These issues are introduced here and discussed in more detail in Chapter 17.

Dualism

Some resistance to drug therapy has derived from the philosophical and semantic custom of distinguishing the mind from the body. Because of this custom, many people are uncomfortable with the fundamental assumption underlying drug treatment, that mental illness is brain illness.

In our everyday speech, we habitually speak of psychological problems as if they were different from "organic," "biological," or "medical" illnesses. Depression, anxiety, and paranoia seem to be "in the mind" and hence not in the body. Psychological problems are treated in separate "mental" hospitals, often by people who have not had extensive training in biological science. Many health insurance policies that cover medical illnesses will not pay for psychiatry, as if treatment for mental illness were not a legitimate medical expense. Within the medical community, psychiatrists may not be looked upon as "real doctors"; they do not seem as "medical" or as "scientific," and they do not treat "organic" diseases. In colleges and universities, psychology departments keep a safe distance from biology departments. Biology majors are required to study physics and organic chemistry in order to lay a foundation for their major subject, but psychology majors are not required to study any of the natural sciences, not even neuroscience.

Occasionally, critics of psychiatry have exploited the customary distinction between mind and body as an ideological battle cry. In an influential book entitled *The Myth of Mental Illness*, Dr. Thomas Szasz, a psychiatrist, attacks the medical status of his profession on the grounds that mental patients are not really ill.[4] Schizophrenia is not an illness, he argues, because it is not caused by any biological or anatomical defect of the body. He says that, in the absence of such a defect, calling schizophrenia an illness is just a semantic fiction promulgated by psychiatrists for their own benefit, not for the benefit of their patients.

Since ancient times, many people have believed that the mind is distinct from the body. One of the most thoughtful proponents of this belief was the French philosopher Rene Descartes, who lived from 1596 to 1650. Descartes saw clearly that the body, including the brain, was an elaborate physical machine. Therefore, like other machines, the body had to obey the laws of physics. In Descartes' day, mechanical clocks were the most elaborate machines whose operation was well understood. Clocks consisted of wheels, levers, and springs that pushed and pulled on each other. But to Descartes, the mind did not seem to respond to physical forces; it did not seem to contain parts that were pushed around like the wheels of a clock. In contrast, he believed that the mind responded to the nonphysical "forces" of reason and purpose. In Descartes' opinion, the laws of causation that control the flow of ideas through the mind are fundamentally different from the laws of physics that control the movements of a machine.

Modern neuroscience has amply demonstrated that the mind is produced by physiological activity in the brain. This important conclusion contradicts the conventional wisdom that properties of the mind, such as reason, purpose, and will, do not come from the body. Furthermore, it implies that mental illness and mental health result from distinct physiological states of the brain. Poor mental health is a state of the brain that is psychologically represented as misery and incapacitation. Good mental health is a state of the brain that allows an individual to express fully his capacity for emotion and intellect. The final objective of treatment for mental illness is to change the state of the brain to relieve misery and restore capacity. Unless the state of the brain is changed, the treatment cannot be successful.

The Tradition of Talk Therapy

Another source of resistance to biological psychiatry has been the vigorous tradition of psychoanalysis and other forms of talk psychotherapy. In the first half of the twentieth century, following the leadership of Freud, it became first fashionable and then customary to think that mental illnesses arose from psychological processes acquired during childhood as a result of problematic relationships with parents and siblings. Among these processes were oedipal conflicts, infantile fixations, and repressed hostilities. Freud thought that the patient had to gain insight into the specific experiences that caused the problematic psychological processes. Consequently, the patient had to laboriously recollect, with the help of a psychoanalyist, the critical experiences of early childhood.

Although Freud's outlook was biological in the sense that he thought the mind obeys the dictates of the "instinctual drives" for sexual gratification and bodily security, he did not theorize about possible brain mechanisms. Knowledge of brain biology was irrelevant to the treatment he recommended. At the time of his seminal work, about 1895, knowledge about the brain was so scant that he could not even speculate about biological mechanisms. He had to formulate his theories at the psychological level. He had to hope, for the sake of his patients, that physiological knowledge would not be necessary for the development of practical treatments for mental illness.

Freud's influence has been very great. To many mental health workers and the public in the United States, it has seemed sensible and correct to think of mental illnesses as unfavorable psychological reactions to stressful problems. For example, a friend of ours, who is a neurophysiologist, recently expressed this belief when he remarked, "She just overreacts psychologically to minor frustrations." With these words he sought to comprehend and explain the frantic tirades of a woman who later was treated successfully with lithium. On another occasion we were talking with a psychotherapist about drug treatments for depression. During the conversation, she remarked, "Yes, it could well be that some depressions result from a biochemical imbalance, but I've found that in 90 percent of the cases, when you really probe in therapy, when you really dig deep, you always find hostility." In yet another conversation, a psychoanalyst whom we first knew as an Oregon graduate student but who now practices in New York recently said to us, "The man [Freud] said it all! He constantly puts me in a state of amazement and admiration. His insights are a wholly sufficient explanation for how we act and think. Others merely rediscover what he saw clearly fifty years ago."

A common opinion among defenders of talk therapy is that drugs yield only superficial relief of symptoms. The charge is not that drugs are ineffective but that their benefits are of less value than the benefits of psychotherapy. The fact that drugs get patients out of the hospital is discounted by saying that the patients do not stay out of the hospital. Those who believe in talk therapy say that modern mental hospitals have revolving doors—patients leave only to return a few months later. The unspoken implication is that patients would stay out if they were treated properly with psychotherapy.

Another common opinion is that psychiatric drugs, including those used for schizophrenia, turn mental patients into "zombies" who are so sedated they cannot participate productively in the psychotherapy they need. A few years ago, we heard a neuroanatomy professor at an ivy league university express this opinion. A journalistic version of this view may be found in *The New Republic* of December 8, 1979, in an article entitled "Psychiatry's Drug Addiction." The fact that some of the drugs are called tranquilizers encourages the idea that the drugs are nothing more than powerful sleeping pills.

Further, opponents of drug therapy sometimes charge that medication subverts mental patients by tempting them with a cheap and easy escape from the hard work of psychotherapy. We once heard about a young woman in New York who had been seeing her analyst four times a week for four years. During this time, she had made a great deal of progress, but she needed more analysis. When we suggested that drug treatment might be appropriate, we were told, "Well, maybe, but then she might leave therapy before she completes the work she is going to have to do." Advocates of drug treatment have sarcastically referred to this attitude as "psychiatric Calvinism"—the harder the patient works, the better the cure.

We believe that the effectiveness of drug therapies and talk therapies can be compared only by evaluating the results of properly conducted research. One needs to ask, *what is the evidence* that a particular therapy is the most effective way to provide relief from a particular illness? Are drugs better for some mental illnesses, while talk therapies are better for others? Maybe, unlikely as it seems, psychotherapy and drug therapy are about equally effective for certain illnesses. What are the bad side effects of the various forms of treatment? What are the social and monetary costs? Such questions will be settled only by data, not by polemics or tradition.

Psychiatry as an Oppressor

Other sources of resistance to biological psychiatry have been the civil rights movement and the counterculture. During the 1960s and early 1970s, rapid social reform and widespread frustration with the government's war policy in Vietnam led many Americans, especially young Americans, to become suspicious of established authority. The psychiatric establishment was not spared. A popular opinion among intellectuals was that people who suffered from so-called mental illnesses were actually suffering from the effects of social injustice under the heel of an unfair political and economic system. For example, the psychiatrist Hugh Drummond, in the antiestablishment magazine *Mother Jones*, wrote: "Whatever madness is, it is deeply rooted in social and sexual inequality. Without a cultural revolution we will continue to have madness; as the contradictions of capitalism become more immensely chaotic, we will have more of it."[5]

In *The Myth of Mental Illness*, Szasz charged that psychiatrists and other mental health workers call schizophrenia an illness to acquire the power to control and oppress the patient. Szasz wrote, "It has become customary to use the term 'mental illness' to stigmatize, and thus control, those persons whose behavior offends society—or the psychiatrist making the 'diagnosis.' "[6] Szasz also wrote, "Who . . . are the people persecuted and victimized in the name of 'health' and 'happiness'? They are legion. In their front ranks are the mentally ill, and especially those who are so defined by others rather than by themselves. The involuntarily hospitalized mentally ill are regarded as 'bad' and valiant efforts are made to make them 'better.' "[7] Szasz provided no data to support his charge that psychiatrists and other mental health workers call deviant people ill solely to gain the power to make them conform. He took this point to be self-evident. Needless to say, conscientious psychiatrists and other mental health workers, who had thought they were relieving suffering, found Szasz's remarks offensive.

One of the most significant charges made by the antiestablishment critics is that drug treatments can deprive mental patients of civil rights guaranteed by the Constitution. If psychiatric drugs are considered to be agents for mind control, then psychiatric treatment is a truly outrageous tyranny. This tyranny would be more odious by far than the mere abridgment of free speech, brainwashing, or coercion through torture. With drugs, the authorities might deprive their victims of the capacity for will power; they might render their victims passive, incapable of autonomous thinking, and incompetent to resist oppression. This view of psychiatric treatment is expressed in *One Flew Over the Cuckoo's Nest*, the novel by Ken Kesey.[8] In the novel, a healthy "patient" was given pills. His offense was that he was mischievous. He used naughty language and excited the other patients with gambling and smutty cards. When the authorities failed to control him with drugs, they tried electroconvulsive shock. When that failed, they performed a lobotomy!

One Flew over the Cuckoo's Nest is just a story. Yet, it makes the important point that powerful institutions, including psychiatric hospitals, are tempted to abuse their power. There are probably a few psychiatrists and nurses who, like Kesey's Big Nurse, are patently unethical and enjoy abusing their power over helpless patients. Some may merely be lazy. In state institutions that are strapped for funds, staff members are often tempted to substitute control of behavior for humane care. Even conscientious psychiatrists in well-equipped and well-staffed hospitals are faced with genuine dilemmas. When a depressed patient threatens suicide and refuses to take antidepressant drugs because he believes he does not deserve to get better and just wants to die, should the psychiatrist heed the patient's bidding, or should he inject the drug against the patient's will? In general medicine, physicians can give drugs only with the patient's informed consent. Do psychiatric patients also have the right to refuse treatment?

Side Effects

Another objection to drug treatment springs from fear that the side effects of the drugs may be worse than the mental illness being treated. This is a realistic concern. Some psychiatric drugs can lead to addiction and dependence. The drugs used for schizophrenia can impair vision and occasionally cause blindness. They can cause a form of brain damage that is expressed as a debilitating movement disorder called *tardive dyskinesia*. Sometimes tardive dyskinesia is irreversible and incurable.

Bad side effects, of course, are not unique to drugs used to treat mental illness. They can also result from drugs used in general medicine. For example, some people become gravely ill or even die from an allergic response to penicillin. Nonetheless, penicillin is a profoundly beneficial drug. Many thousands of times more lives are saved by penicillin than are taken by it. Exploiting a drug's good effects while guarding against its bad ones is an accepted task of the physician. This task is no more difficult for a psychiatrist than for a physician in general medicine. Many mental illnesses are as distressing and debilitating as the diseases treated in general medicine. When combating misery and incapacitation, risking side effects is often justified.

The decision about whether or not to use drugs to treat mental illness should not, in our opinion, depend on the philosophical legacy of Descartes and Freud. The treatment of mental illness should not be controlled by outdated superstitions and customs. Victims often lose their families and livelihoods. They may commit suicide. We think these patients are entitled to the best treatment modern medicine can offer. The important questions to ask about a treatment are: Is there evidence that it works? Do the probable benefits outweigh the risks? If drugs contribute to the return of mental health, we think they should be used.

2

How Drugs Work
on the Brain

The most important assumption underlying our contention that drugs may be used effectively to treat mental illness is that the thoughts, emotions, and behaviors of animals, including humans, result from the activity of nerve cells in the brain and spinal cord (Figure 2-1).[1] The activity of nerve cells depends, in turn, on a complex system of chemical reactions and movements of molecules. We believe that, without these chemical reactions and molecular movements, thoughts, emotions, and behavior could not exist. Indeed, mental phenomena are the result of a very highly organized collection of molecular activities carried out by the nerve cells of the brain. Though these assumptions are essentially unprovable, they have become our credo because they are the foundation for the progress that neuroscience has made in understanding the brain.

A change in behavior signifies a change in brain chemistry. This change in brain chemistry is usually not drug induced; it results from ordinary, everyday experiences. Although many people know that changes in brain chemistry cause changes in behavior, such as falling asleep and making love, they may not appreciate that brain chemistry also produces more subtle alterations in behavior. Chemical reactions in the brain produce your ability to balance on a bicycle and your desire for orange juice in the morning. You stand

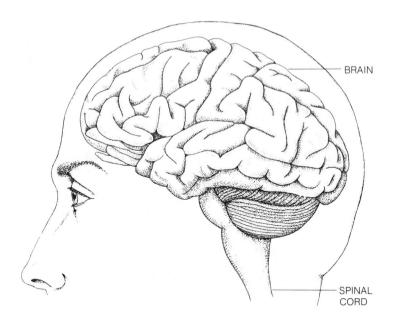

Figure 2-1. The human brain inside the skull. Note how the lower portion of the brain is continuous with the spinal cord. Both the brain and spinal cord are made up of nerve cells and supporting cells. (From "The Brain" by David H. Hubel. Copyright © 1979 by Scientific American, Inc. All rights reserved.)

in awe of a sunset in the mountains because the scene initiates chemical reactions in your brain. The brain is the ultimate provider of "better living through chemistry."

A person develops a mental illness when the brain chemistry changes in a way that affects his ability to function well. The goal of treatment is to modify the brain's chemical reactions in a way that produces good health. Taking drugs is one way to alter brain chemistry. When drugs reach the brain, they alter ongoing chemical reactions. A drug is an effective treatment if it alters brain chemistry so that the symptoms of mental illness are relieved.

But drugs are not the only way to improve a malfunctioning brain. Psychotherapy can also alter brain chemistry. Just as the sunset caused chemical reactions in the brain, so can the advice of a psychotherapist. Effective psychotherapy initiates chemical reactions that counteract the reactions causing the illness.

Although neuroscientists know more about how drugs work than about how psychotherapy works, they do not know the fine details of how either changes brain chemistry to alleviate mental illness. They understand many of the immediate effects of drugs on nerve cells, but these effects are only the first in a cascade of drug-initiated chemical changes. Neuroscientists do not understand the entire sequence of changes.

You will make better judgments about the appropriate role of chemical treatment in mental illness if you have some understanding of the effects of drug molecules on brain chemistry. People are aware that the brain is complex and delicate. Thus, they are reluctant to tamper with it. When the brain is working well, this reluctance is appropriate. Even though the brain may not be functioning perfectly, "let well enough alone" may be the best advice. Chemical intervention is likely to do more harm than good. But when serious mental illness strikes, the situation is quite different. Then the brain is no longer "well enough." At this point, you may agree that some intervention, perhaps drug treatment, is justified. But you will probably be more at ease if the treatment is not capricious, if logical reasons exist for thinking drugs might help. Of course, all treatments have risks. The risks as well as the benefits derive from the effects of the drugs on body chemistry.

Certain misconceptions about psychiatric drugs can be dispelled by learning how the brain works and how drugs influence brain activity. One common misconception is that these drugs are chemical straightjackets or chemical scalpels wielded to prevent socially undesirable behavior. A second misconception is that psychiatric drugs are all the same. Proponents of this view usually refer to all psychiatric drugs as tranquilizers. These two misconceptions can be countered by understanding how each drug affects brain chemistry and behavior.

A third misconception is that a drug ought to cure the disease that it treats; taking medication indefinitely ought not be necessary. When continued use of the drug is required, people tend to conclude that it has attacked only the symptoms, not the disease. The idea that an effective drug cures a disease has developed from the successful treatment of bacterial infections with antibiotics. However, most medical illnesses, such as diabetes, arthritis, and heart disease, are managed rather than cured. They cannot be cured because the basic abnormality, usually a chemical one, remains.

For example, physicians cannot correct the abnormality that prevents a diabetic's pancreas from making insulin; they can only supply the insulin that the pancreas fails to make. Understanding how psychiatric drugs can compensate for chemical abnormalities in the brain can help you understand how drugs can effectively treat these abnormalities, but not eliminate them.

Understanding the action of drugs on the brain requires that you know something about the normal brain. You need to know what brain cells look like and how they work. You also need specific information about how the molecules and chemical reactions in the brain are affected by psychiatric drugs.

The brain has three basic functions: It gets information from the outside world, it uses this information to decide on a course of action, and it implements the decision by commanding muscles to move and glands to secrete. If you look at a brain and spinal cord with your naked eye, you get no hint about how it performs these functions. All you see is a squishy, pink material squeezed tightly into the skull. But if you were to examine small pieces of the tissue under a microscope, you would begin to understand the structure of the brain. You would see that the brain is composed of individual elements called nerve cells, or neurons. These cells are specialized to exchange information with one another in a vast communications network. Understanding the messages that these nerve cells send to each other requires some knowledge of physiology and chemistry.

Brain and Computer: Similarities and Differences

We can draw an analogy between the brain and a computer. The analogy is helpful for understanding the function of the brain and the complexity of its communications network. Of course, the analogy can be carried too far. Obviously, nerve cells are different from the electronic components of a computer. A computer cannot be repaired with drugs, and a brain cannot be repaired with electronic chips.

In both computer and brain, the function of logical processing is performed by a central processing unit that is responsible for combining information and making decisions. The central processing unit of a computer is composed of electronic devices called integrated circuits. Information is transmitted from one integrated circuit to another by conductors. The central processing unit of the nervous system consists of the network of nerve cells in the brain and the spinal cord. This network is called the central nervous system. Information is transmitted from one region of the brain to another over specialized parts of nerve cells called *axons*, which are long, thin extensions of the cell body.

Both the brain and the computer use complex sets of rules to make their decisions. Although the actual rules are usually far more complex than any we could describe here, an example of the decision-making process is as follows. "A grapefruit requires 100 units of space in a fruit bowl, a plum requires 10, and a grape requires 1. If a particular selection of fruits requires at least 50 units of space, signal that a large fruit bowl is needed. If fewer than 50 units of space are required, signal that a small fruit bowl is needed. If, however, the total number of pieces of fruit is less than 3, signal that no fruit bowl is needed." Extremely complex networks of integrated circuits or nerve cells can be put together to perform very sophisticated decisions.

Like the computer, the nervous system has input and output devices for communicating with the outside world. A computer might receive input from a typewriter keyboard or from magnetic tape; the brain receives its input from the sense organs. A computer might produce output with a printer or with a television screen; the brain uses the muscles and glands to express the results of its information processing. Both computer and brain have communications lines for carrying information back and forth between the central processor and the input and output devices. Wires serve this function in computers; axons transport information between the central nervous system and the other organs of the body.

Each message that the brain or the computer sends to an output device is the result of thousands of small decisions, but the brain and the computer use radically different hardware to make these decisions. The computer performs its logic with integrated circuits. The brain uses synapses, the junctions between nerve cells, as decision-making devices. Each output from the computer to the printer is the net result of decisions made by many individual electronic devices. The printer, however, receives only the final decision. Similarly, each output from the nervous system to the muscles is the result of decisions at thousands of synapses, but the muscles receive only the final commands. The muscles are ignorant of how the nervous system arrived at that command.

Innate and Learned Programs

The brain and computer differ not only in the hardware they use to process information but also in the way they are programmed. A modern general-purpose computer is truly like John Locke's *tabula rasa*, a blank slate. A computer comes off the assembly line without a program. The programmer determines which programs are run on the computer and hence all the computer's functions. But the brain of the newborn infant is not a *tabula rasa*. At birth, it is already elaborately "programmed." Some of the innate "programs," such as those controlling breathing and suckling, are necessary for survival. Others limit the abilities of the adult that the infant will become. For example, innate "programs" may dictate that a person will be left-handed or will not become a violin virtuoso.

However, the brain of the infant does not contain all the "programs" that will eventually reside in the brain of the adult. New programs are developed as the child matures, and this development is called learning. Learning results from interactions between the brain and the environment. The environment influences brain function in yet another way. Environmental inputs are often required to run inborn "programs." The breathing "program" cannot run without knowing how much carbon dioxide is in the blood.

Differences in people's behavior reflect differences in their brains. Species-specific behaviors present dramatic examples of such differences. For instance, humans find it difficult to make a nest out of twigs and straw, whereas the robin can do it easily. No amount of training will teach robins to talk, but humans learn without special instruction. Robin behavior and human behavior are different because robin brains and human brains are different. Although behavioral variations among individual humans are less dramatic, these variations also reflect biological differences in individual human brains. Thus, some humans are mentally ill because they have abnormalities in their brains. In some cases, intervention from the social environment may effectively treat the brain's abnormality. In other cases, this intervention is not successful. Then drugs or some other physical intervention may be required.

Nerve Cells

A clear understanding of how the brain functions requires an understanding of individual nerve cells. Nerve cells in different parts of the brain have different functions and look different from each other when seen under a microscope. Nevertheless, all nerve cells have basic similarities in structure, as illustrated in Figure 2-2.

A *cell membrane* separates the contents of each cell from the fluid that surrounds it. Just as skin is the boundary between what is inside the body and what is outside, the cell membrane is the boundary between the inside and the outside of the cell. The membrane also controls the chemical contents of the cell. Because the membrane is primarily fatty material, water and water-soluble molecules cannot pass through it unless special gates or channels are opened.

The metabolic center of the nerve cell is called the *cell body*. It ranges in size from about 0.005 to about 0.100 millimeter in diameter, depending on the type of cell. The cell body contains the nucleus and the chemical machinery needed to keep the cell alive. Many thin extensions diverge from the cell body. Most nerve cells have numerous short extensions called *dendrites*, and a single longer one called the *axon*. The dendrites and the cell body are the parts of the nerve cell that usually receive signals from other neurons. The dendrites range from 0.001 to 2.0 millimeters in length, and they usually branch profusely, giving the cell a bristly appearance when seen under the microscope.

The axon is the part of the cell that sends signals from the region of the cell body to regions of the nervous system a considerable distance away. Axons are often much longer than dendrites and do not branch except very near their ends. The axon illustrated in Figure 2-2 is folded like an accordion so that it fits within the diagram. In the brain it is straighter. If the cell were involved in controlling the feet of a tall man, its axon might reach from the top of the brain to the end of the spinal cord. It would be about 1.0 meter long, though only about 0.01 millimeter in diameter. By contrast, if the cell communicated only with neighboring cells in the brain, its axon might be only 0.1 millimeter long and less than 0.001 millimeter in diameter.

At the tips of the small branches at the end of the axon are small bulblike swellings called *axon terminals*. Axon terminals are

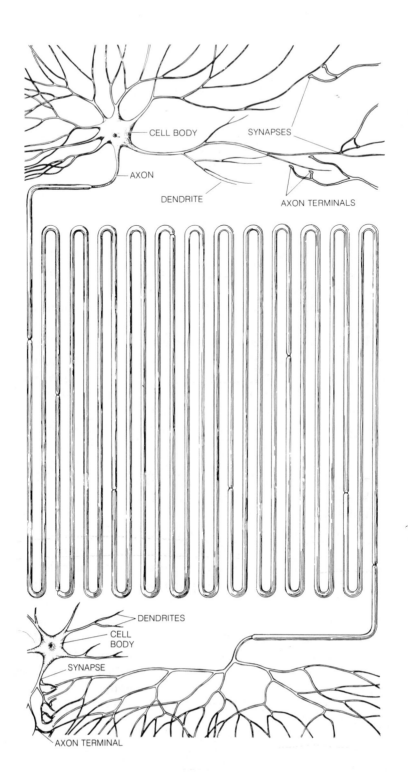

CELL BODY

SYNAPSES

AXON

DENDRITE

AXON TERMINALS

DENDRITES

CELL BODY

SYNAPSE

AXON TERMINAL

almost always found close to a dendrite or cell body of another nerve cell. The junction between an axon terminal of one nerve cell, and a dendrite or cell body of another nerve cell is called a *synapse*.

The vast majority of nerve cells are completely confined to the central nervous system. Of course, the input and output cells must have axons that reach beyond the central nervous system to the sense organs and muscles. Many of the nerve cells involved in sensory input have their cell bodies located in clumps just outside the spinal cord.

The Transmission of Information

Each individual nerve cell must perform many of the same tasks that are performed by the brain as a whole. The cell must receive information, usually at its cell body and its dendrites. It must use that input to make decisions, usually the job of the cell body. The decision must be communicated to other nerve cells, usually by sending a signal down the axon. Because most psychiatric drugs do not affect the transmission of information from the cell body down the axon to the axon terminals, we will discuss this aspect of nerve cell function only briefly.

Nerve Impulses

To send a signal to the spinal cord, a nerve cell in the brain generates a *nerve impulse*. The nerve impulse is a momentary change in the electrical conductivity of the axon membrane. This change lasts only about 0.001 second. Signaling with nerve impulses is like signaling with a Morse code that has only dots and no dashes—the message that travels down the axon is conveyed by the rate of nerve

Figure 2-2. Diagram of typical nerve cells. Cell bodies for axon terminals at the top are beyond the edge of the diagram. Axon of cell body at lower left runs off diagram. Most of the axon terminal branches extend beyond the edge of the diagram, and their synapses are not shown. (From "The Neuron" by Charles F. Stevens. Copyright © 1979 by Scientific American, Inc. All rights reserved.)

impulses. Nerve cells can generate as many as 200 impulses per second. A nerve impulse travels rapidly down the axon from the cell body to the axon terminal. It never travels in the reverse direction. The speed of the nerve impulse is different in different types of nerve cells. It can be as fast as 100 meters per second or as slow as 0.1 meter per second. A fast-conducting axon would send a message from its cell body in the brain to synapses in the tail of the spinal cord in only 0.01 second.

Synapses

How does a nerve cell know when to generate a nerve impulse, and how does it tell other nerve cells to do so? The simple answer is that a cell generates a nerve impulse when instructed to do so by signals that it receives from other nerve cells at synapses. But to understand the action of psychiatric drugs, you must have more detailed knowledge. Psychiatric drugs work by modifying specific events that occur at synapses in both normal and ill brains. Understanding drug action requires a fairly detailed understanding of transmission across synapses. Figure 2-3 shows the detailed structure of a typical synapse as it looks under an electron microscope. A synapse is so tiny that examination of the detailed structure requires a magnification about 100 times greater than the magnification of the cells in Figure 2-2.

The axon terminal of the neuron sending a message is called the *presynaptic terminal* (*pre* meaning "before" or "in front of"). *Synaptic vesicles* are clustered close to the membrane. They are approximately spherical in shape and appear as circles in the presynaptic terminal. These vesicles contain molecules of *transmitter*, the chemical that carries the message to the postsynaptic cell. Depending on the type of transmitter used by the presynaptic cell, the vesicles may appear clear or may appear to be filled with dense material. The receiving portion of the synapse is called the *postsynaptic membrane* (*post* meaning "behind" or "after"). The postsynaptic membrane is a patch of membrane on the cell body or dendrite of the receiving or postsynaptic cell. The presynaptic and postsynaptic regions of the membrane appear slightly thicker and darker than the neighboring regions because they have special proteins inserted into the fatty material of the membrane. These proteins are important for the functioning of the synapse. Notice that

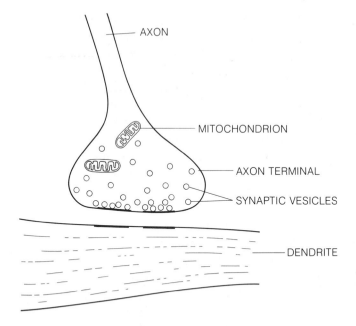

AXON

MITOCHONDRION

AXON TERMINAL

SYNAPTIC VESICLES

DENDRITE

Figure 2-3. Diagram of a synapse as seen with an electron microscope. The synaptic vesicles contain transmitter. The mitochondria supply the energy needed for synthesis and release of transmitter.

the presynaptic and postsynaptic membranes are very close to each other but do not quite touch. The space between them, called the *synaptic cleft*, is about 20 millionths of a millimeter wide.

It is important to realize that the terms *presynaptic* and *post-synaptic* do not refer to entire nerve cells but only to their roles at a particular synapse. At a particular synapse between a brain cell and a spinal cord cell, the brain cell may be presynaptic and the spinal cord cell postsynaptic. But at another synapse, the same brain cell may be receiving information and hence is postsynaptic. When the spinal cord cell transmits information to another spinal cord cell or to a muscle, the spinal cord cell is presynaptic.

Transmitters

How do signals cross the cleft between the presynaptic terminal and the postsynaptic membrane? A nerve impulse cannot cross the cleft because nerve impulses travel only in membrane and no membrane spans the synaptic cleft. Instead, the signals are carried across the cleft by chemical transmitters that are released from vesicles in the presynaptic terminals. The transmitter diffuses across the cleft and attaches to special protein molecules, called *receptors*, embedded in the postsynaptic membrane. This process of attachment is called *binding*. The thickening of the postsynaptic membrane probably represents the protein molecules that form the receptors. The binding of transmitters to receptors constitutes the signal that triggers a change of activity in the postsynaptic nerve cell. Many drugs affect brain function by altering the binding of transmitters to receptors.

To understand the many ways that drugs can affect synapses, it is useful to follow the path of the transmitter molecules moving from a presynaptic terminal to the postsynaptic receptors. In the absence of a nerve impulse in the presynaptic neuron, the transmitter is stored in the synaptic vesicles. When a nerve impulse arrives at the presynaptic terminal, some of the vesicles fuse with the presynaptic membrane and rupture at the point of fusion, releasing their contents into the synaptic cleft (Figure 2-4). Less than 0.0005 second elapses between the arrival of the nerve impulse at the presynaptic terminal and the receipt of the message by the postsynaptic receptors.

What happens to the postsynaptic cell when a transmitter binds to a receptor? The binding of transmitter activates chemical changes in the postsynaptic membrane. At some synapses, the change in the postsynaptic membrane encourages the production of nerve impulses in the postsynaptic axon; at other synapses, the changes induced by binding are different and discourage the production of nerve impulses. When the binding of a transmitter to a receptor encourages the production of nerve impulses, the process is called *synaptic excitation*. Without synaptic excitation, information cannot travel through the nervous system. When the binding discourages the production of nerve impulses, the process is called *synaptic inhibition*. Inhibition prevents inappropriate production of nerve impulses. For example, it prevents two muscles that pull in opposite directions from contracting at the same time and tearing the tendons off the bones.

Different nerve cells use different molecules as transmitters, but a given nerve cell probably releases the same chemical trans-

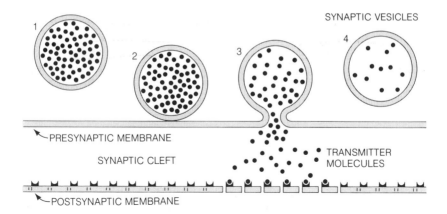

Figure 2-4. Diagram of the rupturing of synaptic vesicles and release of transmitter into the cleft. The transmitter diffuses across the cleft and attaches to the receptor. The vesicle membrane is reclaimed by the presynaptic terminal. (From "The Neuron" by Charles F. Stevens. Copyright © 1979 by Scientific American, Inc. All rights reserved.)

mitter or transmitters at each of its presynaptic terminals. The predominant chemical is called the *transmitter* for that nerve cell. At many synapses, other molecules, called *cotransmitters*, are released along with the predominant transmitter. Some of these other molecules may be just as important as the predominant transmitter, but they have been discovered only recently and comparatively little is known about their function.

Although a particular transmitter is often described as excitatory while another kind of transmitter is described as inhibitory, a single transmitter does not always produce the same effect on all its postsynaptic cells. Whether a given transmitter is excitatory or inhibitory is not determined by the transmitter alone. It depends on the postsynaptic machinery that the receptor controls. For example, acetylcholine is the transmitter released by axons onto muscles controlling the arms and legs. Acetylcholine excites these muscles, causing them to contract. This transmitter is also released by axons controlling the heart. However, it inhibits the heart muscle, causing the heartbeat to slow down.

We do not know how many different kinds of chemicals are used as transmitters in the central nervous system. At present, there is good evidence for about twenty different kinds. There may be many more. The psychiatric drugs affect mainly synapses that use one of five different transmitters: norepinephrine, dopamine, serotonin, acetylcholine, and gamma-amino butyric acid (GABA). But we must always keep in mind the possibility that even the drugs we understand best might have actions we are unaware of at synapses using transmitters that we know nothing about.

The Binding of Transmitters and Receptors

Usually the dendrites and cell body are studded with synapses (Figure 2-5). Each postsynaptic cell receives input from many different presynaptic cells, perhaps twenty, perhaps several hundred. Collectively, these presynaptic cells release several different kinds of transmitters, but each kind of receptor molecule is specialized for binding to one particular transmitter. Some other transmitters will bind to the receptor, but the attachment is weak. Still others will not bind at all. Therefore, a single postsynaptic cell must have several different kinds of receptors to match the several different transmitters it receives. Each kind of receptor is located where it will receive the proper transmitter, that is, across the synaptic cleft from a presynaptic terminal releasing that transmitter. A few thousandths of a millimeter away, another kind of receptor, located across from another presynaptic terminal, will respond to a different kind of transmitter.

The result of this structure is that every cell continuously receives a fluctuating barrage of excitatory and inhibitory synaptic signals. Each nerve cell must evaluate all of its inputs on a moment-to-moment basis and decide whether there is enough net excitation to generate a nerve impulse. At one moment, excitation may be greater than inhibition, and the cell will send nerve impulses down its axon. A few hundredths of a second later, the opposite may be true, and the cell will stop sending impulses. This seems complex enough, but now imagine a human brain consisting of 100 billion nerve cells. At every moment, each cell is deciding whether to produce an output while depending on thousands of other cells for help in making its decision. No computer, no social organization can rival this complexity.

Some kinds of transmitters—for example, dopamine, norepinephrine, and serotonin—have another kind of effect on postsyn-

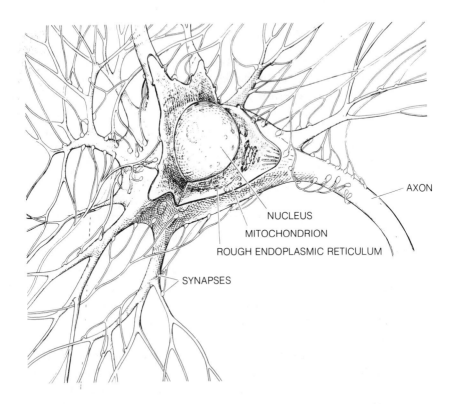

AXON

NUCLEUS
MITOCHONDRION
ROUGH ENDOPLASMIC RETICULUM

SYNAPSES

Figure 2-5.   Nerve cell covered with synapses. The nucleus contains the genetic material of the cell. The rough endoplasmic reticulum is part of the protein-synthesizing machinery. Cell bodies of the presynaptic cells are off the diagram. (From "The Neuron" by Charles F. Stevens. Copyright © 1979 by Scientific American, Inc. All rights reserved.)

aptic cells: They change the cells' biochemistry. When these transmitters bind to receptors, they activate an enzyme. This enzyme causes the cell to synthesize a compound called cyclic AMP (cAMP). Scientists do not understand the significance of cAMP synthesis as thoroughly as they understand the significance of excitation and inhibition, but they do know that cAMP facilitates many biochemical reactions, including some that are involved in neural signaling. Increasing the synthesis of cAMP can alter the cell's ability to send out impulses for several minutes or hours. In contrast, excitation or inhibition that is not mediated by the synthesis of cAMP lasts only a few thousandths of a second.

The Removal of Transmitter

A receptor cannot respond to another nerve impulse until the transmitter is removed from both the receptor and the cleft. Fortunately, the union between receptor and transmitter is reversible. Transmitter molecules easily become unattached from a receptor. No special mechanism is required because all molecules in solution move continuously. They vibrate even when attached to a receptor. By chance, some of these vibrations have enough force to pull the transmitter off the receptor.

Once the transmitter has left the receptor, it is removed from the cleft in one of two ways. First, some types of transmitters are split into two smaller molecules by an enzyme in the postsynaptic membrane. Any transmitter molecule that happens to hit the enzyme is split. Neither of the two molecules formed by this split can function as a transmitter. Second, other types of transmitters leave the cleft by reentering the presynaptic terminal. The membrane of the presynaptic terminal, as well as the membrane of the postsynaptic terminal, has receptors for the transmitter. When a transmitter molecule binds to a presynaptic receptor, the transmitter is taken inside the terminal. This process is called *reuptake*, even though the implied preceding "uptake" is nonexistent. After reuptake, the transmitter either reenters a vesicle so that it can be released again or is destroyed by an enzyme inside the presynaptic terminal.

A Summary of Brain Function

1. The brain must receive information from sense organs, use this information to make decisions, and instruct muscles and glands to implement its decisions.

2. The decisions depend both on the information received from sense organs and on the brain's programs. Some of these programs are learned from experience; others are inborn.

3. Communication between nerve cells occurs at synapses. A synapse consists of an axon terminal (the presynaptic terminal), a postsynaptic receptor (located in a patch of postsynaptic membrane), and an intervening synaptic cleft.

4. A nerve impulse in the presynaptic terminal causes synaptic vesicles to fuse with the terminal membrane and release their transmitter into the cleft.

5. The transmitter binds to postsynaptic receptors, and the post-synaptic membrane responds with either excitation or inhibition.

6. A nerve cell produces nerve impulses on the basis of moment-to-moment evaluations of the excitation and inhibition it is receiving over its synapses.

7. The binding of transmitter to receptor can also alter the biochemistry of the postsynaptic cell.

8. Before the synapse can be used again, the transmitter must be removed from the cleft in one of two ways. Either an enzyme splits the transmitter, or the transmitter is taken up inside the presynaptic terminal.

How Drugs Affect the Transmission of Information

Drugs are known that can alter virtually every step in synaptic transmission. For example, they can prevent the synthesis of the transmitter. They can increase or decrease transmitter release. They can bind to the postsynaptic receptor and thus prevent the normal transmitter from binding. Drugs can alter the shape of the receptor so that it becomes more or less difficult for the transmitter to bind. They can increase or decrease the number of receptors manufactured. They can inactivate enzymes that destroy transmitters. They can prevent reuptake. Most of the drugs used to treat mental illness affect transmitter–receptor binding, reuptake of transmitters, and the manufacture of receptors. In later chapters, we will discuss in more detail how specific psychiatric drugs affect synapses. Here we present a brief preview.

Drugs used to treat schizophrenia block receptors for the transmitter dopamine. Dopamine usually causes inhibition of nerve impulses and increases the synthesis of cAMP, but the drugs used for schizophrenia bind to dopamine receptors without causing either of these effects. As long as a drug molecule occupies a receptor, dopamine cannot bind to it. Thus, the receptor is blocked. Receptor-blocking drugs prevent transmission of synaptic signals from dopamine-secreting presynaptic terminals. Such drugs are called *dopamine antagonists*. Other drugs bind to dopamine receptors but do not block them. These drugs mimic the effects of dopamine by producing excitation and inhibition and by stimulating cAMP synthesis. The dopamine-mimicking drugs are called *dopamine ago-*

nists. Amphetamines are agonists for both dopamine and norepinephrine. Amphetamines are sometimes used briefly to treat hyperactive children and, for short periods of time, to treat depression, but the primary use of dopamine agonists is in research.

Drugs used to treat depression alter norepinephrine and serotonin synapses. They prevent the reuptake of both transmitters. They also decrease the sensitivity of some postsynaptic receptors for norepinephrine and serotonin. These effects are complex and not yet well understood, partly because most transmitters have several different types of receptors and a drug may not have the same effect on each type.

Finally, drugs used in the treatment of anxiety interact with receptors for the transmitter GABA. Antianxiety drugs bind to a molecule that is closely associated with the GABA receptor. When bound, the antianxiety drug changes the shape of the GABA receptor and causes the postsynaptic cell to respond more intensely to GABA.

Any particular psychiatric drug acts primarily on synapses using one particular transmitter. For example, the transmitters dopamine and norepinephrine are very similar chemically, but a drug that affects dopamine synapses usually does not have much effect on norepinephrine synapses, and vice versa. Dopamine-receptor blockers bind only weakly to norepinephrine receptors, and blockers of norepinephrine reuptake have almost no effect on dopamine reuptake. The specificity is not absolute, however. Sometimes, the deviations from specificity are important therapeutically. For example, dopamine antagonists also block certain acetylcholine receptors. The blocking of acetylcholine receptors causes some of the side effects of the dopamine antagonists used to treat schizophrenia.

Whether we focus on the specificity or the deviations from specificity, it is clear that psychiatric drugs are not generalized poisons that merely prevent mental illness by turning the brain off or, worse, by destroying large parts of it. It is also clear that psychiatric drugs are not all the same. Different drugs act on different kinds of synapses and will have different effects on behavior and mental life. For example, all psychiatric drugs are not tranquilizers.

Finally, we can now understand how taking a drug might compensate for a biochemical abnormality in the brain. Suppose that some people have nerve cells that manufacture too many dopamine receptors. The excess receptors would result in excessive synaptic action at synapses using dopamine as a transmitter. In the proper dose, a drug that blocks dopamine receptors could compensate for the abnormality by preventing dopamine from binding with the extra receptors and thus restoring brain function to normal. In later chapters, we provide more evidence for both the therapeutic and the biochemical specificity of these drugs.

Diagnosing Mental Illnesses

The Function of Diagnosis

When you do not feel well, you go to the doctor to find out whether you have a recognized illness, what kind of illness it is, and whether it can be treated. To provide answers, the doctor must have a valid system of diagnosis; that is, he must have a method of naming your illness. He does this by classifying your symptoms according to their similarity to symptoms in other cases. Classification allows physicians and patients to communicate, physicians to prescribe treatments that control or cure diseases, and researchers to study the causes of diseases and to invent more effective treatments.[1]

To appreciate the importance of communication, just imagine how uninformed you would be if you heard that a relative had a nervous breakdown or had become emotionally disturbed. You would not know what symptoms she had; you would have no idea whether treatment was available or desirable, and you would know nothing about the seriousness of her condition. About the only thing you would know is that something was wrong. The words *emotionally disturbed* and *nervous breakdown* fail to communicate because they do not name a mental illness that has a distinct set of symptoms. Everyone defines the terms differently. *Nervous breakdown* and *emotionally disturbed* are words people use because they lack more precise terms. By contrast, if you heard that the same relative had rheumatoid arthritis or mumps, you would be well informed about the nature of the illness. You would know something about the symptoms she had, something about the seriousness of her disease, whether effective treatments were available, and whether the prognosis was good or bad. A reliable system of diagnosis allows people to agree about definitions of diseases.

A reliable system of psychiatric diagnosis is required before researchers can study mental illnesses, discover their causes, and invent treatments. Suppose that two psychiatric researchers, Dr. Nader and Dr. Watt, each decided to investigate whether nervous breakdowns are related to automotive air pollution. Each would measure automotive air pollution in various centers of human population. The definition of automotive air pollution and the methods of measuring it are well known from previous research. Dr. Watt and Dr. Nader would then sample the same populations to determine the rate of nervous breakdowns. At this point, they would begin to disagree. They would find that there is no agreed upon definition of *nervous breakdown* and no agreed upon method for measuring it.

Dr. Nader, whose work was sponsored by the Political Action Coalition for Cleaner Air, would probably find that air pollution is indeed associated with a higher incidence of nervous breakdowns, while Dr. Watt, whose work was sponsored by the International Consortium of Gasoline Refiners, would find that automotive air pollution had no relationship to nervous breakdowns. The researchers would not have made any scientific progress. Because Dr. Nader and Dr. Watt had not come to a prior agreement on the definition of *nervous breakdown,* each researcher defined it to serve his own purposes. Without standard definitions, honest experts can continue to disagree, and people can retain their preexistent conflicting opinions.

Contrast these results with the likely outcome of research by the same two researchers on the relation between automotive air pollution and the birth rate and death rate in the exposed populations. In this study, the researchers would agree about what is being measured, and although they might disagree on the implications of their results for public policy, they probably would agree on whether birth and death rates are correlated with levels of automative air pollutants.

A valid system of diagnosis is also required to prescribe an effective treatment. In the prescientific era, diagnosis had little bearing on treatment. All sick patients were treated in approximately the same way, and the treatment corresponded to the therapeutic superstitions prevailing at the time. During one period, exorcism was in vogue; during another, bloodletting. Today, physicians try to match specific treatments to specific diseases—antibiotics for bacterial infections, insulin for diabetes, surgery for appendicitis, and so on. The specific treatment is chosen because research has proven it effective for the particular disease, diagnosed from specific symptoms.

Psychiatry is just emerging from its prescientific era when only one treatment was used for all illnesses. During the twentieth century, until about 1960, the commonly accepted treatment for nervous breakdowns, emotional disturbances, inferiority complexes, oedipal conflicts, alienation, lack of self-actualization, neurosis, and so on was some kind of psychotherapy in which the therapist tried to help by talking with the patient. Usually, the therapist tried to show how problems evolved from the patient's personal development. Most talk treatments were based on the teachings of great authorities, such as Freud, Jung, and Sullivan, and owed little debt to empirical research. No one tried to collect statistics on whether the treatment was actually having the desired effect. Therapists relied on insight and observation, which gradually became dogma.

Recently, the advent of psychotherapeutic drugs and the developments in clinical psychology challenged this tradition by demanding empirical evidence that a psychiatric treatment is effective. Drug laws in the United States demanded that new psychiatric drugs be proven both safe and effective for a given illness before being marketed. Clinical psychologists demanded that the effectiveness of psychotherapy also be proven. Because of these demands, evidence for treatment effectiveness must be obtained through careful diagnostic categorization of psychiatric illnesses and precise descriptions of treatment methods. Only then can researchers find out which treatments work for which illnesses. Typically, to test treatment effectiveness, the particular treatment being studied is given to patients with a certain illness. The recovery of these patients is then compared to the recovery of patients receiving a different treatment or no treatment at all.

Despite the recent broad interest in diagnosis and the accumulating evidence that accurate diagnosis spawns effective treatment, some psychiatrists and psychologists continue to believe that diagnosis is not important in psychiatry. Generally, these people fall into two groups, which we might call the one-factor theorists and the nonmedical theorists.

The one-factor theorists believe that a single cause underlies all mental illness. They do not think in terms of abnormal brain function. These theorists believe that the cause is "at the psychological level," wherever that is. A Freudian psychoanalyst is a one-factor theorist who believes that all problems are caused by frustration of instinctual motives, and only one treatment is appropriate—psychoanalysis. The cure is always "know thyself," no matter what the symptoms. If only one treatment and one cause exist, then obviously diagnosis is irrelevant.

The nonmedical theorists deny that psychiatric patients are ill and that psychiatrists are healers. Thomas Szasz, a leader among the nonmedical theorists, thinks that people with psychological problems such as schizophrenia are not really ill. They just have trouble solving their problems of living. Thus, without illness, diagnosis is irrelevant.

The best rebuttal to one-factor theorists and nonmedical theorists would be the development of a widely agreed upon diagnostic system together with effective treatments for each diagnosis.

Contemporary Diagnosis

Granting that correct diagnosis is essential for good psychiatry, we ask whether effective diagnostic techniques are currently in widespread use. To answer frankly, we have to say no. Although practices are improving, psychiatrists have not yet fully agreed upon an objective and standardized system of psychiatric classification. If you have had any encounters with psychiatric illness, this fact will probably be painfully obvious to you.[2]

Jill is an example of a patient whose illness was incorrectly diagnosed. Though Jill wanted desperately to be an efficient housewife and a loving mother, each day her good intentions were somehow lost within a half hour of getting out of bed. Day after day, she refused to get breakfast, lunch, or dinner. She said she was "just not up to it." Sometimes, out of an unsubstantiated fear that her family would become poverty-stricken, she refused to give her children lunch money. At such times, she was frightened and weepy. She had to be comforted even though nothing threatening or sad had happened. When she repented of her stinginess and passivity, she went to the opposite extreme, insisting that the whole family eat in expensive restaurants that they could ill afford. At these times, she was too busy and impatient to cook.

At her husband's insistence, Jill visited a psychiatrist, who diagnosed her illness as a personality disorder. He prescribed a benzodiazepine drug (Valium) and insight psychotherapy. Jill continued to weep. Two years later, her husband insisted that she consult another psychiatrist. Neither Jill nor her husband ever found out what her diagnosis was, but this psychiatrist prescribed phenothiazines, drugs usually reserved for schizophrenia, along with more insight psychotherapy. Though Jill wept less often, she was still sick. A year later, in desperation, Jill went to a third psychiatrist. She diagnosed Jill as having unipolar depression and prescribed an antidepressant drug and rationalemotive psychotherapy. Jill improved somewhat but continued to have trouble. After six more months, the same psychiatrist changed the diagnosis again, this time to bipolar affective disorder, and prescribed lithium. The lithium worked, and Jill improved dramatically. She said to her husband, "I feel normal for the first time in years."

Only four classes of drugs are commonly used in psychiatry today: benzodiazepines, antipsychotics, antidepressants, and lithium. It is an embarrassment to the art of psychiatric diagnosis that Jill received the correct drug only after drugs from all three of the other classes had been incorrectly prescribed and had failed.

The attempt to evaluate John Hinkley's mental health also exemplifies the imprecision of diagnostic techniques. On March 30, 1981, Hinkley shot and injured President Reagan and three other members of the president's party as they were leaving the Washington Hilton Hotel.[3] At Hinkley's trial, psychiatrists for the defense testified that Hinkley had schizophrenia and, because of the illness, was not rational when he shot President Reagan. The psychiatrists said that Hinkley was driven to shoot by the delusion that killing the president would win him the love of teenage actress Jodie Foster. Psychiatrists for the prosecution disagreed. They testified that Hinkley did not have schizophrenia and that he could rationally control his behavior. They said that he planned the shooting to become famous without working hard. A jury had to decide which psychiatrists were right.[4] It appears that if lawyers do not like what one psychiatrist says, they just call another until they find one who will give the testimony that fits the clients' needs.

It is hardly surprising that many people regard psychiatry as unscientific or even fraudulent. Just imagine the low regard you would have for nonpsychiatric medical doctors if they routinely disagreed about the appropriate name for your illness and even argued about whether or not you were sick. At the very least, psychiatry needs a uniform system of nomenclature so that professionals will agree about the meaning of such terms as *neurosis, psychosis, insanity, schizophrenia, depression,* and even *mental illness.* Moreover, a psychiatrist should not assign a name to a particular patient's illness when there is no broad professional agreement about what that name should be. Sometimes the psychiatrist should say, "I don't know what to call your illness. I don't even know whether you're ill or not." Although the patient may not be comforted, this honesty is vastly superior to assigning names that will be misunderstood.

Different psychiatrists use the same name to represent different kinds of illnesses. Dr. Gerald Klerman and several associates from the National Institute of Mental Health recently reviewed the use of the term *neurotic depression* in the psychiatric research literature. They found that various psychiatric researchers used the term to represent six different kinds of psychological disorders. Some psychiatrists, for example, used *neurotic depression* to mean depression that is a reaction to a saddening environmental event, such as a death in the family or a divorce. Other psychiatrists used the same term to mean mild depression, distinguishing it from psychotic depression, which is more severe.[5]

Different psychiatrists call the same illness by different names. Dr. R. E. Kendell, Dr. J. E. Cooper, and several other psychiatrists from the United Kingdom and the eastern United States published a paper in 1972 that reported the outcome of an important study comparing the diagnostic practices of American and British psychiatrists. In their study, they showed videotapes of diagnostic interviews with patients to large groups of psychiatrists on both sides of the Atlantic. After viewing exactly the same tapes, the British psychiatrists diagnosed manic depression and personality disorder much more often than the Americans, and the Americans diagnosed schizophrenia much more often than the British. After observing one of the taped diagnostic interviews, 92 percent of the Americans diagnosed schizophrenia while only 2 percent of the British did so; 72 percent of the British psychiatrists diagnosed personality disorder while only 8 percent of the Americans did so.[6]

You can imagine the confusion this disagreement over nomenclature creates at international psychiatric conventions. Calling the same illness by different names also creates problems for a researcher who wants to find out if a particular drug—for example, "Mindclear"—is effective in treating schizophrenia. He may find that, according to British psychiatrists, "Mindclear" works for 90 percent of the cases, but according to American psychiatrists, for only 30 percent of the cases.

Different psychiatrists use different procedures for obtaining diagnostic information. Psychiatrists of Freudian persuasion may use free association to help patients uncover repressed, threatening memories. Those psychiatrists impressed by modern statistical methods may give patients a written test that is designed to identify certain personality traits. Some psychiatrists may simply ask questions about patients' mental states currently and in the recent past. Still others may use a structured psychiatric interview with a fixed sequence of questions to identify patients' symptoms. All these procedures yield different kinds of information, which in turn yield different diagnoses.[7]

A reliable system of diagnosis will achieve at least two goals. First, it will clearly define each illness by specifying its symptoms. Second, it will specify the methods for determining whether a patient has a particular symptom. Only after these goals are achieved will psychiatrists be able to agree with one another in naming a patient's illness.[8]

Although these fundamental goals have not yet been reached, psychiatric diagnosis is improving. In fact, the progress made in the past ten years is truly impressive. Several discrete illnesses have been differentiated, and rules have been established for diagnosing them so that nearly all psychiatrists will agree about their diagnoses. As you will read in later chapters, some illnesses do yield to specific drug therapies and psychotherapies. Sometimes in psychiatry, the correct diagnosis does beget the correct treatment.

Distinguishing Illness from Health

To promote mental health, it is essential to have a concept of how illness can be distinguished from health. In the domain of the mind, this distinction is not always obvious. As we mentioned in Chapter 1, Dr. Thomas Szasz proposed that mental illness exists only when the condition is caused by an anatomical, physiological, or biochemical defect in the brain. If there are no such defects, he said it is a myth to call the condition an illness. Of course, Dr. Szasz's definition of illness does not help people decide whether they have a mental illness and need to see a psychiatrist. We do not think that this definition of illness is consistent even with the use of the term in general medicine. For example, a patient with low back pain has a legitimate reason to receive treatment even though he has no detectable anatomical or biochemical defect. Furthermore, even if psychiatrists understood the anatomical and biochemical defects in mental illness, the defects might be measurable only by invading and further harming the brain. The psychiatrist might not be able to determine whether a particular patient has a particular brain defect. In contrast to Dr. Szasz, we think that illness exists when the patient feels distressed and he is unable to maintain his normal day-to-day activities.

The discovery of anatomical abnormalities in Alzheimer's disease further illustrates the basic flaw in Dr. Szasz's definition of illness. This disease is a form of senility that begins with forgetfulness. In severely ill patients, almost all mental capacities deteriorate, and patients require total care. Anatomical abnormalities in the brains of patients with Alzheimer's disease were first described in 1906.[10] Does Dr. Szasz believe that Alzheimer's disease was just a myth until 1906? We do not think that any disease, psychiatric or nonpsychiatric, is a myth simply because its anatomical, physiological, and biochemical causes are not understood. Advances in science do not convert myths into reality. Psychiatric patients tell the doctor that they are distressed and disabled; the doctor sees evidence of the patients' suffering and loss of capacity for normal living. These symptoms establish the existence of illness in clinical medicine. Whether physicians know what is wrong with the body has no bearing on whether illness is present.[11]

Brief episodes of psychological distress and disability are an unavoidable and normal part of everyday healthy life. Most episodes do not require treatment; they just go away. If you begin a new job, for instance, it is normal to be anxious at first. But as you become accustomed to your new duties, you begin to relax. You stop feeling anxious in the morning; you begin to enjoy breakfast again. You recover your tolerance for minor irritation. If your mother-in-law criticizes you for letting your nine-year-old daughter wear shorts to school, you learn not to become furious. Instead, you give yourself a lecture about your mother-in-law's religious beliefs and the norms in the small town where she grew up. The distress that accompanies the problems of daily living, as long as it is brief and only mildly incapacitating, is not an illness. The difficult questions that psychiatrists and potential patients must try to answer are: How much and what kind of distress and disability indicate mental illness? When is it appropriate to seek medical advice?

Of course, when the distress is severe and the disability is incapacitating, there is no uncertainty about the need for treatment. For example, Mary is in her forties. She was healthy through high school, but when she was about eighteen, she began to have mental health problems. Now she sits or stands for hours at a time frozen rigidly in an uncomfortable posture and refuses to communicate. John is twenty years old. He did well during his freshman year of college, but he had to leave school as a sophomore because he began spending several hours a day making faces in the mirror and talking incoherently, sometimes to imaginary companions. No elaborate diagnostic procedure is required to determine that Mary and John are ill.

More commonly, the disability is less than completely incapacitating and the symptoms are less bizarre than John and Mary's. But how much sadness indicates depression? How much suspicion indicates paranoia? How much self-confidence indicates mania? Such questions make the detection, classification, and treatment of mental illness difficult. If your disability is not severe enough to keep you off the job or to disrupt your family life, and if the distress is not painful enough to make you cry for help, then uncertainty about whether mental illness exists will prevail.

Dr. R. L. Spitzer, in summarizing the problem of defining "clinically significant mental illness," suggested that a psychiatric condition should be called illness only if almost everyone, including the patient, agrees that there is both distress and disability.[12] Thus, Mary and John, or patients who attempted suicide or who sought refuge from imaginary persecutors by going to a police station, would be mentally ill. Patients may not always recognize their need for treatment while in the midst of acute episodes of mental turmoil, but afterward, when the crises have passed, as they almost always do, the patients agree that they are ill. In these clear-cut cases, treatment should be sought even though it may involve some risk, expense, and interference with the patient's established pattern of living.

In many cases, people disagree about whether distress and disability exist. Frequently, a person's family or friends may think that he has an undesirable psychological condition that requires treatment, while the person disagrees. For instance, some people who are heterosexually oriented regard homosexuality as a distressing disability. Yet, homosexually oriented individuals may feel neither impaired nor distressed. Dr. Spitzer recommended that the term *illness* not be applied in these ambiguous cases; instead, it should be reserved for cases in which all parties agree that both distress and disability exist.

Mental illnesses are not simply rare qualities of mind that set an individual apart from the average person. As Dr. Spitzer pointed out, unusual behavior can be admired and rewarded. The unusual psychological conditions of intellectual and artistic genius are not illnesses. Einstein was not considered to be distressed or disabled by his intelligence, nor was Mozart by his musical ability. Van Gogh was considered mad, not because of his artistic talent, but because of his depressions, rages, self-mutilation, and suicide. In fact, the existence of healthy nonconformity helps defend the mental health profession against the charge of surreptitiously enforcing conventional standards of conduct on nonconformists by branding them as ill and then coercively using drugs and psychotherapy.[13]

Although Dr. Spitzer defined only those conditions that unambiguously cause distress and disability as clinically significant illnesses, he did not imply that you should seek the services of a psychologist or psychiatrist only if you think you might have such a mental disease. On the contrary, professional mental health services may be appropriate for a wide spectrum of problems in which the presence of distress and disability is ambiguous. But the decision to seek treatment for these conditions must be an individual judgment made by each prospective patient. To help make this judgment, the prospective patient may wish to obtain professional advice about the probable benefits, risks, and costs of treatment. Psychiatrists or psychologists should give the patient an honest appraisal of what he stands to gain and lose by treatment, but they should not diagnose ambiguous cases as illness.[14]

Most psychiatrists see their mission as broader than merely treating the sick. They also want to help those in need who may not be suffering from a clinically significant illness. When a person asks for help, a psychiatrist or psychologist usually will not refuse assistance just because the person's condition does not fit Dr. Spitzer's definition of illness. Physicians practicing general medicine feel the same way as mental health professionals. When a woman goes to the doctor to get birth control pills, she is asking for help in solving a problem. Her doctor can help without considering her to be ill.[15]

Some people think that bearing hardship and pain in silence is admirable. The stoic has little sympathy for complainers and certainly would not consider asking a psychiatrist for help with a mere problem of daily living. A stoic advises himself to "straighten up and fly right" and to "control" himself. Secretly, or not so secretly, he takes pride in not needing a psychiatrist. His first meeting with a psychiatrist, if he ever does meet one, may be in an emergency situation when a small "problem of living" has become a crisis.

There are other people who are always worried that life is not just right. Such a person may seek psychiatric help to assuage even minor unhappiness. "Why doesn't the baby sleep through the night? Why does my two-year-old get into everything? Why does my husband look at girls? Where did I go wrong?" If a psychiatrist can help such a person, then help should be given. Perhaps the asking is reason enough for helping, even when a person is not mentally ill.

Standardizing Diagnostic Techniques

When it is agreed that illness exists and treatment is desirable, how does a psychiatrist determine what kind of illness the patient has? It would be nice if psychiatrists could perform a laboratory test like the one used to diagnose strep throat. The psychiatrist's assistant would wipe some bacteria off the patient's throat with a cotton swab and grow the bacteria in a dish until the colonies were large enough to see. Then the assistant could identify what might be called "schizophrenococcus," "depressococcus," or "neurotococcus" organisms by their particular visible characteristics. If mental illness were a type of infection, the same diagnostic procedures could be used each time the test was performed, no matter who did the test. Also, the same method of interpreting the results would be used each time, no matter who evaluated them. In fact, the psychiatrist would not have to make the diagnoses at all. She would just certify the diagnoses made by her assistant.

The suggestion that mental illnesses could be diagnosed by a throat culture is facetious, of course, but the idea of using a laboratory test to identify mental illness is not unrealistic. In fact, several research groups are developing such tests. One is the dexamethazone suppression test. It measures the response of a patient's hormone system to the injection of a drug called dexamethazone. In some people who have depression, the hormone system fails to respond normally to dexamethazone. However, the problem with the dexamethazone suppression test, and the reason it remains experimental, is that about 50 percent of the people with depression have normal responses to dexamethazone. Thus, in these people, depression would go undetected if psychiatrists used the test as their only diagnostic procedure. A 50 percent detection rate is not as good as conventional psychiatric diagnosis and is vastly inferior to the detection rate of the laboratory test for strep throat.[16]

Varying Symptoms of Mental Illness

Unlike strep throat, in which a few invariant symptoms suffice to establish a diagnosis, psychiatric illnesses are ever-changing, complex sets of behaviors that are somewhat different in each individual. No set of simple observations and no single symptom differentiates one psychiatric disease from another. In many mental illnesses, there is not even a single symptom that all patients have. For example, not all people with depression attempt suicide, just as their hormone systems do not all respond abnormally on the dexamethazone suppression test. Not all people with mania spend money profligately. Not all people with schizophrenia hear voices.

Psychiatrists must try to identify a pattern of symptoms, even when many elements of the typical illness pattern are absent. Often they must use information about how the illness developed in the months or years prior to a patient's current episode. Sometimes, the psychiatrist will be unable to classify the illness, even though the patient is obviously ill.[17]

In mental illness, the brain is the organ that functions improperly. Thus, we expect, solely on biological grounds, that the symptoms of mental illness would be highly variable from one patient to another. The social and psychological functions of the brain are determined by the details of communication in the brain's vast network of synaptic connections. The construction and maintenance of this network are in turn dependent on a person's heredity and environment. Except for identical twins, every person is born with a different set of genes and hence a functionally unique set of brain circuits. Every person grows up in a unique environment that further individualizes the details of his circuitry. Indeed, it has recently become possible, using microscopes and electronic recording instruments, to observe functionally significant environmental and hereditary effects on the synaptic connectivity of brain cells. Of course, other organs are also individualized by the uniqueness of each person's heredity and environment. For example, a woman's heart and lungs will be unusually efficient if her parents gave her genes for a strong heart and lungs and if she jogs regularly. A man's skin will be unusually brown if his parents gave him genes for lots of skin pigment and if he regularly spends time on the beach. But in comparison to other organs, the uniqueness of each person's brain has a more significant impact on the person's life. In the brain, the effects of heredity and environment individualize each person's social and psychological functioning.

Because each person's brain is unique, we must expect that the same type of mental illness will be expressed differently in different people. Suppose, for instance, that two people have the symptom of bizarre delusions. One person is an Eskimo, and the other a New Yorker. The Eskimo may believe she has a fox inside her that is speaking to her and controlling her behavior. She says she can even feel the hair of the fox's tail in her throat. In contrast, the New Yorker may believe he has been chosen by the Supreme One to save the city from invaders. He knows he has been given this role because the Supreme One regularly inserts instructions and commands directly into his brain via microwaves that radiate from television towers. Suppose that two other people are suffering from depression. One patient may be overcome with the mistaken belief that he is penniless and cannot afford the expense of simple pleasures like buying an ice cream cone or going to the movies. The other patient with depression may lie in bed sobbing, day after day, obsessed with the idea that she is incompetent to work and worthless to others. Thus, psychiatric diagnosis is difficult, not because mental illness is a myth, not because mental illness is nonbiological, and not because psychiatry is unscientific, but because the same underlying problem is not always expressed in the same way by individuals who are unique.

The Diagnostic and Statistical Manual

In 1980 the American Psychiatric Association published a book that promises to bring about a significant advance in the art of psychiatric diagnosis. This book, *The Diagnostic and Statistical Manual*, Third Edition, or simply, the *DSM-III*, includes a set of official definitions of 187 illnesses that psychiatrists and psychologists can use to make standard diagnoses of the mental illnesses they encounter in their practices.[18] The illnesses are defined by easily detectable symptoms. This manual also includes a set of descriptive criteria, stated as precisely and objectively as possible, that must be met by a patient's illness before the illness can be called by a particular name. In the *DSM-III* there is no attempt to explain the causes of mental illnesses. The purpose of the manual is merely to reduce diagnostic confusion.[19]

For almost thirty years, the American Psychiatric Association has sponsored efforts to clarify and standardize psychiatric diagnosis. The association published the first edition of the *Diagnostic and Statistical Manual* in 1952.[20] A second edition appeared in 1968.[21] Work started on the third edition in 1974, when the American Psychiatric Association appointed a task force, under the leadership of Dr. Robert L. Spitzer, to prepare a new diagnostic manual reflecting recent developments in diagnostic research. The members of the task force, together with other invited experts, formed small committees, each specializing in a particular family of psychiatric illnesses. The task of the committee members was, in large part, to debate until they could agree on which conditions to consider illnesses, what symptoms to use to diagnose them, and what to call the illnesses. Their arguments, of course, were supposed to be based on the results of diagnostic research.[22]

The committee consulted with representatives of other professional mental health organizations, such as the American Psychological Association and the American Psychoanalytic Association. At a special convention, about one hundred experts in psychiatric diagnosis gave speeches and questioned each other about problems of defining and diagnosing mental illness. Also, the material in preliminary drafts of the manual was tested extensively in field trials. The purpose of the field trials was to demonstrate the practicality and reliability of the information in the new manual for making psychiatric diagnoses in typical clinical settings. Over 12,000 patients, 550 clinical psychiatrists, and 212 psychiatric facilities were involved in testing the material presented in the successive drafts of the *DSM-III*.[23]

At many times during the project, the task force's work was more akin to treaty negotiation than to scientific deliberation. The experts represented many different theories of psychiatry, from Freud to Skinner. Psychiatrists and psychologists, of course, valiantly protect and defend their theories as if they are monarchs defending kingdoms. Therefore, compromises had to be made. For example, in an early draft of the *DSM-III*, mental conditions were defined as "medical disorders." Objections from the American Psychological Association led the task force to change the definition to "psychological disorders." Also, the word *neurosis* was not used in early drafts because it was considered too ambiguous. But vigorous objections from the psychoanalytic lobby restored this esteemed word in the final draft, though it was placed in parentheses.[24]

The inclusion of diagnostic criteria in the third edition of this manual is perhaps the most pioneering departure from earlier diagnostic manuals. Although diagnostic criteria were used in research as early as 1972, their clinical use had never before been advocated by an official body of clinical psychiatrists, such as the American Psychiatric Association.[25] The recommendation that psychiatrists make their diagnoses by referring to explicit, published criteria rather than by relying on professional judgment, insight, and empathy moves psychiatry closer to other branches of medicine than it has been in the past.[26]

The *DSM-III* is not a final statement about diagnosis. On the contrary, many of the definitions and criteria are based only on the collective opinion of the task force members in 1979. Collective professional opinion is better than individual professional opinion, of course, but it is no substitute for knowledge based on well-designed research. To adequately define a disease, its cause and course of development must be known. This kind of information is simply not available for most psychiatric illnesses. As research proceeds, *The Diagnostic and Statistical Manual* will probably be revised again and again.[27]

The Structured Interview

Because the *DSM-III* specifies criteria for distinguishing among different kinds of illnesses, psychiatrists try to collect the information that the criteria require. The *DSM-III* does not, however, guarantee that different psychiatrists will collect the diagnostic information in exactly the same way. To standardize information acquisition, research psychiatrists have recently begun to use a diagnostic procedure called the structured interview. The structured interview is a standardized set of questions that the diagnostician asks the patient. The questions are organized so that all the information required by the criteria will be obtained efficiently and in the same way for every patient.[28]

One objection to structured interviews is that they are too inflexible. Many psychiatrists are uncomfortable asking all their patients exactly the same questions. They feel they cannot be sensitive to the patient's unique needs when constrained by such a rigid protocol. A possible solution for psychiatrists would be to have a trained diagnostician conduct the standardized interview, much as a family doctor has a laboratory technician take a throat culture. This approach would allow the psychiatrist to deal more exclusively with aspects of the treatment in which judgments and personal relationships are beneficial.

We recently discovered that some psychiatrists have already begun to delegate responsibility for conducting the structured interview. Standing in the checkout line at the supermarket one evening, we met a psychiatrist friend of ours, Dr. Care.

"I've been down at the office playing with my new computer," he said.

This stimulated our interest because we had just purchased a small computer to use as a word processor in writing this book, and we like to compare notes on equipment. "What do you use it for, bookkeeping and word processing?" we asked.

"No, I have a diagnostic program on it," he answered.

Now we were really interested. "Do you do a structured interview and then submit the patient's answers to the computer for a diagnosis?" we asked.

"No, the computer does the interview," Dr. Care explained. "The patient sits down at the console and answers the questions that the computer puts on the screen. After the patient is finished, the computer prints out a psychiatric-medical history in readable English and then gives a *DSM-III* diagnosis. Then I follow up on the computer diagnosis with a personal interview. It's good for patients because they don't have to pay me so much for an hour-and-a-half personal diagnostic interview, and I like it because I can get comparable information about all my patients. Without the computer, I'm always worried that I'll get committed to the wrong diagnosis early in the interview and then fail to obtain all the information that might tell me my initial diagnosis was a mistake."

It is too early to predict whether computers will improve the reliability of psychiatric diagnosis, but we think diagnosis by computer is an exciting development with many potential benefits. For example, patients may develop more confidence in psychiatrists. If we were going to a psychiatrist, we would be more confident that we were getting conscientious, up-to-date treatment if we first received a computer diagnosis. We would be reluctant to depend on the doctor to remember all the questions and to ask them in a way that would not bias our answers. Another benefit, the most important one, is that using a reproducible, uniform diagnostic procedure will encourage mental health professionals to use disease categories in a uniform way. (Incidentally, many health insurance policies now require that patients' claims for mental health services include *DSM-III* diagnoses.)

In Chapter 4 we take a close look at the *DSM-III* criteria for schizophrenia, and in Chapter 9 we examine the criteria for mania and depression. We selected these illness categories for discussion for three reasons. First, they are clinically significant illnesses in that they are prevalent and debilitating. Second, the diagnoses of illness in these categories are supported by a considerable amount of diagnostic research. Third, schizophrenia, mania and depression are the categories of mental illness that are frequently and successfully treated with drugs.

Excessive and inappropriate anxiety is another condition that is often treated with drugs. In fact, many more people receive treatment for anxiety than for schizophrenia, mania, and depression. We discuss the drug treatment of anxiety in Chapters 15 and 16. Usually, anxiety is not a distinct illness. Rather, it is a symptom of stress. The stress may come from an illness or from environmental circumstances. Anxiety is like the fever that accompanies the flu. Fever is a distressing symptom of the illness, and the doctor may suggest treating it with aspirin to make the patient feel better, but the fever is not the illness. Similarly, though treating anxiety may make the patient feel better, anxiety is not the illness. Sometimes, however, anxiety seems to be the principal symptom and to have a life of its own. Then, patients have anxiety disorders, as defined in the *DMS-III*. However, because most patients given drugs to treat anxiety do not suffer from these anxiety disorders, we do not discuss their diagnosis in detail.

4

Diagnosing Schizophrenia

Schizophrenia is probably not a single illness but a group of similar illnesses. The different types of schizophrenia may show some variation in cause, symptoms, course of development, and response to treatment. The existence of several different types is not firmly established, however, so we concentrate here only on the diagnosis of the larger class of schizophrenic disorders. This entire class is commonly referred to as schizophrenia.[1]

Symptoms

In the *DSM-III*, great emphasis is placed on the fact that people with schizophrenia usually suffer from profoundly false beliefs, called delusions, and equally false perceptions, called hallucinations. Emotions and motivations are also disordered, but these symptoms are less useful diagnostically because they are more difficult to describe and observe objectively. Schizophrenic delusions and hallucinations are not just peculiarities; they are not false beliefs commonly held by many people, such as superstitions or eccentric political philosophies. Unlike superstitions and philosophies, delusions are not learned. People with schizophrenia invent them. These delusions are so strange, bizarre, magical, and unrealizable that healthy people are usually amazed that the patient does indeed believe them. Schizophrenia patients cannot be dissuaded from their delusions by reasoned argument. When a patient is asked how he knows that his beliefs are true, he often answers, "I just know."

We can illustrate the nature of schizophrenia most easily by describing a fictionalized patient who exhibits many typical delusional and hallucinatory symptoms. Judy, a twenty-three-year-old college graduate, was brought to the hospital by her parents because she had developed a severe mental illness. About six months earlier, she had quit her first job as a proofreader and had become withdrawn and uncommunicative. This behavior was astonishing because Judy had never before been unusually shy or anxious.

When Judy left her job, she knew that something was happening to her, but she did not know quite what. She became more and more preoccupied with her thoughts. She ruminated on the meaning of existence and religious matters. Her personal appearance deteriorated. She stopped taking care of her hair, using cosmetics, and keeping her clothes clean. Then, a few weeks before she was brought to the hospital, she became convinced that her mission was to save the world from cataclysmic destruction. According to Judy, other people did not know about the imminent threat and did not appreciate the necessity of taking action. Judy said she knew because the information had been directly implanted in her mind by a supernatural power.

She remembered the exact moment when she realized that she had to assume her mission. One morning she had awakened early. She stood in her room, looking out the window at the early light of dawn. An unusually bright planet was still visible near the eastern horizon. As she watched, the top edge of the sun broke over the horizon, and she saw a ray of orange light reach from the sun to the planet. The planet disappeared and the steeple clock began to toll six. She knew then that she had been chosen.

Her enemies knew of her mission because they could read her mind. She tried to occupy herself with trivia to prevent their clairvoyant espionage. They had placed writhing, coiling snakes in her abdomen to stop her. She frequently heard their voices talking about her, swearing at her, and plotting how they could thwart her secret plans. Sometimes, Judy talked back to her enemies. Many times a day, she received new proof of her role in the great cosmic struggle. She knew that certain events, which others thought were meaningless, were really signs. For example, just before she entered the hospital, a fly had landed on the television and started cleaning its wings while Barbara Walters was reporting on the satellite pictures from Jupiter. Judy knew then that not much time was left.

Judy spoke in complete sentences and could usually be understood, but some people with schizophrenia have trouble making their thoughts comprehensible to others. Patients may jump from one idea to another before completing any one sentence. They may also use made-up words. In extremely ill patients, speech may deteriorate into a random string of words that do not form sentences. Psychiatrists often use the term *formal thought disorder* to refer to this disorganization in the thinking process.

The effects of schizophrenia on a person's emotions and motivation are an important part of the illness, even though they are less useful for diagnostic purposes than abnormal thoughts and perceptions. A patient with schizophrenia may express emotion only faintly or not at all. He may have a monotonous, stony, unrevealing facial expression most of the time. He may not laugh at jokes, cry at funerals, or smile when receiving a present. Psychiatrists call this deficit in emotional expression *flat affect.* When a person with schizophrenia does express emotions, he may do so inappropriately; he may laugh when nothing is funny, cry when nothing is sad, or act pleased when telling of a relative's death. The schizophrenia patient often retreats into his private world of fantasies and hallucinations. He ignores his work, family, and social responsibilities. If severely ill, he ignores his basic needs—he will not dress, wash, eat, or use the toilet.

The symptoms of schizophrenia are seldom apparent in childhood. Usually, they first appear in adolescence or young adulthood. The disease lasts at least six months and commonly recurs intermittently throughout a lifetime. With the benefit of hindsight, people can often realize that the patient had strange, eccentric ways even before he became actuely ill.

Schizophrenia is not rare. According to various estimates, between 0.5 and 1.0 percent of the people throughout the world suffer from an episode of the illness at some point in their lives. The illness is about equally common in men and women.

Diagnostic Criteria

Six diagnostic criteria for schizophrenia are presented in the *DSM-III*. To make the diagnosis, all six of the criteria must be satisfied, but several of them can be satisfied in more than one way. These criteria, labeled A through F, follow.

Criterion A

At least one of the following must occur during a phase of the illness:

1. Bizarre delusions (content is patently absurd and has no possible basis in fact), such as delusions of being controlled, thought broadcasting, thought insertion, or thought withdrawal.

2. Somatic, grandiose, religious, nihilistic, or other delusions without persecutory or jealous content.

3. Delusions with persecutory or jealous content if accompanied by hallucinations of any type.

4. Auditory hallucinations in which either a voice keeps up a running commentary on the individual's behavior or thoughts, or two or more voices converse with each other.

5. Auditory hallucinations on several occasions with content of more than one or two words, having no apparent relation to elation or depression.

6. Incoherence, marked loosening of associations, markedly illogical thinking, or marked poverty of content of speech if associated with at least one of the following:
    a. blunted, flat, or inappropriate affect
    b. delusions or hallucinations
    c. catatonic or other grossly disorganized behavior.[2]

Each of the six ways of satisfying this criterion involves false beliefs, false perceptions, or disorganized thought processes. Because every healthy person sometimes has disorganized thinking and mistaken beliefs, this criterion attempts to distinguish the confused and mistaken thoughts of the schizophrenia patient from those of the healthy person and from those of people suffering from other forms of mental illness.

Element 1 says that schizophrenia is indicated by delusions that have the distinct quality of being bizarre, magical, or utterly impossible. Judy had magical, utterly impossible delusions. She believed that thoughts had been placed directly into her mind by telepathic communication (thought insertion) and that others could read her mind (thought broadcasting). She believed that her behavior and thinking were controlled by an outside power (delusion of being controlled) and that she had snakes in her abdomen (utterly impossible somatic delusion). Sometimes, the patient believes that thoughts have been removed from his mind (thought withdrawal).

Element 2 of Criterion A refers to a second category of delusion in which the false beliefs are less bizarre, less magical, and perhaps not impossible. The afflicted person may erroneously believe that one of his legs has gangrene and is rotting away (nonbizarre somatic delusion). A woman may wrongly believe that she is engaged to an heir of the Spanish throne (a grandiose delusion, but not an impossible one). Judy believed incorrectly that she occupied a position of great responsibility (grandiose delusion, not impossible) and that the world was soon coming to an end (nihilistic, not impossible). Nonbizarre delusions of jealousy and persecution are excluded from the second element because, by themselves, they do not always signify schizophrenia. They can occur in other illnesses, for example, depression. Thus, a depressed wife might falsely believe that because of her sexual inadequacy her husband has rejected her for another lover. Or a divorcée might believe incorrectly that her ex-husband is purposely persecuting her by being nice to the children and making them love him more than her.

Element 3 specifies that persecutory and jealous delusions can satisfy Criterion A if they are accompanied by hallucinations. Suppose, for instance, that the divorcée, while on vacation by herself in another city, hears her children talking to each other about what a bad mother and a good father they have. This delusion of persecution satisfies Criterion A for schizophrenia, but without the hallucinated voices, one is unsure whether this delusion of persecution is a symptom of schizophrenia.

Elements 4 and 5 deal with the common symptom of hallucinated voices. Visual hallucinations are much less common than auditory hallucinations. Other sensory hallucinations (those involving touch, taste, or smell, such as the belief that one smells an alien being) are more rare still. Element 4 specifies that a hallucinated voice must speak rather elaborately. A hallucinated voice that speaks no more than a word or two on only a few occasions does not, by itself, qualify because such simple auditory hallucinations also occur in nonschizophrenic mental illness. In Element 5 simpler auditory hallucinations are included as a qualifying symptom if they are clearly not accompanied by emotional depression or elation. When emotional depression or elation also exists, the patient's abnormally intense emotions may be triggering the hallucinated voices. In genuine schizophrenia, according to the *DSM-III*, the patient can hear voices even when he is not experiencing extremes of emotion.

Element 6 focuses on a class of symptoms that has been regarded as a signature of schizophrenia ever since the illness was first described by Emil Kraeplin in 1896. These symptoms are the formal thought disorders. As we described earlier, the patient's speech may make no sense or contain little meaning. The patient may jump from one idea to the next with little continuity. She may repeat the same words over and over or make up new words. She shows no signs of being aware that her thinking is strange or that her listeners can not understand her. In fact, she may believe that her thoughts are profoundly significant.

In the *Comprehensive Textbook of Psychiatry* Dr. Heinz E. Lehmann described a patient who had a formal thought disorder. This patient, who had been diagnosed as having schizophrenia, was nevertheless well enough to retain a part-time job as a secretary. She was generally preoccupied with ideas about religion, invisible forces, radiation, psychology, and other esoterica. One day she typed the following memo:

Mental health is the Blessed Trinity, and as man cannot be without God, it is futile to deny His Son. For the Creation understands germ-any in Voice New Order, not lie of chained reaction, spawning mark in temple Cain with Babel grave'n image to wanton V day 'Isreal.'

Lucifer fell Jew prostitute and Labeth walks by roam to sex ritual, in Bible six million of the Babylon woman, infer-no salvation.[3]

Dr. Lehmann also presented another example of schizophrenic writing, one even more difficult to decipher:

The seabeach gathering homestead building upon the site of the bear mountains. Time placed of the dunce to the recovery of the setting sun, upon the stream, poling paddleboat, Mickey, Rooney, Bill. Proceeded of, to the enlivenment. Placed upon the assiduous laboriousness of keeping aloof, yet alive to the forest stream. Haunting the distance of the held possession, requiring means of liberty to sociability. . . .[4]

Of course, meaningless speech often occurs temporarily in people who do not have schizophrenia—for instance, in people who are intoxicated with alcohol or some other drug, or in people who have other illnesses that cause extreme excitement and delerium. Even a perfectly healthy teenager can sound disordered at a football game if his team scores the winning touchdown in the last seconds of the game. A normal parent may be a bit confused at a child's wedding. Therefore, Criterion A requires that the disordered thought be accompanied by the additional symptoms of (a) blunted, flat, or inappropriate affect, (b) delusions or hallucinations, or (c) catatonic or other grossly disorganized behavior.

"Blunted, flat, or inappropriate affect" refers to the abnormalities in the expression of emotion that often occur in schizophrenia. As we mentioned previously, many people with schizophrenia show little emotion at all. Their faces remain expressionless most of the time, and they do not respond to events that would normally cause pleasure, amusement, or sadness. Other patients show emotions at inappropriate times, laughing while telling of a child's death or becoming enraged when greeted with, "How are you?"

We have already adequately discussed delusions and hallucinations. We have not, however, described "catatonic or other grossly disorganized behavior." *Catatonia* refers to abnormal movements as distinguished from abnormal thoughts and speech. One well-known catatonic symptom is assuming a fixed, often uncomfortable posture and remaining motionless for an extremely long time. A patient might stand for hours with one arm raised or sit rigidly in one position for so long that pressure sores develop. The patient seems to be in a stuporous state, unresponsive and silent. Paradoxically, injecting the patient with a small dose of barbiturate, a drug that causes relaxation and sleep in normal people, will often release the catatonic patient from his statuelike pose. A second catatonic symptom is "waxy flexibility." A patient with this symptom holds any posture that she is put into. If the hospital attendant raises the patient's arm, she will hold the arm up indefinitely; if the attendant turns the patient's head to the right, she continues looking to the right, and so on. A third symptom, excited catatonia, is excessive, purposeless, and disorganized movements. A patient with excited catatonia can become so hyperactive and uncontrolled that he becomes a danger to himself and others. Fortunately, because of drug treatments for schizophrenia that have been developed during the past twenty-five years, catatonic symptoms are no longer often seen in patients with schizophrenia.

Other examples of grossly disorganized behaviors that may accompany incoherent speech include posturing and grimacing in front of a mirror for hours, failing to use the toilet, eating feces, taking off all one's clothes, and dressing in weird ways. In a recent journalistic account of a schizophrenia patient, Susan Sheehan described a woman named Sylvia Frumkin who adorned herself by knotting silverware into her hair and by tying a tee shirt around her neck and periodically wearing it around her head like a headband.[5]

Criterion B

Deterioration from previous level of functioning in such areas as work, social relations, and self-care.[6]

As in Judy's case, the onset of schizophrenia is marked by clear-cut changes from previously established patterns of thought, emotional expression, and behavior. Thus, the patient's family and friends may remark, "Judy has changed," or "Judy didn't used to be this way." Furthermore, if working, the schizophrenia patient may lose his job or be transferred to a position of lesser responsibility. He also may alienate his friends or cease responding to them. If married, he may begin having new difficulty getting along with his spouse. Of course, some people exhibit eccentric behavior almost from birth. Some never learn to speak coherently. And some are passive, shy, or withdrawn. Such lifelong traits, distressing though they may be, are not symptoms of schizophrenia, according to the *DSM-III*. Both personality traits and lifelong illnesses that have no clear onset are excluded from the category.

Criterion C

Duration: Continuous signs of the illness for at least six months at some time during the person's life, with some signs of illness at present. The six-month period must include an active phase during which there were symptoms from Criterion A, with or without a prodromal or residual phase, as defined below.

Prodromal phase: A clear deterioration in functioning before the active phase of the illness not due to a disturbance in mood or to a Substance Use Disorder and involving at least two of the symptoms noted below.

Residual phase: Persistence, following the active phase of the illness, of at least two of the symptoms noted below, not due to a disturbance in mood or to a Substance Use Disorder.

Prodromal or Residual Symptoms

1. Social isolation or withdrawal.

2. Marked impairment in role functioning as wage-earner, student or homemaker.

3. Markedly peculiar behavior (e.g., collecting garbage, talking to self in public, or hoarding food).

4. Marked impairment in personal hygiene and grooming.

5. Blunted, flat, or inappropriate affect.

6. Digressive, vague, overelaborate, circumstantial, or metaphorical speech.

7. Odd or bizarre ideation, or magical thinking, e.g., superstitiousness, clairvoyance, telepathy, 'sixth sense,' 'others can feel my feelings,' overvalued ideas, ideas of reference.

8. Unusual perceptual experience, e.g., recurrent illusions, sensing the presence of a force or person not actually present.[7]

The main purpose of this criterion is to establish that schizophrenia is a long-lasting illness. Symptoms as severe as those specified in Criterion A, however, do not have to be present continually. Schizophrenia waxes and wanes in severity. The time spent in the severe phase plus the time in less severe phases must total at least six months.

A "prodromal phase" refers to a period of lesser severity that precedes the outbreak of an intense episode. A "residual phase is a period of less intense illness that follows an intense episode. Judy had a prodromal phase which preceded the outbreak of delusions and hallucinations. During this phase, she quit her work (sympton 2), became socially withdrawn (symptom 1), and let her personal appearance deteriorate (symptom 4). She also became preoccupied with thoughts about the meaning of existence and other religious matters (perhaps symptom 7). Note that symptoms thought to result from excessive drug use (called substance abuse disorder) or from a disturbance of mood do not contribute to a diagnosis of a prodromal or residual phase of schizophrenia.

Though all these symptoms seem like disturbances of mood, psychiatrists make a subtle distinction between disturbances of mood and disturbances of thought and perception. Illnesses due to changes in mood are called affective disorders and are distinct from schizophrenia. The word *affect* often means "emotion" or "mood." The illness of depression, with its unjustified feelings of hopelessness and sadness, is a disorder of affect. Mania, with its overconfident excitement, is also a disorder of affect. But, according to the *DSM-III*, schizophrenia is primarily a disorder of thinking and perception, not an affective disorder. Mood changes occur in schizophrenia, but they are thought to be a result, not a cause, of the delusions and hallucinations. Criterion C, therefore, instructs psychiatrists to discount symptoms that seem to be caused by mood changes. Sometimes, this distinction is difficult to make with certainty. How can a psychiatrist know, for instance, that a patient's social withdrawal is not being caused by a depressed mood?

Criterion D

The full depressive or manic syndrome (criteria A and B of major depressive or manic episode), if present, developed after any psychotic symptoms, or was brief in duration relative to the duration of the psychotic symptoms in A.[8]

Again, the focus is on differentiating schizophrenia from mania and depression. This is an important distinction because of the tendency for American psychiatrists to overdiagnose schizophrenia and underdiagnose affective disorders. As we mentioned in Chapter 3, American psychiatrists have diagnosed schizophrenia much more frequently and manic depression much less frequently than have British psychiatrists. A catchy slogan that became popular in the

American psychiatric community in the 1950s is, "Even a trace of schizophrenia is schizophrenia."[9] Obviously, the attitude expressed in this slogan would lead to the excessive diagnosis of schizophrenia.

The *DSM-III* task force tried to restrict the diagnosis of schizophrenia to those patients in whom the schizophrenic symptoms clearly predominate over the symptoms of affective disorders. To predominate, the schizophrenic symptoms must occur before and last longer than the symptoms of mania or depression. If the psychiatrist cannot determine which symptoms predominate, then according to the *DSM-III*, she should call the illness a Schizoaffective Disorder, meaning that clear symptoms of schizophrenia are present together with clear symptoms of an affective disorder.[10]

Criterion E

Onset of prodromal or active phase of illness before age 45.[11]

This criterion is as clear as it is brief. If schizophrenia is going to occur, according to the *DSM-III*, it will occur in the young adult. Symptoms often first appear in the late teens or early twenties. One effect of this criterion is to exclude from schizophrenia illnesses with similar symptoms that occur in the elderly as a result of deterioration of blood vessels and nerve cells in the brain. The *DSM-III* calls these diseases *dementias*. It is interesting that even though some symptoms of schizophrenia and dementia are similar, the two classes of disease do not appear to have the same biological causes. Visible anatomical deterioration of the brain's blood vessels or nerve cells occurs frequently in the dementias but seldom in schizophrenia. Of course, biochemical deterioration that is not visible anatomically might frequently occur in schizophrenia.[12]

Criterion F

Not due to any Organic Mental Disorder or Mental Retardation.[13]

The purpose of this brief criterion is to rule out the possibility that the symptoms are caused by another known illness that is not schizophrenia. Mental retardation, of course, would be easily

5

Causes of Schizophrenia

In the first four chapters we presented the view that mental illness is brain illness; we presented some fundamentals of neuroscience; and we discussed psychiatric diagnosis, including the diagnostic criteria for schizophrenia. In the next four chapters, we discuss the causes and treatment of schizophrenia. We consider the evidence that schizophrenia is a genuine biological entity and that it can be effectively treated with drugs.

Research on Brain Biochemistry

If the biology of schizophrenia were really understood, we would be able to describe precisely how the brain of a person with schizophrenia differs from the brain of a healthy person. The discussion of the biology of the brain in Chapter 2 suggests that there are many possible ways in which the function of a healthy brain might be disrupted. An entire region of the brain might be missing. The neurons in a schizophrenic brain might fail to produce a particular transmitter. The neurons might produce too much or too little transmitter. Or, they might make the wrong transmitter. Another possibility is that a particular class of receptors does not function normally. There are, of course, many other possible causes of mental illness.

Unfortunately, neuroscientists do not yet know exactly what causes schizophrenia. They are fairly certain, however, that the biochemistry of schizophrenic brains is abnormal. In conjunction with their work on how drugs that are used to treat schizophrenia affect the brain, researchers are obtaining some hints about the nature of the defects causing the disease. One of the most probable hypotheses is that schizophrenia involves a malfunction of synapses using dopamine as a transmitter. We further discuss the biochemistry of schizophrenia in Chapter 7 when we examine the biochemical consequences of treating schizophrenia with drugs.

Consider some of the difficulties in determining the nature of the defect in a schizophrenic brain. The usual procedure in biomedical research is to conduct experiments on laboratory animals which have either the disease being studied or a very similar disease. But only humans suffer from schizophrenia. Therefore, researchers cannot compare the brain biochemistry of normal and schizophrenic rats like cancer researchers compare the cells of normal and cancerous rats. Research on living human patients is, of course, severely restricted by ethical considerations. Scientists can analyze samples of human blood and urine, and in some cases they can analyze the cerebrospinal fluid (the fluid surrounding the brain and spinal cord). But because schizophrenia is probably caused by a defect that exists in only a few small regions of the brain, researchers would have to be extremely lucky to learn much from blood or urine that has picked up chemicals from all over the body, or from cerebrospinal fluid that has washed the entire brain. Therefore, data from experiments using these methods cannot fully describe the biochemical differences between a schizophrenic brain and a healthy brain. Nonethless, even relatively crude biochemical experiments can provide some leads about the causes of schizophrenia.

Another research approach is to biochemically analyze the brain of schizophrenia patients immediately after their death. In these postmortem studies, scientists compare the brains of schizophrenia patients with brains of healthy people or with brains of people suffering from other psychiatric diseases. But this approach does not always produce reliable information. The chemicals in the brain begin to deteriorate rapidly at the moment of death. Biochemical studies of dead brains are meaningless unless pieces of both healthy and schizophrenic brains can be removed within seconds of death under the same conditions. In addition, most schizophrenic patients have received drug treatment for many years. Scientists have no way of knowing whether changes in patients' brains result from the disease or from the drugs used in treatment.

Despite our ignorance of details, we have three sound reasons for thinking that schizophrenia is a biological entity with biochemical causes. First, drug treatments that alter the biochemistry of the brain often cause a dramatic improvement in the symptoms. (In Chapter 6, we discuss the drug treatments in more detail.) Second, some recent research suggests that the anatomy of schizophrenic brains may not be quite normal. Using an x-ray technique called computerized tomography, a researcher can view the outlines of a patient's brain. Although brain scans of patients with schizophrenia seem normal on casual inspection, some researchers believe that these brains have a variety of subtle abnormalities. For example, the fluid spaces in the brain may be enlarged, the structure of the cerebral cortex may be abnormal, or the asymmetry between the right and left sides of the brain may be quite different from the asymmetry in a healthy person's brain. While these findings are tantalizing, they are controversial, especially since some researchers have been unable to replicate them.[1]

Third, we believe that a predisposition to schizophrenia is inherited. The importance of heredity does not mean that the environment is unimportant. Both heredity and environment contribute to many aspects of normal human development. For instance, excellence in musical performance requires both innate talent and training; tallness requires both tall ancestors and adequate nutrition.

Influence of Heredity and Environment on Disease

Among diseases that affect the brain and behavior, all degrees of genetic transmission and environmental causality exist. For example, Huntington's chorea is a neurological disease of purely genetic origin.[2] Patients carrying the gene for Huntington's chorea usually seem healthy until they are between thirty and fifty years old. About this time, the first symptoms, involuntary, jerky movements, appear. Mental deterioration and death follow. Physicians know that the disease is inherited because they understand its mechanism of transmission. Half the children of an affected parent will develop the disease.

Wilson's disease, a disorder of copper metabolism, is another genetically transmitted neurological disease.[3] A person who inherits Wilson's disease genes from both parents (even if neither parent actually suffers from the disease) will always develop it. The abnormal accumulation of copper may cause a variety of psychiatric symptoms, including some typical of schizophrenia or manic-depressive psychosis. A normal environment cannot prevent the disease, but a drug that increases the excretion of copper can. (You may or may not want to call the use of a drug an environmental change.)

Phenylketonuria (PKU) is another genetic disease that affects the brain.[4] A baby born with PKU is unable to metabolize the amino acid phenylalanine, a substance that is part of most proteins and exists in many foods. In a PKU baby the incompletely metabolized phenylalanine builds up to toxic levels in the blood. These toxins affect the brain, causing mental retardation. But if a PKU baby is diagnosed at birth by chemical tests, the parents can avoid these dire consequences by feeding the baby a special diet containing no phenylalanine. Although the effects of PKU can be prevented, we would not want to say that a parent with an undiagnosed, mentally retarded PKU baby is guilty of providing a bad environment for the child.

Deprivation dwarfism is a brain disease with proven environmental causes. In this syndrome, children who receive little love, cuddling, or attention actually stop growing normally and are, therefore, extremely small for their age. The release of the hormones responsible for growth is controlled by the brain, and lack of normal social stimulation prevents the child's brain from calling for the proper amounts of these hormones.

A dramatic example of deprivation dwarfism is an infant who, because of a birth defect, had to be fed through a tube in her esophagus.[5] The mother religiously followed the doctor's feeding instructions but was so fearful of dislodging the tube that she rarely picked up or fondled her daughter. By fifteen months of age, the child's physical development was only that of a normal eight-month-old. When she was admitted to the hospital, she began to receive considerable attention from the hospital staff. Thus, she began to grow rapidly even though the staff and the mother fed her, still through the tube, precisely the same food.

Older children diagnosed as deprivation dwarfs exhibit some bizarre behaviors.[6] They wander about the house in the middle of the night. They eat and drink inappropriately, for example, drinking water out of toilet bowls. Upon entering the hospital, their behavior improves rapidly. They begin to grow even more rapidly than their healthy peers, indicating that they are not genetically small. You might suspect that this improvement results from improved nutrition, but these children are not malnourished when they enter the hospital. The attention they receive in the hospital probably triggers the brain to function normally, just as neglect probably triggers the brain to malfunction.

The relative influences of heredity and environment in schizophrenia have been more difficult to distinguish. Schizophrenia is neither purely hereditary, like Huntington's chorea, nor purely environmental, like deprivation dwarfism. Researchers still have not succeeded in discovering either the mechanism of genetic transmission or the environmental factors that precipitate the disease. Nevertheless, scientists do know that both heredity and environment are involved in the development of schizophrenia.

The fact that schizophrenic parents frequently have schizophrenic children suggests, but does not prove, that schizophrenia is genetically transmitted. Because families share their environments as well as their genes, the shared environment, rather than the shared genes, might cause the disease to run in families. As the well-known psychiatrist Seymour Kety pointed out, the disease pellagra exemplifies the importance of a shared environment in the development of disease within a family.[7] Pellagra, a vitamin deficiency disease, runs in families not because it is inherited but because all family members eat the same food.

Study of Heritability

To show that schizophrenia is heritable, one must distinguish the effects of genes from the effects of environment. This distinction can be made by demonstrating that genetic children of schizophrenic parents have a high risk of developing schizophrenia even when they are raised in a healthy family. Of course, children cannot be assigned to parents at the whim of psychiatric geneticists, but by studying adopted children, the effects of heredity can be separated from the effects of the environment without disrupting families. Adopted children receive their genes from their genetic parents but their environments from their adoptive parents. Therefore, if the genetic parents of schizophrenic adopted children have an abnormally high incidence of schizophrenia but their adoptive parents do not, then one could conclude that schizophrenia is heritable. (The prevalence of schizophrenia in the general population is between 0.5 and 1.0 percent, which means that slightly fewer than 1 out of every 100 people will have the disease at some point during his lifetime.)

The prevalence of schizophrenia in adopted children and in their genetic and adopted parents can be studied only in countries such as Denmark where adoption records are not sealed by the courts. Therefore, the American psychiatrist Seymour Kety went to Denmark to obtain evidence for the heritability of schizophrenia. Kety studied both healthy and schizophrenic adopted "children."[8] (We call them children even though most were grown up by the time the study was done.) The two groups were as similar as possible in age, sex, socioeconomic class of adoptive family, time spent with biological relatives before adoption, and time spent in institutions or foster homes.

After locating the adoptive and genetic relatives of each adopted child, Kety's team interviewed each relative. Then, from these interviews, psychiatrists diagnosed each person as healthy, suffering from schizophrenia, or having a nonschizophrenic psychiatric illness. They found that about 6.4 percent of the genetic relatives of the schizophrenic adopted children had suffered from schizophrenia. In contrast, only 1.4 percent of the adoptive relatives had had the disease.

How do these statistics translate into the probability that schizophrenia will occur in any one family? If the genetic family of a schizophrenic child includes two parents and two additional siblings, there is a 25 percent chance that at least one member of this family will suffer from schizophrenia. If the adoptive family includes two adoptive parents and their two genetic children, there is only a 6 percent chance that at least one of these relatives will suffer from schizophrenia. Not surprisingly, neither the genetic nor adoptive relatives of the healthy adopted children had a high prevalence of schizophrenia. Less than 2 percent of these relatives ever suffered from the disease.

We can infer from these results that a person with schizophrenic genetic relatives is at risk for schizophrenia even though he is raised in a family that is free from schizophrenia. Kety's results provided excellent evidence that a predisposition to schizophrenia is genetically transmitted.

Before Kety's conclusions can be accepted, a number of other interpretations of the data must be ruled out. First, the hypothesis that schizophrenic parents are more likely than healthy parents to give their children up for adoption explains, without recourse to genetics, Kety's finding that schizophrenia is prevalent in the genetic relatives of adopted schizophrenic children. Nevertheless, the hypothesis is probably wrong because it makes another prediction that is false. Because schizophrenic parents would give up both children destined to develop schizophrenia and children destined to be normal, the hypothesis predicts that schizophrenia would be prevalent in the genetic relatives of healthy adopted children. However, Kety's group found that the genetic relatives of healthy adopted children do not have an abnormally high prevalence of schizophrenia.

Second, Kety's data might be explained by the hypothesis that schizophrenia is transmitted by the biological mother, but not genetically. Perhaps the environment inside the uterus is responsible for the disease. Or, the mother's behavior toward the baby during his first few weeks of life, before adoption, might cause schizophrenia. To eliminate this possible cause of schizophrenia, Kety searched for paternal half-siblings of the schizophrenic adopted children—half-siblings who had the same genetic father but not the same genetic mother. These children not only developed in a different uterus from the schizophrenic children, they also lived with a different mother immediately after birth. However, the schizophrenic adopted children and their paternal half-siblings inherited genes from the same father, and the paternal half-siblings, like the schizophrenic adopted children, had a high prevalence of schizophrenia. Clearly, the uterine environment and the environment of the first few weeks after birth are not the sole causes of schizophrenia.

Third, perhaps Kety's team used biased diagnostic procedures. Maybe the interviewers were more lenient in diagnosing schizophrenia when they interviewed relatives of a schizophrenic adopted child than when they interviewed relatives of a healthy adopted child. However, Kety and his colleagues were aware that psychiatric diagnosis is not an exact science. Therefore Kety's researchers took great care not to let their own biases affect their results. They conducted blind psychiatric interviews so that the researchers would not know whether they were interviewing a relative of a healthy child or a relative of a schizophrenic child. Then, transcripts of the interviews were carefully edited to remove any inadvertent hints about the relation of the interviewed relative to a particular adopted child. Three psychiatrists who had never seen the relatives or read the unedited transcripts each provided diagnoses from the interviewees' transcripts. After the three psychiatrists reached a consensus among themselves about the relatives' mental health, each genetic and adoptive relative was identified with either a healthy or a schizophrenic adopted child.

Because these security procedures were used, bias cannot account for the results, unless you believe in extrasensory perception and mental telepathy. We think that Kety's procedures were extremely important. When a task requires some subjective judgment, and the judge has a vested interest in the outcome, honesty, education, and experience cannot ensure against bias. Proper experimental procedures are the only safeguard.

A fourth explanation for the data is that, though unbiased, perhaps Kety's diagnostic procedures were inadequate. Clearly, he was measuring some genetically transmitted behavior, but it might not have been schizophrenia. After all, Kety conducted his research several years before the *DSM-III* was published. His diagnostic criteria were less precise than those used today. However, an independent team of psychiatrists recently rediagnosed all the relatives from the transcripts of Kety's interviews, using *DSM-III* criteria.[9] Again the diagnoses were blind; the psychiatrists did not know whether or not the person interviewed was a genetic relative of a schizophrenic or healthy adopted child. This second evaluation confirmed Kety's conclusion: The genetic relatives of the schizophrenic adoptive children were more likely than any of the other groups to suffer from either schizophrenia or a less severe variant called schizotypal personality disorder.

With Kety's results, one can argue convincingly that the causes of schizophrenia cannot all be found in the environment. The disease is not just "a special strategy that a person invents in order to live in an unlivable situation," the view advocated by the prominent British psychiatrist R. D. Laing.[10] Laing's view implied that for each patient there is a guilty party or parties who caused his illness by making his situation unlivable. It also implied that the mind of the newborn baby is a blank slate and that all thoughts can reside equally easily in all brains; no brains are predisposed to schizophrenic thought. Using Kety's data, one can also argue against Thomas Szasz's idea that schizophrenia is just a myth. In Kety's words, "If schizophrenia is a myth, it is a myth with a strong genetic component."[11]

If you have schizophrenia in your family and are considering having children, you should be sobered but not panicked by this information. Some authorities believe that the grandchildren of a person with schizophrenia are not at risk if the children (prospective parents) are still healthy at about age twenty-five.[12] It would probably be wise to assess your risks realistically by seeking the advice of a genetic counselor.

Studies of Environmental Factors

The strongest evidence that the environment also contributes to schizophrenia comes from studies of identical twins.[13] Identical twins originate from a single egg that splits after fertilization. Therefore, both twins have identical genes. If schizophrenia were determined solely by genetics, we would expect that either both twins or neither of them would be schizophrenic. But, in about 50 percent of the pairs in which one twin has schizophrenia, the other is healthy. Therefore, the genes cannot be the only factor influencing the development of schizophrenia. The environment must contribute as well.

The effect of the environment, like that of the genes, must involve the brain. The brain gathers information from the environment, information which can change behavior and cause sanity or madness. Yet, scientists have not been able to determine what features of the environment are critical for the development of schizophrenia. Studies of the families of schizophrenia patients and of the societies they live in have not provided good clues.

Psychiatrists have come up with many conflicting theories about the characteristics of families that produce schizophrenic children. For example, mothers who supposedly produce schizophrenic children have been alleged to be both dominating and passive.[14] The role of the parents' personalities is particularly doubtful when one twin develops schizophrenia and the other remains healthy. In this situation, both children have the same parents and very similar family environments.

In any event, studies of the behavior of parents of schizophrenic children cannot elucidate the effects of the environment if only genetic parents are examined. Though the parents of a schizophrenic child may have some bizarre behaviors, these behaviors need not be the cause of the child's illness. The abnormal behavior of both the child and the parents may result from common genes. Only an adoption study can separate genetic and environmental effects.

To study the effects of a schizophrenic environment, Kety's team compared the prevalence of schizophrenia in three groups of adopted children: those who had a genetic parent with schizophrenia, those who had an adoptive parent with schizophrenia, and those who had healthy genetic and adoptive parents.[15] The researchers found that only children with a schizophrenic genetic parent had a high prevalence of schizophrenia. Children with a schizophrenic adopted parent or with healthy parents had the usual 1 percent rate of schizophrenia. Apparently, even growing up with a schizophrenic parent does not cause schizophrenia in children who are not genetically susceptible. Some feature of the environment may precipitate the disease, but at present, that feature has not been identified.

Perhaps this information can allay some of the guilt that often burdens the parents of a child who has schizophrenia. Parents often ask, "What have I done?" Sometimes, mental health professionals are all too eager to tell them. But the fact is that parents probably cannot cause schizophrenia in a child who is not genetically susceptible. Furthermore, psychiatrists do not know any way to prevent the disease in a susceptible child. Genes determine susceptibility, and you are not responsible for your genes. You received them from your ancestors at the moment you were conceived, and you pass on half of your genes to your child at the moment he is conceived.

The Labeling and Oppression Theories of Schizophrenia

There are two versions of the notion that society causes schizophrenia. The labeling theory claims that labeling deviant people mentally ill creates a self-fulfilling prophecy; that is, because of the label, deviant people are encouraged to behave in an even more deviant manner.[16] The oppression theory admits that mental illness is real but contends that it is caused, not by a genetic defect in the brain, but by social and/or economic oppression.

If the labels do not describe preexisting phenomena but rather create patterns of deviant behavior, similar patterns of behavior labeled mental illness would not exist in widely different cultures. Yet, both the Eskimos and the Yoruba, a rural African culture, have words for a cluster of symptoms that bears an uncanny resemblance to our European–American description of schizophrenia.[17] The Eskimo word *nuthkavihak* describes people who scream at someone who does not exist, refuse to talk, refuse to eat, make strange grimaces, and hide in strange places. However the content of the symptomatic delusions is culturally determined. For example, a *nuthkavihak* Eskimo might believe that a fox lives inside her, whereas an American with schizophrenia might believe that he is possessed by a powerful electromagnetic force. Eskimos and Yorubas also recognize as sick those people with symptoms that American psychiatrists call severe anxiety and depression, even though these two cultures do not have a label for these symptoms.

Healthy Eskimos and Yorubas respond to mental illness in others much as Americans do. The mentally ill are considered sick and are treated by society's healers. The Eskimos and Yorubas do not treat all deviants or even all who claim supernatural powers. Evil deviants are "witches." Good deviants are faith healers. They have no difficulty distinguishing between a person with schizophrenia and a witch or faith healer. The fact that these very diverse cultures believe that very similar behaviors are symptoms of illness suggests that the illness existed before the label, not vice versa. We do not know whether mental illness is ever created by labeling, but we are quite sure that it is not always created by labeling.

If schizophrenia were a product of social oppression in Western society, it ought not to exist in non-Western societies. But, in fact, all societies that have been studied in Asia, Africa, Europe, and the Americas have a prevalence of schizophrenia between 0.2 and 1.0 percent. Non-Western societies have approximately as much schizophrenia as do Western societies.[18]

We do not think that industrialization and its associated psychological stress have increased the incidence of schizophrenia. The rate of first hospital admissions for young and middle-aged psychotics in Massachusetts did not increase from 1840 to 1940.[19]

Oppression theorists usually point out that schizophrenia is more common in the lower than in the higher socioeconomic classes. Socioeconomic class is measured by education and occupation; people in lower classes tend to have little education and unskilled jobs. Oppression theorists believe that poverty causes schizophrenia. An alternative explanation is that schizophrenia causes poverty. This explanation is intuitively reasonable. Most patients leaving the hospital have residual symptoms. Many of these patients are young adults who have not yet completed their education, and their residual symptoms may prevent them from completing it. Their illness may also rob them of the subtle social skills that are required for success in a high-paying career.

A study examining the social class of schizophrenia patients and their parents supports the notion that schizophrenia causes downward social mobility. In families without schizophrenia, the children's social class is similar to the parents' social class, but schizophrenia patients tend to have a much lower social class than their parents. This downward mobility is a specific effect of schizophrenia, not a general effect of psychiatric illness or hospitalization. The social class of schizophrenia patients is much lower than the social class of other hospitalized psychiatric patients, yet the social class of the parents of schizophrenia patients does not differ from the social class of parents of patients with other psychiatric illnesses.[20]

Psychiatrists know that both heredity and environment are important in the genesis of schizophrenia, but they do not know precisely how either acts on the brain to encourage or retard the development of the disease. They do not know how to change the environment to reduce the incidence of schizophrenia. Schizophrenia cannot be cured; it is a chronic illness. But it can be treated. To work, the treatment must change the patient's brain chemistry.

Treatment of Schizophrenia

The Discovery and Acceptance of Phenothiazines

Phenothiazines are the class of drugs most commonly used to treat schizophrenia.[1] The most familiar drug in this class is chlorpromazine (trade name, Thorazine). Phenothiazines were not discovered through research designed to find a treatment for schizophrenia. Rather, the history of phenothiazines reads like a story of a drug in search of a disease. The molecule on which the modern drugs are based, the phenothiazine nucleus, was first synthesized by the German dye industry in 1883. All phenothiazines currently in use are chemical modifications of this parent compound. No one thought that this molecule might have important medical uses until 1944, when several phenothiazine variants were tested as antimalarial agents in both France and the United States. These tests were inspired by the fact that some chemically related dyes were known to have antimalarial value. Therefore, variants of the phenothiazine molecule were tested on the chance that they would be more effective in treating the disease.

Phenothiazines failed as a treatment for malaria, but during this research, their potential value as sedatives and antihistamines was discovered. Rhone-Poulenc, the French pharmaceutical firm that had synthesized the compounds, became interested in developing a phenothiazine that was an effective antihistamine but had minimal sedative effects. Chemists at Rhone-Poulenc synthesized several variants of the phenothiazine nucleus and tested their effects on rats. The chemists looked for drugs that would be effective antihistamines but would not make the rats sleepy and would not impair their muscular coordination.

In 1949, while Rhone-Poulenc was testing phenothiazines for antihistaminic properties, the French surgeon Laborit was working on the theory that antihistamines would prevent surgical shock. To test this theory, he began giving phenothiazines to surgical patients. Although his theories about shock turned out to be wrong, Laborit described dramatic effects of the drug on the central nervous system. Like the Rhone-Poulenc scientists, he found that most phenothiazines had sedative effects. Because he was working with people rather than rats, Laborit also had the opportunity to observe another effect of phenothiazines: in low doses the drugs calmed anxious surgical patients without making them fall asleep.

Probably, Laborit's work in conjunction with their own animal research made the scientists at Rhone-Poulenc do an abrupt about-face and start searching for a phenothiazine variant with maximal rather than minimal effects on the central nervous system. In December of 1950, these researchers synthesized chlorpromazine, and tests on animals suggested that it had considerable clinical potential. But it is not clear that the Rhone-Poulenc scientists could have answered the question, potential for what?

Rhone-Poulenc began testing chlorpromazine on patients in March of 1951—only three months after it had been synthesized. This quick transfer from the chemistry laboratory to the hospital would, of course, be impossible today. Extensive animal trials showing both efficacy and safety are now required before a new drug can be tested on humans.

At first, chlorpromazine was used in conjunction with barbiturates in both surgical anesthesia and in psychiatric treatment. (For want of any better treatment, barbiturates were often used to sedate violent and uncontrollable mental patients.) Until chlorpromazine was used alone, its antipsychotic properties—that is, its ability to suppress psychotic thoughts and behaviors—were not obvious. In 1951, two French psychiatrists, Delay and Deniker, used chlorpromazine alone to treat six manic patients. Shortly afterward, they published the first paper on the antipsychotic properties of chlorpromazine. Delay and Deniker claimed that chlorpromazine caused rapid improvement in their patients. Yet, several years passed before the physicians in the French psychiatric hospitals made any substantial use of the drug. Their reluctance to use chlorpromazine may have resulted from the low scientific standards of psychiatric research in the 1940s. Although French psychiatrists had a tradition of faith in physical and chemical treatments for mental illness, they had been assailed too many times by worthless drugs touted as cures. The drug companies had cried "saviour" too often.

Chlorpromazine was first introduced to the United States when Rhone-Poulenc asked the Smith, Klein, and French Corporation, a large U.S. drug company, if it would be interested in a licensing agreement to market the drug in the United States. Smith, Klein, and French was very interested. The company performed laboratory tests and clinical trials for two years and in May, 1954, began to market chlorpromazine under the trade name Thorazine.

The development of other antipsychotic drugs followed rapidly. Some, like chlorpromazine, were members of the phenothiazine family. Others, such as haloperidol (trade name, Haldol) were chemically unrelated to chlorpromazine. Sixteen effective antipsychotics are currently described in a standard pharmacology text, and that list includes only a small fraction of all the drugs with antipsychotic effects (see the Appendix).[2]

Deniker commented that the initial resistance to chlorpromazine in the United States had quite different origins from the resistance in France. In the United States, the psychoanalytic tradition originating with Freud led many psychiatrists to believe that psychotherapy was the only proper treatment for mental illness. Although Freud himself never claimed that psychoanalysis could cure schizophrenia, his disciples in the United States were more Freudian than Freud. Loyalty to his theories required them to resist the use of drugs. Nevertheless, by 1955, antipsychotics were commonly used to treat schizophrenia in U.S. mental hospitals. Consequently, the population of these hospitals began to decrease.

Behavioral Changes Produced by Antipsychotics

Antipsychotics are so effective in treating schizophrenia that many patients in mental hospitals appear quite healthy. If you were to visit a psychiatric hospital, particularly one providing primarily short-term care, you might wonder why many of the patients were hospitalized at all. It may even appear to you that psychiatrists cannot tell the difference between the sane and the insane. David L. Rosenhan, a psychologist at Stanford University, expressed this opinion in his article entitled "On Being Sane in Insane Places," published in *Science* magazine.[3] Rosenhan and some of his colleagues gained admittance to a psychiatric hospital by claiming that they were having hallucinations and hearing voices. After admission, they reported that their symptoms disappeared. However, they were not released. The pseudopatients claimed that the staff merely assumed that all patients were "crazy" and refused to recognize any evidence to the contrary.

Rosenhan and his associates did not consider the possibility that antipsychotic drugs might have been helping many schizophrenia patients to behave normally much of the time. The absence of florid psychotic behavior does not mean that a patient is cured and ready to leave the hospital. Rosenhan interpreted his experience as evidence that psychiatrists are incompetent. We interpret it as evidence that antipsychotic drugs effectively control the symptoms of schizophrenia.

If you were to observe the behavior of a floridly schizophrenic patient during his first few weeks in the hospital, you would see some dramatic changes in his behavior. Upon entering the hospital, the patient excitedly converses with his voices, broadcasts his thoughts to the president, or proclaims that enemy forces are poisoning his food. His first few doses of antipsychotic probably make him somewhat sleepy, but the sedative effects of the drug wear off after a few days or weeks. After a week or two, the patient's psychotic symptoms begin to improve. Although the initial sedative effect may be somewhat useful for a violent or excited patient, sedation is neither the main effect of antipsychotics nor the reason they are so effective in treating schizophrenia.

As treatment progresses, the patient stops conversing with his voices. He is no longer harassed by their psychotic commands to harm himself or others. External forces no longer instruct him to be hostile and belligerent, so these behaviors, too, decrease. As paranoia and suspiciousness fade, the patient no longer accuses the hospital staff of trying to harm him. If the patient has been incoherent, his speech becomes connected and comprehensible.

Not only do symptoms of illness decrease, but symptoms of health return. The patient becomes emotionally more responsive.

He begins to listen and respond to the staff and fellow patients, perhaps because he is no longer completely absorbed by the demands of his hallucinations. He begins to care for himself. If he has rarely spoken, he may now engage in conversations. His sentences become more grammatical and complex. If he has rarely moved, he now begins to walk around and participate in activities. Catatonic patients no longer stand or sit in their fixed positions; their pressure sores begin to heal.[4]

Mental health workers have vividly described the changes in hospitalized psychiatric patients brought about by antipsychotics:

The opinion seems to be almost unanimous that patients who exhibit psychomotor activity, assaultiveness, hostility, and negativism show a reduction in their motor output [movements] with the administration of the drug. They are less restless, are quite ready to sit quietly, are less assaultive and destructive, are orderly and well-behaved. Subjectively, they exhibit a marked reduction in anxiety. They are clear mentally, in good contact with their surroundings, and are able to discuss their hallucinations and delusions calmly and with a considerable degree of objectivity.[5]

In another report, a hospital official said, "It is a distinct pleasure to think of the patients . . . who formerly paced about more like caged animals than any group of patients that I have ever seen, now going to the general dining room and eating with silverware."[6] Such changes in the patients' behavior have caused dramatic changes in the hospital environment. Hospitals can now provide more recreational and therapeutic programs, and the patients can take advantage of them. Patients, no longer catatonic, violent, or incoherent, can learn social and occupational skills.

Case Studies

In his autobiographical book *The Eden Express*, Mark Vonnegut poignantly documented his own recovery from schizophrenia.[7] When Vonnegut became ill, he was living on a communal farm in British Columbia, trying hard to be a "good hippie" during the peak of the counterculture period (1969–1970). Even his hippie friends, admiring as they were of deviant behavior, recognized that he was ill. Vonnegut vividly described the hallucinations and delusions of his schizophrenic episodes. But his descriptions of schizophrenic thought, even though culled from his own memory, cannot quite capture the aberrant quality of schizophrenic thought that is so obvious in a direct quote from a schizophrenia patient (as we cited in Chapter 4).

Vonnegut's recovery, like that of most patients, took several weeks. The first sign of improvement was that he began to notice his surroundings. Vonnegut explained: "I was all taken up with voices, visions and all. I vaguely knew I was in a mental hospital, but it wasn't any different from being anywhere else. Where I was was beside the point. Little by little with the help of massive doses of Thorazine in the ass and in my milkshakes (which was all they could get me to eat), little by little it started mattering to me where I was and what was going on."[8] Though Vonnegut does not like Thorazine, he admits that he needed it.

Vonnegut's first episode was not his only one. He was rehospitalized twice before he enjoyed a lasting recovery. (Vonnegut attributes his permanent recovery to orthomolecular psychiatry, a treatment consisting primarily of large doses of vitamins. We discuss orthomolecular psychiatry later.) At the end of *The Eden Express*, Vonnegut said that he had recovered. He began to write, studied biochemistry, and applied to medical school. He wrote that he "got more and more disgustingly healthy." Interestingly, the healthier he got, the more convinced he became that schizophrenia is a biochemical disease.

Mark Vonnegut is among the most fortunate of recovered schizophrenia patients; he seems to have recovered fully and permanently. Vonnegut's compelling and elegant book is in itself evidence of his recovery.

A word of caution is in order before we become too encouraged by Mark Vonnegut's recovery. Mark Vonnegut and the heroes of other narrative accounts of recovery from schizophrenia were diagnosed without the benefit of the *DSM-III*. Thus, we do not know whether these patients would have satisfied the *DSM-III* criteria for schizophrenia. That most of the narrative accounts of schizophrenia (*I Never Promised You a Rose Garden*, for example) document recovery rather than chronic illness and psychiatric deterioration should perhaps make us suspicious. In fact, in a recent article in the *Archives of General Psychiatry*, the authors analyzed the symptoms described in several such narratives. They concluded that none of the protagonists actually suffered from schizophrenia.[9] Furthermore, the authors suggested that these books gave the public an unrealistically optimistic view of the prognosis for schizophrenia patients. In particular, they concluded that Mark Vonnegut had bipolar affective disorder rather than schizophrenia. Unless Vonnegut relapses, we will never be certain what his diagnosis would have been under *DSM-III* criteria. In spite of the possibility of incorrect diagnosis, we think that Mark Vonnegut's recovery is a good illustration of the ability of Thorazine to alleviate hallucinations and confusion and restore rational thought processes.

Another patient, Paul, also recovered from schizophrenia, but his recovery was less complete than Mark Vonnegut's. As a child, Paul spent a lot of time with his parents but little with friends his own age. His adolescence was uneventful, but a skilled observer would have noticed that his emotional development was not normal. At the age of seventeen, he often told, with great relish and amusement, foolish stories and jokes appropriate to a six-year-old. He did not respond to the obvious boredom of his listeners, which is just what is meant by blunted affect. He never went out with girls. However, he worked hard at school and was a brilliant student. He went to a prestigious college, and, although he was somewhat demoralized by the competition, he continued to do well academically. Nonetheless, he still showed no signs of maturing emotionally.

After college, he went to graduate school in biology for a year. At this time, he became both discouraged with academic work and piously religious. He became convinced that he did not have the ability to succeed academically and professionally. Devoting himself to God, he believed, was his only alternative. Consequently, he enrolled in a fundamentalist bible college. At first, his involvement with the supernatural did not seem abnormal in the context of the religious community in which he lived. But gradually, Paul began claiming to receive direct messages from heaven. Paul's messages came from the apostle whose name he bore. One morning, Paul's roommate found him under his desk, naked, proclaiming something unintelligible about "orders from Paul and Jesus, and the frauds of the devil and Communism." The college officials persuaded Paul to enter a psychiatric hospital, where he was treated with phenothiazines. After a few months in a halfway house, Paul was well enough to live on his own. He obtained a good job as a laboratory technician and has kept it for over ten years. He continues to take phenothiazines. Occasional experiments with drug-free periods have resulted in psychotic relapses.

Antipsychotics worked effectively for Paul. Without them, he would probably have spent his entire life in the hospital. But Paul is not completely well. His affect is still blunted; he still fails to respond to other people's facial expressions or words. His own expressions oscillate between stony and giggly. In a conversation, Paul responds to his own remarks, never to the words of another speaker. When he tells a story, Paul's performance is as immutable as a tape recording: the responses of his listeners do not alter his speech. Yet, Paul does not appear sedated. His soliloquies are lively. He is energetic. In many ways, Paul behaves very much like he did before his schizophrenic episode. He is still emotionally immature and self-centered. He does not have relationships with women. He still has intellectual ability and perseverance.

In some ways, Paul typifies the recovered schizophrenia patient. He can provide his own food, clothing, housing, and personal hygiene. He probably will never marry or develop intimate friendships. Even a short conversation with a recovered schizophrenia patient like Paul would probably cause you to think that he is not quite healthy. Paul might stand too close or too far away. He might laugh inappropriately or continue to talk when no one is listening. However, Paul's occupational success is greater than that of most recovered schizophrenia patients. He holds a job requiring professional expertise, whereas most patients with a history like his cannot handle the complexity and stress of such a position.

The overall adjustment of the recovered schizophrenia patient can be fairly well predicted from his adjustment before he became ill. Antipsychotic drugs cannot create a new personality or solve the problems of living that the patient had prior to his illness. Treatment with antipsychotic drugs will not create a social butterfly out of a wallflower. Mark Vonnegut was socially adept and perceptive before his illness and his illness did not destroy these skills. Paul's social competence was always marginal and so it remains marginal. To exaggerate this point, one psychiatrist said that you cannot expect a patient to write the great American novel after taking antipsychotics if he could not construct a paragraph before. In short, miracles are not recorded in the annals of psychiatry.

Unfortunately, some schizophrenia patients improve very little or not at all. Sylvia Frumkin, whom we mentioned in Chapter 4, was such a patient.[10] Miss Frumkin's struggle with schizophrenia began when she was about fourteen years old. Her parents were forced to hospitalize her a year later when she asked her uncle to adopt her. She insisted that she did not belong to her parents anyway. Miss Frumkin, like many schizophrenia patients, could not take care of herself. She could not eat without smearing food on herself and others. When she attempted to cook at home, she plastered the kitchen with food and dirty dishes. She would not clean her room, shower, or change clothes. She dressed inappropriately. On one occasion she attended the hospital's Jewish services in a t-shirt, half-slip, and high-heeled gold sandals. During one of her brief periods out of the hospital, she danced in the streets and gave away phonograph records while wearing only a bra and half-slip.

Because she repeatedly struck the hospital attendants and other patients, she was often put in a padded seclusion room for hours. While in seclusion she did not control her bowel movements; the hospital attendants had to hose down both Miss Frumkin and the seclusion room before they could release her.

Miss Frumkin never recovered enough to live independently. By 1980, sixteen years after her first admission to the hospital, Sylvia Frumkin had been admitted ten times to the Creedmoor Psychiatric Center, a New York state hospital. But did antipsychotic drugs help Sylvia Frumkin? When she received medication in sufficiently large doses, she was able to avoid seclusion. Sometimes she could even participate in the hospital's sheltered typing workshop. When taking antipsychotics, she wore a skirt with a matching blouse, properly buttoned, and spoke civilly with the staff and other patients. On one occasion, she stayed out of the hospital long enough to complete a medical secretary course but relapsed the day before graduation. Whenever her medication was reduced, Miss Frumkin's symptoms returned. She believed she carried Paul McCartney's baby. She also alternately became a Buddhist and a born-again Christian. She cut up her pillowcase because demons were dancing in it. Though Miss Frumkin's condition improved at times, even at her best she could not live and work on her own. Therefore, even though the drugs decreased her symptoms somewhat, we think that antipsychotics failed as a treatment for Miss Frumkin.

The NIMH Study of Antipsychotic Therapy

When a patient enters a psychiatric hospital with symptoms of schizophrenia, the major goal of treatment is to reduce the symptoms so that he can rejoin society. The success of treatment can be measured by the amount of time the patient remains in the hospital and by the reduction in symptoms. So far we have not provided scientific evidence that antipsychotic treatment aids in accomplishing these goals. We have only provided anecdotes about patients who took antipsychotics and got relief from schizophrenia symptoms. These anecdotes are not adequate evidence that the drug causes recovery because schizophrenia, like almost every other disease, sometimes improves by itself. Sometimes, the disease goes away when the patient believes he is taking a useful drug whereas, in reality, he is taking a placebo, a pill containing sugar or starch instead of a therapeutic agent. A few patients will recover with nearly any treatment. Their recover, however, does not prove that the treatment is a specific remedy for the disease.

To show that antipsychotics are effective, researchers have to show that a group of patients receiving the drugs either improves more or leaves the hospital sooner than another similar group receiving a placebo. Because of the unreliability of psychiatric diagnosis, the same physicians must diagnose both drug and placebo patients. The patients must be randomly assigned to the drug group and to the placebo group. Finally, neither the patients nor the doctors and nurses evaluating them must know who is receiving active drug and who is receiving placebo.

In 1964, The National Institute of Mental Health Pharmacology Service Center organized nine hospitals in a collaborative study to find out whether antipsychotics really helped schizophrenia patients.[11] Since this study antedates the *DSM-III*, it appears to have the same problem as the literary narratives describing schizophrenia: all the patients may not have met the *DSM-III* criteria for schizophrenia. We think, however, that the diagnostic problem is less relevant to evaluation of the National Institute of Mental Health (NIMH) study than it is to evaluation of the literary accounts of schizophrenia. Not surprisingly, the patients in the literary accounts recovered. Recovered patients make better stories than deteriorating patients, but they may not be typical. In contrast, the NIMH study did not include patients because of their literary value—

because they recovered or because they responded to drugs. It included all patients who had a certain set of symptoms. Although some of these patients may not have met the *DSM-III* criteria for schizophrenia, their symptoms were similar to those in the *DSM-III*.

The patients in the NIMH study were randomly assigned to one of four groups. Each of the first three groups received a different antipsychotic drug; the fourth group received a placebo. Neither the patients nor the hospital staff knew which pills contained an active drug and which contained a placebo. Three hundred and forty-four patients completed the study, about 90 in each of the three drug groups and 74 in the placebo group.

At the beginning of the study, the hospital staff made a global judgment of the severity of each patient's illness and then placed each patient in one of seven categories ranging from "extremely ill" to "normal." In addition, the staff described the specific symptoms of each patient and noted their severity. For example, a patient could have been described as moderately ill (category four) and suffering from hallucinations, lack of personal hygiene, and incoherent speech.

After six weeks of treatment with either an antipsychotic or placebo, the patients were reevaluated. This time the staff rated each patient's improvement as well as the current severity of his illness. Based on improvement or lack of it, they put each patient into one of seven categories ranging from "very much worse" to "very much improved." As the graph in Figure 6-1 illustrates, the drug patients improved much more than the placebo patients. Over three-quarters of the drug patients were "much improved" or "very much improved" (the two categories reflecting the most improvement) while only one-third of the placebo patients fell into these two categories.

In what ways did the patients show improvement? Did the drugs actually help them to think more normally? To answer these questions, the NIMH group examined the effects of the drugs on specific symptoms of schizophrenia. While virtually all symptoms decreased with the use of antipsychotics, the decrease in symptoms of confusion and disorganization was the greatest. For example, incoherent speech became more connected. Personal hygiene improved; patients dressed themselves, washed, combed their hair, and used the toilet. Patients who had not spoken or responded to others became responsive to questions and requests. The drugs were

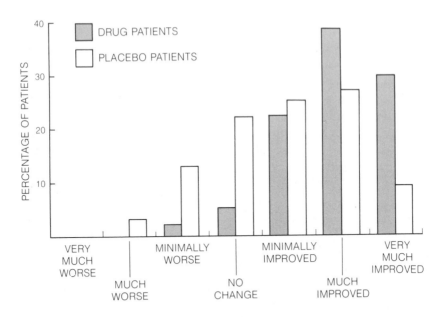

Figure 6-1.   The effect of treatment with antipsychotic drugs or placebo on patients with schizophrenia.

less effective in combating thoughts that, though somewhat grammatical and logical, were unrelated to reality. Antipsychotics do not always eliminate delusions and hallucinations, but the drugs usually permit the patient to recognize hallucinations or delusions as such and to know that they are symptoms of disease.

How healthy were the patients at the end of the treatment? Even if they were not well enough to leave the hospital but were cleaner, calmer, and better nourished, then the drugs were beneficial. Of course, the benefits of antipsychotics are much more impressive if they permit patients to resume a relatively normal life outside the hospital. Because antipsychotics, like all drugs, have risks and side effects as well as benefits, people must know just how great the benefits are. After six weeks of treatment, the hospital staff described almost 50 percent of the drug patients as "borderline ill" or "normal," the two categories indicating the greatest degree of health. Only about 15 percent of the placebo patients fell into these two categories; the rest remained more seriously ill. Because the NIMH study continued for only six weeks, the total length of hospitalization of the drug and placebo patients could not be compared. But in other studies, ample evidence has been gathered indicating that the average hospital stay is greatly decreased by drug therapy. In one of the most detailed studies, the patients receiving drugs stayed in the hospital only about half as long as the patients not receiving drugs.[12]

The actual effectiveness of the drugs compared to placebo is probably underestimated by the NIMH statistics. Some of the placebo patients became so much worse during the treatment period that they had to be eliminated from the study and given some other type of treatment. Had these very ill patients been included in the statistical results, the percentage of improved placebo patients would have been smaller.

The conclusions of the NIMH study have been confirmed by many other researchers. In hundreds of double-blind studies, the effects of antipsychotics and a placebo have been compared. When adequate doses were used, virtually all researchers found that antipsychotics were more effective. In a few early studies, when very low doses of antipsychotic were used, no difference between drug and placebo was detected. The antipsychotics were probably ineffective because the dosage was inadequate.[13]

Use of Antipsychotic Therapy to Prevent Relapse

For a recovered patient to stay out of the hospital, is continued medication required? To answer this question, researchers compare relapse rates of patients who are maintained on antipsychotic drugs after release from the hospital with relapse rates of patients who are maintained on placebo. Gerald Hogarty and his colleagues found that recovered patients maintained on antipsychotics had about a 55 percent chance of remaining in the community for two years after leaving the hospital, whereas patients maintained on placebo had only a 20 percent chance. Thus, maintenance therapy with antipsychotics more than doubles a patient's chances of remaining out of the hospital for two years.[14] Some of the drug patients who relapsed may not have taken their medicine at all or may have decided on their own to reduce their dose. To determine whether these factors contributed to relapses, the same group of researchers compared for two years the relapse rates of patients taking oral antipsychotics with the relapse rates of patients receiving antipsychotics by injection. The researchers had accurate drug records of the patients who received injections but had no way to know whether the patients receiving oral medication took their drugs as directed. During the first year, the relapse rates for the two groups were about the same, but by the end of the second year, 64 percent of the patients receiving injected antipsychotics were still in the community compared to 39 percent of the patients taking drugs orally. This difference was not statistically significant. It suggested, however, that failure to take medication contributes to relapses.[15]

The prevention of relapse seems to be the only benefit of maintenance therapy. The drugs neither help nor hinder patients' adjustment to the world outside the hospital.[16]

Because 20 to 30 percent of recovered schizophrenia patients do not need maintenance antipsychotic therapy, a rationale should exist for deciding who should be given pills upon release from the hospital. To this end, several teams of physicians and scientists have been studying all the obvious features of the patients' lives and illness. However, they have not yet found any consistent patterns that could be used to predict who will relapse if drug use is suspended.[17]

Because antipsychotics can have serious side effects, they should not be taken needlessly. The most disastrous side effect is the neurological disorder called *tardive dyskinesia*, which means "late developing movement disorder." Tardive dyskinesia, discussed in more detail later, attacks primarily older patients who have taken antipsychotic drugs for several years or more. At first, the patient is afflicted with involuntary twitchlike movements of the face and tongue. As the disease progresses, the movements develop in the shoulders, arms, and, finally, throughout the entire body. The patient's face twitches relentlessly; his tongue darts in and out of his mouth. The syndrome is both embarrassing and debilitating. Living a normal life becomes nearly impossible. Obviously, patients who needed antipsychotic drugs to control an acute episode of schizophrenia but who, once recovered, might get along without them should be taken off drugs. Unfortunately, as we have already said, there is no reliable method for identifying these patients.[18]

The only sure way to find out whether a patient needs continuing medication is to withdraw the drug and watch warily for signs of a schizophrenic relapse. Symptoms appearing shortly after the patient stops taking the drug must be interpreted very carefully because tardive dyskinesia sometimes first appears when the drug is withdrawn. The strange movements can easily be mistaken for a schizophrenic relapse. Of course, the proper treatment for a relapse is resumption of drug therapy, whereas the correct treatment for tardive dyskinesia is termination of antipsychotics.

Because of the danger of developing tardive dyskinesia, most patients should have the opportunity to find out whether they can discontinue medication and remain symptom free. Nonetheless, no patient should be taken off drugs as soon as he is released from the hospital. He should first have time to establish a fairly stable life in the community. In addition, he should not discontinue anti-psychotics when a relapse would be disastrous. For example, if relapse would mean the loss of a job and the patient has no other means of support, then he probably should stay on medication until he has more financial security. If a relapse might bring on an out-break of violence or suicidal behavior, perhaps the patient should be hospitalized when he stops taking medication. Unfortunately, many patients require medication for very long periods, perhaps for their entire lives. Sometimes, even a patient who has had no symptoms for several years may relapse when drugs are withdrawn.[19]

Antipsychotic drugs remain in the body for a long time after the patient stops taking the medicine, and relapses occur unpredictably. Therefore, many months must pass before the patient or his family can conclude that the patient can stay off medication indefinitely. Often, patients get along well for several months, and just as they are becoming confident that they do not need medication, they suffer a relapse. Sometimes, psychiatrists gradually reduce the dosage of antipsychotics to find the smallest amount of medication that will prevent a relapse. Because the drugs remain in the body for so long, the effects of small changes in the dosage are hard to detect. Many dosage changes several months apart may be required to determine the minimum effective dosage for a particular patient.

Long-Term Recovery

Can a person who experiences a schizophrenic episode expect to lead a normal life for the following twenty to thirty years? Can drugs help him achieve that goal? Answers to these questions require long-term studies that follow drug and placebo patients for many years. Unfortunately, such studies are difficult to conduct. The research psychiatrist usually has no control over the patient's treatment after he leaves the hospital. Also, many patients disappear after several years, leaving no forwarding addresses. However, researchers have done follow-up studies by first attempting to locate all patients who were diagnosed as having schizophrenia at a given hospital within a particular period and then evaluating the mental health of those people they located. All of these studies antedated the *DSM-III*, so the consistency of the original diagnoses is open to question. To judge the mental health of the patients, the researchers usually used information from psychiatric interviews, and considered patients' marital status, employment status, and ability to live without institutional help. Not surprisingly, the results of such studies are not in precise agreement, so figures for long-term recovery are only rough estimates. The information we present in this section summarizes the findings of several studies.

The most optimistic estimates are that only about 10 percent of the patients fail to respond to drugs and remain chronically ill inside psychiatric hospitals for much of their lives. Approximately 30 percent experience partial recovery; these people remain outside the hospital and are employed much of the time, but they still need some help in caring for themselves. Approximately, 30 percent do not recover completely, but they are not obviously ill. Their occupational level may have decreased because of their illness, or they may be social isolates. Approximately 30 percent appear to recover completely. These people are almost continuously employed and stay out of institutions. Some are married. It is not obvious that they had previously suffered from schizophrenia. More pessimistic authorities estimate that as few as 2 to 4 percent enjoy a full and permanent recovery.[20]

Some authorities believe that long-term recovery is more likely for some types of patients than for others. The prospects are best for patients who have had only one episode of schizophrenia, who were relatively old (over 25) when the illness began, and who had the paranoid or catatonic type of schizophrenia. The prospects are less favorable for patients who have had many schizophrenic attacks, who were in their teens when they first became ill, and who had extremely disorganized thought and speech patterns.[21]

Certainly, long-term recovery rates for schizophrenia have improved over the last fifty years.[22] Emil Kraeplin, who first described the disease in 1896, said that only 13 percent of patients improved even temporarily and that most of these eventually relapsed.[23] In 1941, rates of recovery were reported to be between 1 and 7 percent.[24] Today's long-term recovery rate of approximately 60 percent represents a dramatic improvement, even if many of these recoveries are not complete.

In view of antipsychotics' demonstrable effectiveness over the short term (two years or less), it seems hard to believe that the drugs have not contributed to the increase in long-term recovery rate. However, the contribution of the drugs to long-term recovery cannot be proved rigorously. A rigorous proof requires that patients be randomly assigned to drug and placebo groups and studied for ten to thirty years. Such studies have not been done and are almost impossible to carry out.

Overuse and Misuse of Antipsychotics

Antipsychotics, like other drugs, can be incorrectly and carelessly prescribed. Usually the physician, not the patient, is responsible for overuse and misuse. Here we discuss some of the ways antipsychotics can be misused and how that misuse has led many people to believe that the drugs are nothing more than chemical straightjackets with dangerous side effects.

In *One Flew Over the Cuckoo's Nest*, Kesey illustrated the popular idea that psychiatric drugs make life easier for the hospital staff but do not help the patients.[25] Kesey described a psychiatric hospital, where many of the patients stared at the walls or aimlessly paced back and forth. The more alert patients argued pointlessly over a card game. Their day was marked primarily by the line-up for medication, the perpetuator of their minimal and meaningless activity.

Unfortunately, Kesey's portrayal contains a grain of truth. Many state hospitals are grossly understaffed. Drugs are dispensed mechanically without sufficient regard for accurate diagnosis and without thorough evaluation of their effectiveness for each individual. The staff rarely has time to evaluate each patient individually to determine the best drug therapy for each. In addition, the ward staff may not be adequately trained to recognize overdose and side effects, particularly the beginnings of tardive dyskinesia. Staff members are responsible for running the hospital in an orderly manner, and they are concerned about keeping the patients under control. They constantly fear that a patient will break into psychotically violent or destructive behavior. Under these conditions, it is hardly surprising that the staff may take comfort in overly sedated patients.

When patients receive the proper dosages of antipsychotics, they remain reasonably alert. Although the drugs have a pronounced sedative action during the first few days of treatment, after awhile, they produce antipsychotic effects without sedation. In fact, psychotic symptoms usually begin to disappear just as the sedative effects begin to wear off. At this point, the drugs appear to normalize activity levels. Agitated patients may appear tranquilized, while stuporous catatonic or withdrawn patients become more active and sociable. The drugs, then, decrease abnormally high activity and increase abnormally low activity.[26]

In the United States, about twenty different drugs are used to treat schizophrenia. They vary in their antipsychotic and their sedative potency. Their potency against psychotic symptoms does not always correspond to their potency as sedatives. In fact. some of the drugs most effective in relieving psychotic symptoms are the least effective as sedatives.[27] It is also worth pointing out that sedation, in itself, is not antipsychotic. Barbiturates and other sleeping pills are of little use in controlling psychotic symptoms.

It is unfortunate, we think, that the antipsychotic drugs are often referred to as major tranquilizers. This term probably originated early in the development of antipsychotics, when Laborit used chlorpromazine to calm surgical patients and to improve surgical anesthesia. Moreover, Delay and Deniker's first clinical use was to calm manic patients. Before the antipsychotic properties of the phenothiazines were well understood, the term *major tranquilizer* may have seemed appropriate, but it is inaccurate.

Patients and their relatives may complain that antipsychotic medication makes people emotionally unresponsive or reduces drive and energy. Mark Vonnegut espoused this view about Thorazine while admitting that the drug had its uses. He felt that the drug deprived him of his ability to care or to make judgments. He said, "While I very likely owe my life to Thorazine, I doubt if I will ever develop much affection for it or similar tranquilizers. . . . I knew that Dostoyevsky was more interesting than comic books, or, more accurately, I remembered that he had been. I cared about what happened at the farm [a communal farm that Vonnegut had founded], but it was more remembering caring than really caring."[28]

Thorazine might have produced Vonnegut's emotional wasteland. On the other hand, flat affect, a classic symptom of schizophrenia, might have been responsible for his inability to distinguish nuances of emotions. In such situations, it is difficult to know whether the emotions had been dulled by Thorazine or by the underlying disease, which the drug only partially relieved.

Often, a patient cannot make very good judgments about the effects of a drug, even if he is not suffering from a thought disorder. Patients' reports about the effectiveness of placebos are evidence that judgments about drug effects must be carefully validated. Researchers require double-blind experiments with many trials before they are willing to believe physicians' and hospital staffs' reports about the effectiveness of a given treatment. The patient's self-reports must be received with the same degree of skepticism. If a person with schizophrenia takes snake oil and then gets better, he may conclude that snake oil cured schizophrenia. Furthermore, a patient may feel that a drug has cured his disease merely because it makes him feel better. Alcohol has this capacity but has no genuine therapeutic benefit. In fact, many of the patent medicines popular in this country in the nineteenth century owed their popularity to their high alcohol content.

To reject a treatment because of alleged side effects can be a mistake. In some patients, the alleged side effects may really be exacerbations of the illness and not caused by the drug at all. In other patients, the benefits may compensate for the side effects. For example, we think relief from incapacitating psychotic symptoms compensates for a few weeks of moderate sedation.

Antipsychotics are overused if a physician continues to prescribe them even though they are no longer useful. One situation that encourages this kind of overuse is failure of drug treatment. The physician may continue to prescribe an antipsychotic even when the patient shows no signs of improvement. The physician may continue the medication merely because that is his usual policy. This practice is particularly likely to occur in an understaffed state hospital. Sometimes medication is continued because the patient has a history of violence or extreme excitement. Antipsychotics are usually fully effective in three to six weeks. If a patient fails to improve after six months of treatment, he probably is not going to improve in twelve. The only consequence of continued medication is an increased risk of tardive dyskinesia and other side effects.

Theoretically, overuse can also occur when long-term antipsychotic treatment is prescribed for the few patients who will recover with brief drug treatment or with none at all. In actual practice, this sort of overuse is inevitable because psychiatrists cannot identify these patients except by observing the consequences of withholding drugs.

Even at the risk of prescribing antipsychotics for some patients who do not need them, we think that almost all schizophrenia patients should receive antipsychotics early in their hospital stay. The exceptions would be those patients who show immediate signs of rapid recovery. We make this recommendation because very few patients will recover without drugs, and there are risks in allowing a person to remain in a psychotic state. After the symptoms are relieved, most patients should receive maintenance antipsychotics for six to twelve months.[29] If the patient has been living in the community without relapse for about six months, the physician may decide to risk discontinuing medication.

Antipsychotics are misused, as opposed to overused, when they are prescribed in the absence of an appropriate diagnosis. Schizophrenia is the most common indication for antipsychotic drugs, but there are others. For example, a short course of antipsychotic therapy is often effective for a manic patient who is severely agitated or for a depressed patient with psychotic symptoms. In the early 1960s, chlorpromazine was occasionally misused as a treatment for morning sickness in pregnancy, a clearly inappropriate use, especially since no evidence existed that the drug was safe for the unborn baby. Perhaps because of their designation as tranquilizers, antipsychotics have also been prescribed for all sorts of psychiatric problems involving excessive agitation, including schizophrenia, mania, depression, anxiety, and insomnia. Antipsychotics are not the safest or most effective treatment for anxiety, insomnia, or most types of depression. For these illnesses, other drugs or psychotherapy should be tried before resorting to antipsychotics.[30]

The Effects of Psychotherapy

Because the environment contributes, at some point, to the genesis of schizophrenia, you might think that a well-chosen environmental change would reverse the disease process. Psychotherapy is the traditional change in the environment. Vonnegut elegantly explained the preconception that therapy for schizophrenia should be verbal: "It's such a poetic affliction from inside and out, it's not hard to see how people have assumed that schizophrenia must have poetic causes and that any therapy would have to be poetic as well."[31]

Unfortunately, understanding the environment and changing it may not reverse the damage it causes. When a skier falls on an icy patch of snow and breaks a leg, the damage is done. No lesson in ski safety can undo it; no change in the snow conditions will put on a cast. No understanding of the forces that break bones will cause them to heal any faster. Similarly, there is no reason to assume that, just because schizophrenia is partially caused by environmental factors, psychological treatment will help the patient with schizophrenia. Neither is there any reason to assume that understanding schizophrenic thinking will lead to a curative change in the brain. Vonnegut provides another apt analogy: "People suffering from high fevers also sometimes suffer from hallucinations and delirious thinking, but I have yet to hear anyone suggest that understanding the content of such delirium could bring down the fever."[32]

Rather than jumping to the conclusion that psychotherapy can help the schizophrenia patient, we must look at the evidence. Two questions should be considered separately. First, is psychotherapy alone an effective treatment? Second, is psychotherapy plus drug therapy more effective than drug therapy alone? Attempts to answer these questions are fraught with difficulties.

One difficulty is that psychotherapeutic techniques are almost as numerous as psychotherapists. Three hundred milligrams of chlorpromazine is 300 milligrams of chlorpromazine no matter who hands out the pill. But psychotherapy, particularly the types commonly used with schizophrenia patients, changes with each psychotherapist. If psychotherapy fails, its ineffectiveness can be attributed to the inadequacy of the particular therapist. However, a practical treatment must be useful when delivered by any qualified therapist. A patient cannot evaluate the effectiveness of each practitioner before selecting one to administer psychotherapeutic treatment.

Another difficulty in studying the effectiveness of psychotherapy is that some patients get better without any treatment at all. This means that novels, occasional case histories, and anecdotes cannot provide evidence that psychotherapy (or any other treatment for that matter) actually works. Though a patient might have recovered without any treatment, recovery is credited to the treatment in progress. Like any other medical treatment, psychotherapy can only be evaluated by comparing the progress of patients receiving psychotherapy with the progress of similar patients receiving other treatments or no treatment at all. Obviously, each group of patients must have the same symptoms, diagnosis, and prognosis. This caveat may seem obvious, but it is not always heeded, even in studies that have been published in respected psychiatric journals. For example, in an article published in the *American Journal of Psychiatry*, the recovery of two groups of patients was compared.[33] One group received psychoanalytically oriented psychotherapy and milieu therapy but minimal drug therapy while the other group, in a different hospital, received only drug therapy. The patients receiving the psychological treatment recovered somewhat faster and were somewhat better adjusted two years after leaving the hospital. So far this sounds like substantial evidence for the effectiveness of psychotherapy. But a careful reading of the article revealed that only patients who were well-adjusted prior to their illness were selected for psychological treatment. Many psychiatrists think that these are just the patients who are most apt to recover and have the best post-illness adjustment, regardless of treatment. The authors of the article admitted that their work was not designed to compare drug and psychological treatment. Nevertheless, they implied that they were presenting evidence for the effectiveness of psychological treatment. While admitting the flaws in their research plan, the authors concluded that their "observations in a biologically oriented clinical research program employing psychosocial techniques argue for the feasibility of treating acute schizophrenic patients with minimal use of medication. The experience can be gratifying for patients and staff. Patients in such a program have not fared poorly compared with patients treated in more conventional settings."

We disagree with this conclusion. Comparing the rapid recovery of patients with good prognoses to the slower recovery of patients with average prognoses cannot provide any information about treatment effectiveness. It is like comparing recovery from a cold without treatment to recovery from pneumonia with penicillin treatment and then arguing that the results demonstrate the feasibility of using nondrug techniques in the treatment of respiratory infections and that the experience can be gratifying for patients and physicians.

A third difficulty in evaluating the effectiveness of psychotherapy is that, in many studies, the people evaluating the recoveries are the therapists themselves. Psychotherapy requires hard work and emotional investment. Precisely because they have worked so hard, psychotherapists cannot give an unbiased evaluation of the effectiveness of their own work.

The most thorough comparison of pharmacological and psychological treatments was performed by Dr. Phillip R. A. May, a psychiatrist at the University of California, Los Angeles (UCLA).[34] He studied five treatments for schizophrenia: antipsychotics, milieu therapy, individual psychotherapy, a combination of antipsychotics and individual psychotherapy, and electroconvulsive therapy. (We do not discuss electroconvulsive therapy for schizophrenia.) In milieu therapy, the patient learned occupational skills and improved social competence through recreational activities and group meetings. Patients' illnesses were not treated on individual bases. In psychotherapy, the patient spent several hours each week with his therapist, investigating the psychological origins of his illness and the problems he was going to face outside the hospital.

The 228 schizophrenia patients in May's study were randomly assigned to one of the five treatments. The patients' progress was rated in three ways: evaluation by doctors and nurses, performance on a battery of standardized tests, and length of hospitalization. The evaluation teams did not deliver treatment and were asked not to try to find out what kind of treatment a patient received. The evaluation results were straightforward: psychotherapy and milieu therapy were about equally ineffective when compared to drug therapy, which was quite effective.

May, Tuma, and Dixon studied these same patients two to five years later to find out whether drug therapy or psychotherapy had long-term advantages or disadvantages.[35] (After patients left the hospital, drug treatment was no longer controlled by the researchers, but the patients' physicians could prescribe drugs and/or psychotherapy as needed.) The drug patients were rehospitalized less often than the psychotherapy or milieu patients. The drug patients spent the fewest number of days in the hospital during the two to five years following their initial release. With these facts, the authors could argue against the notion that antipsychotics create "revolving door" mental patients, patients who are released into the community only to be rehospitalized in a few weeks or months. Certainly, many patients relapse, but patients treated with antipsychotic drugs relapse less frequently than patients treated with individual psychotherapy or milieu therapy. We do not know the reason for this difference in relapse rates. Perhaps increasing the amount of time that the brain remains in a schizophrenic state increases the likelihood that it will return to that state; therefore, rapid relief of symptoms may be important.

Critics of May's study argued that his therapists, psychiatric residents, were too inexperienced to provide adequate psychotherapy for schizophrenia patients, but Milton Greenblatt, a professor of psychiatry at UCLA, believes that inexperience does not explain May's results. Greenblatt conducted a similar study using more experienced psychiatrists. He obtained essentially the same result: psychotherapy alone produced little change while drugs produced obvious improvement.[36]

Nowhere in the massive literature on schizophrenia is there any clear evidence that psychotherapy and milieu therapy alone are effective in decreasing schiziphrenic symptoms.[37] Those studies in which positive results are reported had methodological errors; there were no control groups or psychotherapy was given only to patients with good prognoses for spontaneous recovery. Of course, a behavioral or psychotherapeutic technique that is effective for schizophrenia may yet be developed. At the present, however, no psychological treatment for schizophrenia has been proven effective. Vonnegut summed it up: "The poets in the business gave little hope and huge bills."[38]

When May's team compared the patients receiving both drugs and psychotherapy to those receiving only drugs, the researchers found no difference between the two groups. As long as the patient has blatant symptoms of thought disorder, adding psychotherapy to drug therapy accomplishes nothing.[39] This result is obtained whether effectiveness is measured by doctors' and nurses' ratings of patient improvement or by length of hospital stay. In fact, psychotherapy slightly increases the amount of time the patient spends in the hospital. Perhaps, as May explained, the therapist becomes attached to the patient and does not want him to be discharged.

It is hardly surprising that a schizophrenia patient who is catatonic, disorganized, mute, withdrawn, or paranoid does not benefit very much from psychotherapy. Psychotherapy almost requires that a person have reasonably normal thought processes. Therefore, after antipsychotics have restored some degree of rationality, it is again appropriate to ask whether psychotherapy helps. Do patients improve more when psychotherapy and drugs are used together than when drugs are used alone? One would hope that the answer is yes because removal of the most florid schizophrenic symptoms rarely leaves the patient entirely normal. Perhaps the symptoms that cannot be relieved by drugs can be treated through psychotherapy.

During bouts with schizophrenia, patients may develop some behaviors that affect their ability to live normally in society. For example, a patient may have become withdrawn as her compulsion to talk to her voices increased. By the time her symptoms are under control, she may feel that she does not know how to make friends anymore. In addition, many schizophrenia patients become ill as young adults. They have not had the opportunity to learn the skills of adult living. For example, the discharged patient may not know how to find a place to live or how to get a job. Furthermore, he may not know what to tell friends about his illness. Can psychotherapy help the patient solve these problems? The answer is yes. Psychotherapy can benefit a schizophrenia patient, but only psychotherapy that focuses on solving real-life problems is known to be effective. There is no evidence that insight psychotherapy (that is, treatment in which a therapist attempts to find the psychological origins of the illness in the patient's past) is effective.

A team led by Gerald Hogarty thoroughly studied the effectiveness of social therapy in preventing relapse in recovered schizophrenia patients.[40] Social therapy was conducted primarily by psychiatric social workers and consisted of counseling on personal problems and solving practical problems such as finding housing and employment. Hogarty's team described a patient whose schizophrenic symptoms had included hallucinations, delusions of grandeur, and badly impaired judgment. By the time she was released from the hospital, she was no longer psychotic. The hallucinations and delusions had disappeared, but she was now fearful and withdrawn. Her behavior appeared to be studied and to be lacking in spontaneity. She talked very little and did not keep up her personal appearance. Though she did not require hospitalization, she still could not get along very well in the community. If drugs had done all they could for her, could social therapy do more? After two years of social therapy, the patient was able to separate from an exploiting husband, arrange for child care, and become a competent homemaker. She paid attention to her appearance, began to date, secured employment, and was finally able to live in her own home.

Hogarty and his colleagues examined the effects of two years of social therapy on a large sample of recovering patients, both those who continued with drug therapy and those who switched to placebo. During the first six months social therapy had little or no effect on the probability of relapse. But, if a drug patient stayed out of the hospital at least seven months, social therapy increased his chances of staying out for the next eighteen months. In contrast, social therapy was competely ineffective for the placebo group. Perhaps one explanation for these results is that social therapy takes seven months to begin working. Another possible explanation is that those who relapsed during the first six months were too sick to benefit from social therapy—the effects of therapy show up only after these patients have been eliminated by relapse.

If a patient stayed out of the hospital for the entire two years of the study, did social therapy improve his adjustment? The results of patient self-ratings, family ratings, psychiatrist ratings, and social worker ratings all failed to show consistently that those patients receiving social therapy were better adjusted.[41]

If social therapy does not help a patient become better adjusted, how does it keep him out of the hospital? One possibility is that the therapist encourages the patient to take his medicine and thus eliminates a major cause of relapse. By examining the effects of social therapy on patients receiving injected antipsychotics, Hogarty and his colleagues showed that therapy has a value beyond cajoling the patients to take their drugs. Social therapy increased the percentage of patients remaining in the community for two years from 50 to 77 percent even though all patients received their drug injections regularly.[42] Clearly, social therapy works, but precisely how is not known.

The effectiveness of social therapy on recovered patients living in the community suggests that similar treatment ought to help hospitalized patients once their flagrant confusions and bizarre irrational thoughts have been effectively treated with drugs. Indeed, there is some evidence that milieu care and group psychotherapy are effective if they concentrate on real-life problems and on preparing patients for discharge.[43] In view of the financial cost of psychotherapy, we believe that hospital treatment programs should include only those types of psychological care known to be effective.

Megavitamin Therapy

In the early 1950s, Humphrey Osmond and A. Hoffer began to treat schizophrenia patients with large doses of vitamins, primarily niacin (vitamin B_3). A small amount of niacin is required for good nutrition. (Lack of it causes pellagra.) But Osmond and Hoffer used doses many times larger than the amount present in a normal diet, hence the term *megavitamin* therapy. They compared the recovery of patients receiving niacin to the recovery of patients receiving a placebo. About half of both groups also received electroconvulsive therapy. (During the early 1950s, when Osmond and Hoffer conducted their studies, antipsychotics were not yet widely used in this country. Electroconvulsive therapy was an accepted treatment for schizophrenia.)

Osmond and Hoffer reported that, although the niacin patients spent a few more days in the hospital than the placebo patients, many fewer niacin patients relapsed during the three to five years following their release. They also claimed that the niacin patients adjusted better to the community, though the researchers did not explain how they measured that adjustment. Therefore, they concluded that niacin is an effective treatment for schizophrenia.[44]

Osmond and Hoffer accumulated a small but devoted following. Megavitamin therapy appeals to people who oppose drugs because they prefer not to introduce "unnatural" substances into the body. They hope to cure diseases with plant and animal products. We might remind these people that vitamin pills are manufactured in chemistry labs.

Among the most famous converts to niacin treatment are Nobel Prize-winning chemist Linus Pauling and writer Mark Vonnegut. Pauling considers megavitamin therapy to be one type of *orthomolecular psychiatry*, a term that he coined and defined as "the achievement and preservation of mental health by varying the concentrations in the human body of substances that are normally present, such as the vitamins."[45] Although we have great respect for both Pauling and Vonnegut, we disagree with their views on orthomolecular psychiatry.

The medical establishment has opposed orthomolecular psychiatry, and, we think, with good reason.[46] Unfortunately, the debate has often been polemical and emotional and not on the highest scientific plane. When Hoffer disagreed with the way a committee of the American Psychiatric Association interpreted his work, he commented, "It seems more charitable to ascribe this statement [the committee's interpretation] to a deliberate attempt to confuse rather than to accuse the authors of being unable to read."[47]

Osmond and Hoffer's conclusions are not generally accepted because in almost all subsequent studies that included a placebo control group and a reasonable number of patients, researchers found that niacin was ineffective in the treatment of schizophrenia. Hoffer and Osmond never claimed that niacin alone was effective in severe cases; they used niacin in conjunction with electroconvulsive therapy. Ethically, psychiatrists cannot now repeat Hoffer and Osmond's experiment because modern psychiatry does not accept electroconvulsive therapy as treatment for schizophrenia. Antipsychotics are less intrusive and more effective. One psychiatrist, however, examined his records for patients who had received electroconvulsive therapy in conjunction with niacin or in conjunction with placebo. He was unable to find any effect of niacin.[48]

Modern researchers have concentrated on determining whether niacin is a useful addition to antipsychotic therapy. Wittenborn, a psychiatrist at Rutgers University, compared the use of antipsychotics alone to the use of antipsychotics with niacin. Patients were treated for two years. In all measures of effectiveness, such as nurses' ratings, psychiatric tests, and home adjustment, niacin was ineffective.[49] In other studies, this conclusion was corroborated.

Wittenborn did discover one small scrap of evidence that orthomolecular therapy might be effective. His data suggested that patients who were well-adjusted before developing schizophrenia might be helped by niacin.[50] Wittenborn stressed, however, that this hypothesis is only tentative. More data are needed to confirm or deny it. At present, we cannot say that niacin is an effective treatment for *any* schizophrenia patient, but we can say that it is ineffective for *most* schizophrenia patients.

Although niacin is a "natural" substance, very large doses of it are neither natural nor harmless. Megadoses of niacin can cause uncomfortable and unsightly skin conditions, vomiting, nausea, diarrhea, heartburn, liver abnormalities, and changes in heart function and blood pressure. Suffering from side effects may be justifiable if the drug relieves a greater suffering caused by a serious disease, but no one should have to endure side effects produced by an ineffective drug.

If a completely satisfactory treatment existed, recovered schizophrenia patients would be indistinguishable from other people in the community. The death, marriage, and divorce rates of schizophrenia patients would be like those of other members of society. These patients would, on the average, earn as much money as anyone else. All symptoms of the disease would be eliminated without producing any uncomfortable or dangerous side effects. Just as an electronics expert repairs a computer, the physician would restore the ill person to a healthy condition. But current drug treatments for schizophrenia do not come close to achieving these goals. Typically, recovered schizophrenia patients are marginally competent at their jobs. They often have few friends and no intimates. To achieve even a marginally normal life, they must risk developing serious side effects. We think that for patients with schizophrenia the benefits of antipsychotic treatment outweigh the risks, but it would be foolish to pretend that the benefit is normality and that the risks are inconsequential.

Barring another stroke of good luck similar to the one that produced the phenothiazine treatment in 1952, treatment for schizophrenia will not improve until research progresses in two directions. First, scientists must discover how antipsychotic drugs relieve schizophrenic symptoms and cause undesirable side effects. Then they may be able to develop new drugs with increased therapeutic effects and fewer side effects. Second, the biochemical defects in schizophrenic brains must be understood. Because schizophrenia may be a class of diseases rather than a single disease, a number of different brain malfunctions may be involved. Progress in either of these two research areas will aid progress in the other. Finding how the drugs work will provide valuable hints about the nature of the brain defect. Discovering the nature of the defect will suggest how the drugs might work. The ultimate goal is to find treatments that repair the malfunctions in the brain but do not tamper with its normal functions.

7

How Antipsychotic Drugs Work

In our lab, we have a small computer with a troublesome video terminal. Every now and then, the image on the screen begins to dance and jitter, making it hard to read. We can usually fix the problem by giving the terminal a good hard whack with the heel of the hand. Usually, we are satisfied with this expedient solution; it works temporarily. But it is not very elegant, it is not permanent, and perhaps it even damages the terminal. Eventually, we will have to call the repair shop to get it fixed by an expert who can figure out why the terminal does not work and can then replace the faulty components.

In a sense, treating schizophrenia with drugs is similar to whacking the computer terminal. Antipsychotics are an inelegant solution to the problem of schizophrenia. They do not work for every patient. No one knows why they work at all. When they do work, their effects are not permanent. Just as the heel of the hand can damage the terminal, antipsychotics can damage the brain. Here, however, the similarities between the malfunctioning electronic device and the malfunctioning schizophrenic brain end. There is no expert who understands the cause of schizophrenia and can provide a rational and permanent cure. As we mentioned earlier, the treatment of schizophrenia with phenothiazines was discovered accidentally and was used successfully on many patients before physicians had any understanding of the drug's effects on the brain.

The Effect of Antipsychotic Drugs on Synapses

Most of the knowledge about the biology of schizophrenia has come from investigations of how antipsychotic drugs act on synapses. The most definitive result of these investigations is that antipsychotic drugs block postsynaptic receptors for the transmitter dopamine. As we discussed in Chapter 2, the postsynaptic receptors are protein molecules embedded in the postsynaptic membrane. Their function is to attach, or bind, to molecules of transmitter that are secreted by the presynaptic cell. The binding of a transmitter to its postsynaptic receptor triggers electrical and biochemical responses in the postsynaptic nerve cell. At dopamine synapses, the binding of dopamine to the dopamine receptor triggers an inhibitory response in the postsynaptic cell. At some, but not all, dopamine receptors it also triggers an increase in the synthesis of cAMP, an important messenger compound in cells.

The phenothiazines and other antipsychotic drugs bind to the postsynaptic receptors for dopamine. While the drug molecule is bound to the receptor, the dopamine secreted by the presynaptic cell cannot bind to it. The drug molecule actually gets in the way and blocks the access of dopamine to its receptor. But the drug cannot activate the receptor; that is, it neither inhibits nerve impulses nor triggers the enzyme activity that synthesizes cAMP. Therefore, the receptor is blocked. A single synapse, of course, has many receptors molecules, and if all of them are blocked, transmission across the synapse will fail. If only some of the receptors are blocked, transmission will be weakened but will not fail completely.[1]

In the next section of this chapter, we discuss the evidence that antipsychotics block dopamine receptors and the evidence that their antipsychotic effects depend on this blockade. You could simply accept our conclusions about how antipsychotic drugs work and go on to the next chapter, but we urge you not to do so. There is considerable value in examining and understanding the evidence. Before you can really believe that mental illness is a disease of the brain and that drugs are an appropriate treatment, you must be confident that the drugs cause specific changes in brain function, that they do not shut down or slow down the entire brain. We cannot expect you to agree that drugs are an appropriate treatment unless you are first convinced that neuroscientists can observe and measure the effects of antipsychotics on dopamine synapses and can relate the effects on synapses to the effects on schizophrenia.

First, we examine the evidence that antipsychotic drugs block dopamine receptors. Next, we review the experiments showing that receptor blockade is related to the antipsychotic effects of the drugs. Finally, we explain how the findings from experiments on the mechanism of action of antipsychotic drugs have added to scientists' understanding of the brain defects causing schizophrenia.

The Blockade of Dopamine Receptors

Certain regions of the brain are particularly rich in dopamine synapses. In these regions, many of the presynaptic terminals contain dopamine and the corresponding postsynaptic cell membranes have dopamine receptors. Scientists can perform an experiment on rat brains to measure the number of receptors available to the transmitter. Researchers remove cells from a particular region of a rat's brain, separate them from each other, and place them in a dish. Separation of the cells insures that all the receptors are exposed to the fluid in the dish. A large amount of radioactive dopamine is then added to the fluid. Some of this dopamine binds to receptors on the cells' membranes, and some remains in the fluid. After gently washing out the unbound radioactive dopamine, scientists can determine the amount that is bound to the membranes by using an instrument designed to measure radioactivity. The number of molecules bound depends on the number of cells in the dish and the part of the brain that the cells were taken from. The experiment is then repeated, but this time a radioactive antipsychotic is used rather than radioactive dopamine. The antipsychotic also binds to the cell membranes.

This experiment shows that dopamine and the antipsychotic bind to the same types of *cells*, but it does not show that they bind to the same *receptors*. Perhaps the cells in the dish have two different types of receptors. one type that binds dopamine and one that binds the antipsychotic. Perhaps the dopamine or the antipsychotic attaches to all membranes regardless of whether the membranes contain specific receptors for any transmitter. To disprove these hypotheses, biochemists have shown that dopamine and antipsychotics compete for the same receptors. They have demonstrated this competition by comparing the amount of radioactive antipsychotic bound when only antipsychotic is added to the cells with the amount bound when nonradioactive dopamine is also added. When dopamine is present, less antipsychotic binds. This means that dopamine is occupying some receptors that would otherwise be available for antipsychotic. Dopamine and the drug compete for the same receptors.[2]

If antipsychotics block dopamine receptors, they should prevent all the postsynaptic effects of dopamine. This prediction turns out to be correct. The binding of dopamine to its receptor normally causes a number of biochemical and electrical changes in the postsynaptic cell, and all these changes are blocked when antipsychotics bind to dopamine receptors.

One important biochemical response to dopamine binding is the synthesis of cAMP. When antipsychotics instead of dopamine occupy certain dopamine receptors, dopamine cannot initiate the synthesis of cAMP. The following experiment on rat brains demonstrates this action of antipsychotics. Cells from brain regions rich in dopamine synapses are dispersed in a dish. The researcher adds dopamine and measures the amount of cAMP produced. Next, she repeats the experiment, but this time adds an antipsychotic drug as well as dopamine and measures the amount of cAMP synthesized. The antipsychotic decreases the amount of cAMP produced.[3] That antipsychotic drugs have the ability to prevent cAMP synthesis in response to dopamine is more proof that dopamine receptors are blocked by antipsychotic drugs.

This experiment establishes the important fact, not deducible from the experiment demonstrating that antipsychotic drugs bind to dopamine receptors, that the antipsychotics are antagonists at the dopamine receptor. In other words, not only do the antipsychotics prevent the binding of dopamine to its receptor, they also prevent the activation of the biochemical processes normally initiated by dopamine binding. Thus, dopamine synapses are partially incapacitated when some of the postsynaptic receptors are occupied by antipsychotic drugs. In fact, the greater the number of receptors occupied by the drug, the less effective are the dopamine synapses.

Dopamine also affects the electrical activity of postsynaptic cells. If antipsychotics block dopamine receptors, then presumably the drugs would prevent the cell's electrical response to dopamine.

This prediction has been tested by applying both dopamine and antipsychotic drugs to living nerve cells. Chemicals are applied through a tiny glass tube to a living nerve cell in the rat brain. At the same time, microelectrodes record the electrical response of the cell. Many cells with dopamine receptors emit nerve impulses spontaneously at a fairly steady rate in the absence of dopamine. If dopamine is applied to one of these cells, the rate of nerve impulses decreases. If dopamine is applied along with an antipsychotic drug, the drug prevents the response to dopamine—the rate of impulses does not decrease.[4] Just as scientists found through the cAMP experiment that antipsychotics block the biochemical response to dopamine, they discovered through this experiment that antipsychotics also block the cell's electrical response to dopamine. The drug alters the cell's capacity to respond to synaptic input and, hence, alters its capacity to transmit information to other nerve cells.

The Therapeutic Effect of Blocking Dopamine Receptors

Although we have presented evidence that antipsychotic drugs are antagonists at dopamine receptors, we still cannot assume that the blocking of receptors produces relief from the symptoms of schizophrenia. The drugs may have many other effects on nerve cells, effects still unknown to scientists. One of these unknown effects may be responsible for alleviating schizophrenic symptoms.

The wide variety of antipsychotic drugs on the market provides a tool for determining the relation between receptor blockade and relief of schizophrenic symptoms. The drugs vary widely in clinical potency; that is, they vary in the size of the dose required to alleviate schizophrenic symptoms. (If a larger dose is required, the drug is less potent, but less potent drugs are not necessarily inferior to more potent ones. Considerations governing choice of drug for a particular patient are discussed in the next chapter.) The drugs also vary widely in their receptor-blocking ability. If blockade of dopamine receptors is required for therapeutic effectiveness, the drugs that are most potent in the psychiatric clinic should be the best dopamine-receptor blockers. Similarly, the drugs that are least potent clinically should be the poorest dopamine-receptor blockers. On the whole, these predictions are valid.[5]

Surprisingly, researchers can better predict clinical potency by a drug's ability to displace haloperidol (a potent antipsychotic drug) from dopamine receptors than by its ability to displace dopamine from these same receptors. To measure haloperidol displacement, the researcher first measures the amount of radioactive haloperidol that binds to calf nerve cells dispersed in a dish. He then repeats the experiment when the test drug is also added to the dish. If the test drug binds to dopamine receptors, it will displace some of the radioactive haloperidol from the receptors, decreasing the amount of haloperidol already bound. Many antipsychotic drugs have been tested in this way. The graph in Figure 7-1 shows the relationship between drugs' clinical potency and their ability to compete with haloperidol for receptors. If a drug's ability to block haloperidol binding is weak, its clinical potency is low. If a drug's ability to block haloperidol binding is powerful, its clinical potency is high.[6]

To explain why the potency of an antipsychotic is better correlated to its ability to displace haloperidol, an artificial chemical, than to its ability to displace dopamine, the natural transmitter, Dr. Solomon Snyder hypothesized that the dopamine receptor exists in two states: the agonist state and the antagonist state. In the agonist state, the receptor is able to bind agonists, drugs that bind to the receptor and activate it. Activation of dopamine receptors typically causes synthesis of cAMP and a decrease in the rate of nerve impulse production. Dopamine is the natural agonist for the dopamine receptor. (There are artificial agonists as well.) In the antagonist state, the receptor can bind antagonists, chemicals that bind to the receptor but do not activate it. Antipsychotics such as haloperidol and chlorpromazine are antagonists and thus bind preferentially to the antagonist state. Scientists think that, when the receptor changes from the agonist to the antagonist state, the receptor molecule slightly changes its geometric shape, much as an adjustable wrench takes on different shapes when it grips (binds) different sized nuts.[7]

If dopamine binds only to receptors in the agonist state but antipsychotics bind only to receptors in the antagonist state, how do antipsychotics prevent dopamine from binding to the receptor? Dr. Snyder imagined that, when no drug is bound to the receptor, it flips back and forth between the two states rather freely. When molecules of an antagonist drug appear in the vicinity of the recep-

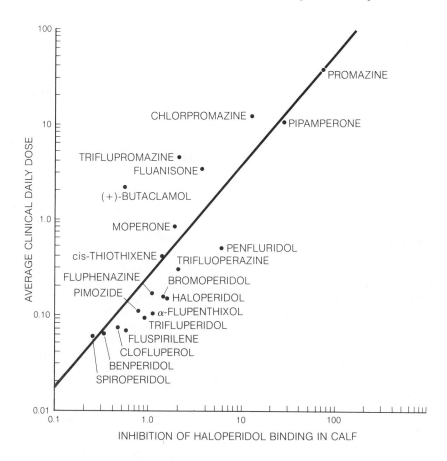

Figure 7-1. Correlation between the ability of antipsychotic drugs to decrease haloperidol binding and their clinical potency. (From S. H. Snyder, D. R. Burt, and I. Creese, "The Dopamine Receptor of Mammalian Brain: Direct Demonstration of Binding to Agonist and Antagonist Sites." In A. J. Ferendelli, B. S. McEwen, and S. H. Snyder, eds., *Neurotransmitters, Hormones, and Receptors: Novel Approaches.* Bethesda, Md.: Society for Neuroscience, 1976.)

tor, they are likely to bind to the receptor while it is in the antagonist state and thus lock the receptor in that state (Figure 7-2).[8] Before long, a large number of the receptors will be locked in the antagonist state and transmission at dopamine synapses will be significantly weakened. Although Dr. Snyder's theory about the two states of the receptor has not been conclusively proven, it is consistent with a very large body of knowledge about the mecha-

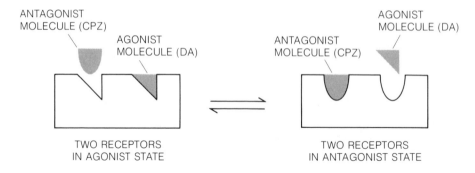

Figure 7-2. The two-state model of receptor binding. The cell membrane has dopamine receptors that can change back and forth between two different states, drawn here as triangular and semicircular. When the receptor is in the agonist state, drawn as triangular, it can bind agonists like dopamine, shown here as a triangle. This receptor cannot, however, bind antagonists like chlorpromazine, shown here as a semicircle. When the receptor is in the antagonist state, drawn as semicircular, the reverse is true: it binds antagonists but not agonists. CPZ: chlorpromazine; DA: dopamine. (After S.H. Snyder, "Neurotransmitter and drug receptors in the brain," *Biochemical Pharmacology*, 1975, 24:1371–1374.)

nism of action of enzymes and receptors other than the dopamine receptor.

According to Dr. Snyder's scheme, dopamine transmission should be most effectively prevented by drugs that bind to the antagonist state of the receptor, increasing the number of receptors in that state. The potency, then, of an antipsychotic should be better predicted by its ability to compete with the powerful antagonist, haloperidol, than by its ability to compete with dopamine. The impressive correlation between a drug's clinical potency and its ability to inhibit haloperidol binding is perhaps the best evidence that the blockade of dopamine receptors is essential to the action of antipsychotic drugs.

The Effects of Excessive Activation of Dopamine Synapses

If blocking dopamine receptors alleviates schizophrenia, then a drug that activates dopamine receptors excessively should produce symptoms of schizophrenia. At the very least, the drug should exacerbate schizophrenic symptoms in people who already suffer from the disease. It might even cause schizophrenialike symptoms to appear in healthy people. In addition, the schizophrenialike symptoms produced by such a drug should be reversed by treatment with antipsychotics such as chlorpromazine and haloperidol.

Amphetamine is a drug that increases the activity at dopamine synapses in two different ways.[9] First, amphetamine causes the release of dopamine from the presynaptic terminal. Second, it blocks dopamine reuptake into the presynaptic terminal, increasing the amount in the synaptic cleft.

Ingestion of high doses of amphetamine (500 to 1000 milligrams) can induce a psychosis that can be easily mistaken for schizophrenia, even by an experienced psychiatrist. Drs. Burton Angrist and Abraham Sudilovsky described a volunteer subject who had no symptoms of schizophrenia before taking amphetamine. After taking the drug, the patient proclaimed that he had become a "prophet" who was being addressed directly by God. He stated: "In my human form he might let me act human for the rest must still wonder at my actions which make them doubt my having been used to enlighten. Every thought that stops me from accepting all knowledge more than man has ever know."[10] It is hard to imagine a more typical example of bizarre schizophrenic rambling.

People who abuse amphetamine sometimes bring such a psychosis upon themselves. Jessica was a 41-year-old divorced pharmacist who took advantage of her easy access to amphetamine. She used the drug to counteract lethargy and boredom. Eventually, she became addicted. Jessica had always been friendly and open, but now she became hostile and suspicious. She accused her son of spying on her and hiring detectives to follow her. One day she told her son that the announcer on the evening news had sent her brain messages in secret code that would enable her to outwit the detectives. At first, Jessica's son was irritated at her suspiciousness. Later, he became angry. Finally, he realized that his mother was seriously ill. Like most people suddenly confronted with serious mental illness, he had no idea what might be wrong or how to get help. He knew nothing of her amphetamine abuse. It took much wheedling to get Jessica to a psychiatrist, and once she did meet with him, she successfully concealed her drug use. The psychiatrist thought she had schizophrenia and needed antipsychotic therapy, but Jessica refused to enter the hospital. Because initiating antipsychotic therapy on outpatients is risky, the psychiatrist could not offer her much help.

Several days later, Jessica walked into a camera store and smashed a movie camera that she believed had been spying on her from the window. She was then hospitalized on a two-physician certificate. (In many states, a person can be involuntarily committed to a psychiatric hospital for a few days if two physicians certify that the person is a danger to himself or others or cannot care for himself.) In the hospital, Jessica had no access to amphetamine and was given antipsychotics. Her symptoms cleared up unusually fast. When medication was removed, she did not relapse. As soon as Jessica stopped taking amphetamine, she stopped suffering from "schizophrenia."

As we discussed in Chapter 4, the proper diagnosis of schizophrenia requires the psychiatrist to rule out the possibility that the symptoms are caused by drug abuse. Amphetamine and similar drugs are the possible culprits in cases of apparent schizophrenia. In Jessica's case, the psychiatrist should have immediately suspected amphetamine abuse because Jessica had no history of schizophrenia, and the disease rarely, if ever, develops for the first time in a person Jessica's age.

A small dose of amphetamine can exacerbate symptoms in patients who are suffering from schizophrenia but does not increase the symptoms of patients with other psychiatric diseases, for example, affective disorders.[11] In addition, amphetamine does not induce symptoms in patients whose schizophrenia is in remission. Dr. D. S. Janowsky and his colleagues at Vanderbilt University described a schizophrenia patient who was dramatically affected by amphetamine.[12] The patient entered the hospital claiming that spirits rose out of people's heads and spoke to him. After treatment with antipsychotics, he admitted that his talk about spirits had been "crazy talk," but within one minute of an amphetamine injection, he again claimed that spirits were rising out of the interviewer's head. This exacerbation of schizophrenia is a specific effect of amphetamine. Other psychoactive drugs do not exacerbate schizophrenia. Caffeine produces anxiety and tremor but not schizophrenia. LSD produces psychotic symptoms, but they are clearly different from those in naturally occurring schizophrenia or the schizophrenialike syndrome produced by amphetamine.[13]

If amphetamine psychosis results from the overactivation of dopamine receptors, amphetamine-induced symptoms, like Jessica's, should be reversed by antipsychotic drugs. Indeed, they are, and the treatment is quite specific to antipsychotics. Thus, sedatives such as barbiturates do not alleviate psychotic symptoms even though they sedate the patient.[14]

Since amphetamine and anti-psychotic drugs pose some risks, researchers do not experiment on humans by inducing amphetamine psychosis and then examining the potency of various antipsychotic drugs in alleviating it. Researchers can, however, experiment on rats. Rats and humans treated with amphetamine exhibit some similar symptoms. People who abuse amphetamine frequently engage in ritualized, stereotyped behavior. They repetitively disassemble complex objects like radios. Not surprisingly, reassembly requires more concentration than they can muster. Rats given high doses of amphetamine develop a similar syndrome called stereotypy. They pace back and forth, sniffing the corners of their cages. They chew repetitively on the bars.

Predictably, the antipsychotic drugs that are most potent in reversing the effects of amphetamine in rats are those that bind best to the antagonist state of the dopamine receptor.[15] Recall that the antipsychotics most potent in treating schizophrenia in humans were also those that bound best to the antagonist state of the dopamine receptor. This finding suggests that similar abnormalities might be present in the brain of a schizophrenia patient and in the brain of an amphetamine abuser. Understanding how amphetamine affects brain cells might yield some important hints about the biochemical defects in the schizophrenic brain.

L-DOPA is another drug known to cause schizophrenialike symptoms. Like amphetamine, it increases dopamine transmission. L-DOPA is normally present in the body and is used in the synthesis of dopamine. If a person is given large amounts of L-DOPA, his brain makes abnormally large amounts of dopamine. The amount of dopamine released from presynaptic terminals in the brain will also be abnormally high. L-DOPA is used to treat Parkinson's disease, a type of palsy caused by deficient dopamine transmission. Occasionally, patients with Parkinson's disease who are treated with this drug develop symptoms of schizophrenia as side effects. When the drug is given experimentally to schizophrenia patients, their symptoms get worse.[16] These facts about L-DOPA support the conclusion that antipsychotic drugs are effective in the treatment of schizophrenia because they can block transmission at dopamine synapses.

The Brain's Response to Receptor Blockade

The conclusion that antipsychotic drugs act by blocking dopamine receptors has led researchers to form the dopamine hypothesis of schizophrenia. It simply states: Schizophrenia is *caused by* abnormalities at dopamine synapses. It is obvious, however, that relief from the symptoms of schizophrenia involves more than changes at dopamine synapses. Cells directly affected by antipsychotic drugs transmit altered messages to other cells. And so, the changes in dopamine synapses spread, domino fashion, throughout the brain. Unfortunately, neuroscientists are ignorant about where the dominoes fall. They do not yet understand the sequences of synaptic events that produce the simplest normal behaviors, much less behaviors as complex as speech. Until they understand how the normal brain can organize thoughts and execute speech, they probably cannot understand how the schizophrenic brain produces delusional and disorganized thought and speech or how blocking dopamine receptors reorganizes thought and speech. If scientists have only the barest outline of how the brain produces normal posture or movement, how can they understand catatonia? If they do not know which synapses fire in which order when we laugh or cry, how can they understand the synaptic changes underlying flat affect? One thing neuroscientists are sure of, though, is that none of these complex, distinctly human behaviors can be produced by just one or even a few types of synapses working alone. Each behavior requires nerve circuits involving many different types os synapses.

While neuroscientists cannot follow the chain of drug-induced events from blockade of dopamine receptors to the relief of schizophrenic thought, speech, and emotion, they do understand two changes that follow closely from the blockade of dopamine receptors. These changes appear to result from the brain's attempts to combat the effects of antipsychotic drugs and to maintain stable dopamine transmission.

Under the influence of antipsychotic drugs, the postsynaptic cells make extra dopamine receptors.[17] Scientists explain this overproduction as the postsynaptic cells' attempt to compensate for the weakening of synaptic transmission, caused by drugs. The extra receptors tend to restore the cells' sensitivity to dopamine in the face of partial receptor blockade. Just as a sensitive photographic film with more silver salt is more likely to "see" an object in dim light than is a less sensitive film with less silver salt, a cell with more dopamine receptors is more likely to "see" a small amount of transmitter than is a cell with fewer receptors. If a photographer switches from a less sensitive film to a more sensitive film and does not reduce the amount of light he allows through his lens, his pictures will be overexposed. Discontinuing an antipsychotic drug after long-term treatment is similar to switching to a more sensitive film—the increased number of dopamine receptors that have been produced in reaction to the drug causes an abnormally large response to dopamine.

This compensatory increase in receptors has been measured in rat brains. The first step in the experiment was to inject rats with an antipsychotic drug for several weeks. Next, the scientists let a few days elapse so that the drug had time to leave the receptors— the number of dopamine receptors could not be measured while the drug was blocking them. Then the scientists removed a region of the brain known to contain dopamine receptors. In order to compare the number of dopamine receptors in treated and untreated rats, they also removed the identical region of the brain from rats that had not been treated with an antipsychotic. Finally, the researchers separated the cells removed from each group of rats and added radioactive haloperidol to each. By measuring the amount of haloperidol bound to cells from each rat, they calculated the number of dopamine receptors on the cells from the treated rats and on the cells from the untreated rats. The cells from the treated rats had more dopamine receptors.[18]

The brain compensates for dopamine-receptor blockade in yet another way: it increases dopamine synthesis. This increased synthesis does not, however, increase the total amount of dopamine in the brain because there is a compensatory increase in the rate at which dopamine is broken down.[19] Nevertheless, increased synthesis probably does increase the effectiveness of dopamine synapses by increasing the amount of dopamine that is in the vesicles, ready for release.

Neuroscientists disagree about whether the therapeutic benefits of antipsychotic drugs depend on increases in dopamine synthesis. Some investigators attempted to estimate changes in dopamine synthesis in patients receiving antipsychotics. Dopamine synthesis did increase, but the increases disappeared after a week or two of medication, about the time it takes for the drug to become fully effective. The short duration of the increased synthesis suggests that it is not required for the therapeutic effect of the drug.[20] But these experiments are not conclusive because studies on humans require that increases in dopamine synthesis be inferred from the amount of dopamine metabolites in the cerebrospinal fluid. This procedure measures only the average change in dopamine synthesis throughout the entire brain. It might not detect permanent increases in particular small regions of the brain.

It seems reasonable, however, to suppose that the important effects of an antipsychotic drug, including a permanent increase in dopamine synthesis, would not occur uniformly throughout the brain but only in particular small regions. This hypothesis cannot be tested on humans but can be tested on experimental animals. Dr. N.C. Bacapoulos and his colleagues at Yale Medical School obtained evidence in support of this hypothesis. First, they gave control monkeys a large dose of the antipsychotic, haloperidol. In response, all regions of the brains of these monkeys increased their rate of dopamine synthesis. Experimental monkeys received small doses of haloperidol for 20 days before they received the large dose. Some regions of the experimental brain increased dopamine synthesis in response to the large dose, but the 20 days of treatment made other regions insensitive to haloperidol. These regions did not increase dopamine synthesis in response to the test dose. The same group of scientists examined various regions of human brains taken from deceased patients who had been treated with antipsychotics. In both the human and monkey experiments, the same regions showed maintained increases in dopamine synthesis.[22] Clearly, the activity in individual regions of the brain cannot be inferred from measurements made on cerebrospinal fluid.

At least one experiment suggested that increased dopamine synthesis is an important part of the therapeutic effect of antipsychotics. Researchers measured both dopamine synthesis and changes in schizophrenic symptoms during the first few weeks of treatment while dopamine synthesis was still elevated. The patients with the greatest increase in dopamine synthesis had the greatest clinical improvement, in spite of the fact that the measurements were made on dopamine metabolites in cerebrospinal fluid.[23]

The brain's ability to combat receptor blocking with increased receptors and increased dopamine production is puzzling. If the brain can counteract receptor blocking, then why is receptor blocking so strongly correlated with the drugs' capacity to relieve the symptoms of schizophrenia? One possibility is that the brain's compensation for receptor blockade is not complete. If this were true, the blockade might be the primary cause of the antipsychotic effects. Another possibility is that the increased rate of dopamine synthesis and breakdown permits more precise regulation of the amount of dopamine in each synaptic terminal. Yet another possibility is that the crucial changes occur in cells that do not use dopamine as a transmitter but are many synapses removed from the synapses directly affected by the drug.

The Schizophrenic Brain

We would hope that understanding what antipsychotic drugs do to synapses would provide some hints about the nature of the defect in the schizophrenic brain. What scientists have learned so far about antipsychotic drugs and amphetamine suggests that overactive dopamine synapses may be a factor in causing schizophrenia. Overactivity at dopamine synapses could result either from the release of too much dopamine at the presynaptic terminal or from an excess of dopamine receptors at the postsynaptic cell.

Although there is no evidence for increased dopamine synthesis and/or release in the unmedicated schizophrenic brain, two different research groups obtained evidence that schizophrenic brains have too many dopamine receptors. Lee and Seeman in Canada and Owen and his colleagues in England measured dopamine binding in samples of human brains obtained at autopsy. They found many more dopamine receptors in brains taken from schizophrenia patients than in brains taken from people who did not have schizophrenia. In some of the patients, antipsychotic drugs probably caused the increase in receptors. But even patients who had never received antipsychotics or who had been off medication for at least a year had an excess of dopamine receptors.[24] This result is, perhaps, the best lead in the search for the abnormality in the schizophrenic brain, but the finding is still tentative because the number of unmedicated schizophrenia patients studied is very small.

The hypothesis that the schizophrenic brain contains excessive dopamine receptors explains some of the effects of antipsychotics. It explains why blocking dopamine receptors alleviates the symptoms. It also explains why antipsychotics control schizophrenia but cannot cure it. As soon as the drugs leave the body and dopamine receptors are no longer blocked, the excess receptors would again be free to do their damage. The analogy with diabetes that we used earlier is instructive here. Insulin does not cure diabetes; it cannot induce the pancreas to make insulin. Similarly, an antipsychotic does not cure schizophrenia; it cannot induce the nerve cells to make normal dopamine synapses. In both diseases, the drug compensates, at least partially, for a biochemical abnormality, but the underlying abnormality is still present.

But there are some facts that cannot be explained by the excess receptor hypothesis. First, the long time lag between the beginning of antipsychotic treatment and the improvement of the patient cannot be explained. The putative excess dopamine receptors are blocked almost as soon as treatment begins. Second, scientists cannot explain why patients do not become tolerant to antipsychotics. Because the drugs themselves induce synthesis of dopamine receptors, we would expect the patient to require increasing doses to block his increasing dopamine receptors. Third, the scientists cannot explain why discontinuing a drug does not make the disease worse than it was before treatment. During treatment with antipsychotics, the patient becomes extremely sensitive to dopamine because both the old and the new dopamine receptors are exposed. Surprisingly, removal of the drug does not worsen the disease. Relapses of schizophrenia after drug holidays are not obviously worse than the initial episodes or relapses occurring while the patient is on medication. Clearly, neuroscientists do not completely understand what is wrong with the schizophrenic brain. But progress has been made. Studying the effects of antipsychotic drugs has taught us that dopamine synapses are an important factor. Refining the research methods and investigating other transmitter systems may tell us more precisely how the schizophrenic brain differs from the healthy one.

8

Side Effects of Antipsychotic Drugs

If you were to look up the side effects of the antipsychotic drugs in a standard medical pharmacology text, you would be appalled at the number listed and at the severity of some of them.[1] You would find that these drugs can affect virtually every organ of the body, from the skin to the liver. The severity of these side effects ranges from just annoying to life threatening. We discuss only the most common ones because many are so rare that, while physicians need to watch for them, it is unlikely that any particular patient will experience them. If you do consult a complete list, try to keep the information in perspective. A cloud of side effects hangs over every significant drug, but that cloud should not obscure the benefits. For instance, patients with bacterial infections are treated with penicillin even though on occasion a person is allergic to the drug and dies from it. Before deciding whether to use a particular treatment, the physician and the patient must weigh both its risks and its benefits. How damaging is the disease? Is the patient willing to live untreated even if treatment is available? How serious are the side effects? How likely are the most serious side effects?

Our discussion of the side effects of antipsychotic drugs emphasizes the neurological side effects because they are the most common, and one of them, tardive dyskinesia, is among the most dangerous. Furthermore, your knowledge of how antipsychotic drugs affect the brain will help you to understand, at least partially, why these side effects occur.

Movement Disorders

Parkinsonian Side Effects, Dystonia, and Akathisia

Antipsychotic drugs can cause several different kinds of movement disorders.[2] One of these disorders is very similar to Parkinson's disease. Patients with Parkinson's disease typically have an expressionless face, move very slowly with a shuffling gait, and have a severe tremor. One cause of Parkinson's disease is a deficiency of transmission at dopamine synapses in the basal ganglia, brain structures involved in the control of posture and movement. When schizophrenia is treated with antipsychotic drugs, the dopamine receptors in the basal ganglia are partially blocked and synaptic transmission is impaired. It is not surprising, then, that Parkinsonian symptoms result as a side effect of the drugs.

As we mentioned in Chapter 7, L-DOPA is an effective treatment for Parkinson's disease. This drug increases the amount of dopamine in the basal ganglia and relieves the symptoms. But L-DOPA cannot be used to treat Parkinsonian symptoms that are a side effect of antipsychotic therapy. L-DOPA enhances transmission at dopamine synapses throughout the brain. Therefore, it counteracts the effect of the antipsychotic drug and may exacerbate schizophrenia.

Parkinson's disease can also result from an excess of activity at acetylcholine synapses (acetylcholine is a common transmitter). In fact, a more complete explanation of the cause of Parkinson's disease is that it results when the balance between activity at dopamine synapses and activity at acetylcholine synapses shifts in favor of acetylcholine synapses. This balance can be restored either by decreasing transmission at acetylcholine synapses or by increasing transmission at dopamine synapses. Therefore, Parkinsonian symptoms caused by antipsychotics are usually treated effectively with drugs that partially block acetylcholine synapses. Two of the drugs most commonly used to alleviate these symptoms are Artane and Cogentin (trade names).

Sometimes abnormal movements that look like drug-induced Parkinsonism are actually symptoms of schizophrenia that are not controlled by the antipsychotic drug. Slow and reluctant movement may be schizophrenic withdrawal. The expressionless face may be a manifestation of flat affect. Schizophrenia patients often assume peculiar postures and make grimaces. Therefore, these symptoms are not always Parkinsonian side effects of the drugs. Even a psychiatrist may have difficulty distinguishing between Parkinsonian side effects and a reemergence of schizophrenia. Merely observing the patient may not suffice. Usually, but not always, a psychiatrist can make this distinction by giving the patient anti-Parkinsonian medication. If this treatment helps, the patient is suffering from side effects of medication and not from an increase of schizophrenic symptoms.

Some patients suffer from *dystonia,* defined as "involuntary muscle contractions that cause bizarre and uncontrolled movements of the face, neck, tongue, and back." A particularly distressing form of dystonia is *oculogyric crisis,* in which the eyes roll uncontrollably. Like the Parkinsonian side effects, dystonia can be confused with an increase in the symptoms of schizophrenia because schizophrenic patients often assume peculiar postures. Dystonia can also be mistaken for seizures. When dystonic symptoms are, in fact, a side effect of antipsychotic drugs, they respond dramatically to anti-Parkinsonian drugs.

Other patients suffer from akathisia. At first glance, akathisia looks like severe restlessness and agitation. In fact, akathisia is sometimes mistaken for schizophrenic agitation. The patient complains of severe discomfort in his arms and legs; he moves them about continually. He cannot describe or localize any specific pain, but no position—sitting, standing, or lying down—is comfortable for very long. He continues to move about in the vain hope of finding a comfortable position. Anti-Parkinsonian medication is the usual treatment but is not always successful. Reduction in the dose of the antipsychotic medication may be necessary.

Dystonia and akathisia, like Parkinson's disease, probably result from subnormal synaptic transmission at dopamine synapses in the basal ganglia, but it is not known why some patients experience Parkinsonian side effects, others dystonia, and yet others akathisia. Most of the neurological side effects occur early in treatment, decreasing in severity after a few weeks. Again, it is not known why the side effects diminish while the drugs continue to block dopamine receptors throughout treatment.

Tardive Dyskinesia

Schizophrenia is usually a chronic disease. Antipsychotic medication is the only effective treatment for it. Unfortunately, the treatment has one devastating side effect that prevents many victims of schizophrenia from taking medication indefinitely.[3] The patients are haunted by the specter of tardive dyskinesia. *Tardive dyskinesia* means "late appearing movement disorder." Unlike most neurological side effects of antipsychotics, tardive dyskinesia usually does not appear until a patient has taken antipsychotics for many years. It begins as jerky, ticlike movements in the tongue and face.[4] As the disease progresses, the entire body may become affected, making either ticlike or writhing movements. These movements are virtually continuous during waking hours but cease during sleep. A patient with tardive dyskinesia may flick her tongue in and out of her mouth as often as 20 times in 30 seconds. Her gait becomes unsteady as the disease progresses. If the disease becomes extremely severe, she may start rocking back and forth at the hips. Irregular breathing gives her the appearance of gasping for breath. Fortunately, she will not lose complete control of the muscles used in breathing. Patients with tardive dyskinesia do not die of respiratory failure. This fact may be small consolation, though, for tardive dyskinesia can be so socially debilitating that it is to be feared nearly as much as schizophrenia itself. On the other hand, some cases of tardive dyskinesia are mild and are diagnosed by the psychiatrist before they are noticed by the patient or his family. Some cases do not progress beyond mild tongue flicking even if antipsychotic medication is continued.

Estimates of the prevalence of tardive dyskinesia vary widely. As the use of antipsychotic drugs has become more prevalent, so has tardive dyskinesia. In 1960, probably less than 5 percent of chronically hospitalized schizophrenic patients developed the disease. By 1980, this estimate had increased to about 20 to 25 percent.[5] Older patients are more likely than younger ones to get tardive dyskinesia. Only about 10 percent of chronically hospitalized patients under 40 develop the condition, whereas 35 to 40 percent of those over 55 suffer from it. Also, a patient's chances of getting tardive dyskinesia probably increase with the number of years that she takes antipsychotics; the disease is rare in patients who have been taking the drugs for less than two years. Although it seems obvious that patients taking higher drug doses would be more likely than those taking lower doses to develop tardive dyskinesia, there are no controlled studies demonstrating this pattern. It seems reasonable that intermittent drug holidays of a few months might provide some protection, but there is no evidence that they do.[6]

What causes tardive dyskinesia? The best hypothesis, and it is only a hypothesis, is that tardive dyskinesia results from a drug-induced production of extra dopamine receptors. The extra receptors make the postsynaptic cell supersensitive to dopamine.[7] In a sense, tardive dyskinesia may be the converse of Parkinson's disease. Both diseases result from abnormalities in the basal ganglia. In Parkinson's disease, dopamine transmission is inadequate and acetylcholine synapses dominate. This imbalance causes slow and shaky bodily movements. In tardive dyskinesia, extra dopamine receptors increase the strength of dopamine synapses to the point where they dominate acetylcholine synapses. Dopamine domination causes the writhing and twitching of tardive dyskinesia. According to this hypothesis, tardive dyskinesia results when the basal ganglia overcompensate for the partial dopamine blockade caused by the antipsychotic drug.

A number of facts about tardive dyskinesia are consistent with the dopamine supersensitivity hypothesis.[8] First, tardive dyskinesia gets worse if antipsychotic drugs are suddenly terminated. Presumably, drug withdrawal unblocks receptors, increasing the number available to dopamine. Second, tardive dyskinesia gets worse if the patient is given L-DOPA, which causes the brain to make extra dopamine. The increased supply of dopamine increases the number of receptors activated. If the patient receives much smaller doses of L-DOPA for a long time, his tardive dyskinesia may actually improve.[9] Perhaps this improvement occurs because chronic stimulation with extra dopamine causes a compensatory decrease in the number of receptors. Third, tardive dyskinesia can be temporarily suppressed by increasing the dose of antipsychotic drug. The increased amount of drug available to the dopamine receptors may block a higher proportion of the receptors and counteract their excessive number. As we mentioned earlier, however, a higher dose of antipsychotic drug only postpones the inevitable return of symptoms. The higher dose probably causes the slow development of even more dopamine receptors and a corresponding worsening of the underlying condition.[10]

From time to time, articles appear in medical journals claiming successful pharmacological treatments for tardive dyskinesia. Unfortunately, rigorous testing has failed to show that any of these provide reliable help. The only effective way to treat tardive dyskinesia is to prevent it. Psychiatrists and nurses should be on the lookout for the first signs of tardive dyskinesia in hospitalized patients. They should check outpatients before renewing their prescriptions for antipsychotic drugs. The families of outpatients should be alerted to watch for symptoms.

If antipsychotics are withdrawn at the first signs of tardive dyskinesia, the symptoms may eventually disappear.[11] As we already mentioned, the symptoms may worsen during the first few weeks after drug withdrawal. These symptoms are relieved by restoring antipsychotic medication, and increased doses can often suppress them entirely.[12] Nevertheless, patience is essential; drug therapy should not be reinstated. If the patient is fortunate, the uncontrolled movements will abate a few weeks after she stops taking medication. If, however, she continues to take antipsychotics after the first twitchlike movements of the face and tongue are noticed, the symptoms may become worse and irreversible. Once an elderly person develops dramatic symptoms throughout the entire body, removal of antipsychotics will probably not result in much improvement.

The appearance of tardive dyskinesia presents a dilemma. If antipsychotics are withdrawn at the first signs, tardive dyskinesia often improves or disappears.[13] If antipsychotics are continued, the tardive dyskinesia may become worse. On the other hand, withdrawal of the antipsychotic may cause a relapse of schizophrenia, and continuing the antipsychotic does not always lead to a debilitating case of tardive dyskinesia. Often the psychiatrist, patient, and patient's family must make a choice between schizophrenia and tardive dyskinesia.

Other Neurological Side Effects

Another neurological side effect of antipsychotic drugs is the secretion of milk from the breasts, occasionally even in men. The blockade of dopamine receptors in a portion of the brain called the hypothalamus can increase production of prolactin, the hormone controlling milk secretion. Sometimes the increase in prolactin is so great that milk is produced. Although this side effect of antipsychotic medication is annoying and embarrassing, it is not dangerous. It can even be useful to the physician because the level of prolactin in the blood is an indicator of how effectively an antipsychotic drug has blocked dopamine receptors. Interestingly, blood prolactin increases almost immediately after antipsychotic therapy begins, demonstrating again that antipsychotic drugs block dopamine receptors immediately, even though their therapeutic effects are not fully expressed for about two weeks.[14]

When a physician prescribes a drug, he usually would like to confine its action to a specific target. Unfortunately, this is rarely possible, and antipsychotics are no exception to this rule. In addition to blocking dopamine receptors, they can also block certain norepinephrine receptors and some, but not all, acetylcholine receptors.[15] Fortunately, antipsychotic drugs do not block the acetylcholine receptors on skeletal muscles and, hence, do not cause muscle weakness or paralysis. They do, however, block acetylcholine receptors at the junctions between nerve fibers and internal organs. Blockade of these synapses causes many side effects known collectively as anticholinergic side effects. For example, blockade of synapses at the salivary glands causes dry mouth, and blockade of synapses at the iris of the eye causes blurred vision. Anticholinergic side effects are usually more annoying than serious. They complicate the treatment of movement disorders because the anti-Parkinsonian drugs also decrease transmission at acetylcholine synapses and, therefore, exacerbate anticholinergic side effects.

Some side effects are caused by the blockade of norepinephrine receptors.[16] One such side effect is orthostatic hypotension. Orthostatic hypotension is a sudden decrease in blood pressure when the patient stands up suddenly after having been sitting or lying down for a while. The drop in blood pressure prevents the brain from receiving enough blood, and, hence, enough oxygen. The patient feels dizzy or faint and may experience a partial blackout of vision. These effects usually disappear in a few seconds. Healthy people experience orthostatic hypotension from time to time, but the antipsychotic drugs make it occur more often. Furthermore, the decrease in blood pressure can be dangerous to people with cardiovascular disease and to people whose blood pressure is already low. Older patients are at greatest risk. Obviously, people taking antipsychotic drugs should avoid situations where loss of balance is particularly dangerous. Also, they should not stand up suddenly in a situation where a fall would be disastrous. They should not paint the gutters while squatting on a steeply pitched roof. They may be unable to stand up slowly enough to avoid dizziness and a dangerous fall.

The sedative effect that patients and their relatives so often complain about is probably caused by the blockade of receptors for transmitters other than dopamine. Several different transmitters and receptors may be involved. Most antipsychotic drugs cause some sleepiness at first, but in most patients, this sedation gradually disappears after the first few weeks of therapy. Nevertheless, patients and their relatives may continue to insist that medications turn patients into "zombies." You recall Mark Vonnegut's complaint that drugs had impaired his ability to make judgments and feel emotion. Sometimes these complaints are justified. If the drug dose is large enough, the sedative effects will be incapacitating and may not disappear completely with time. Often, however, symptoms that appear to arise from drug overdose are, in fact, a reassertion of the active disease. Patients suffering from schizophrenia often do not have normal emotional expressions. They may look more like "zombies" when not taking the drug than when taking it. Before concluding that a patient has been overmedicated, you need to know how she behaved in the absence of medication and whether her psychosis could be controlled with a lower dose.

Addiction and Tolerance

Because many patients take antipsychotic drugs for months or years, it is appropriate to ask whether the patient may become addicted as people become addicted to alcohol, tobacco, and opiates. Although we present a detailed discussion of addiction in Chapter 16, a brief definition is in order here. A person suffers from addiction to a drug if he (1) uses the drug in greater amounts than can be medically justified, (2) brings harm to himself or others as a result of his excessive use, and (3) cannot voluntarily stop his excessive use. Most addictive drugs produce physiological dependence;

that is, withdrawal from the drug causes the addict to become ill. In addition, most addictive drugs produce tolerance; that is, the addict must increase his dose over time or the drug loses its effectiveness.

The behavior of cigarette smoking fits this definition of addiction. The smoker uses more tobacco than is medically justified. He harms his health and the health of others as a result of his excessive use. He usually finds it difficult or impossible to quit smoking. Over several months or years, he increases his consumption from a few cigarettes a week to a pack, or even two packs, a day. The definition also encompasses the addictive behaviors associated with heroin, alcohol, sleeping pills, and many other substances. It does not apply, however, to the pattern of use associated with antipsychotic drugs. First, the patient with schizophrenia does not tend to increase his drug use beyond that which is medically required. In fact, the side effects of the antipsychotic drugs are sufficiently unpleasant that many patients are inclined to defy the doctors' orders and refuse to take the drugs. Second, although it could be said that the side effects of the drug harm the patient, the therapeutic effect prevents even greater harm, both to the patient and to others. Third, patients taking antipsychotic drugs have no difficulty discontinuing their drug use when the psychiatrist instructs them to do so. They feel no craving for the drug. Neither do they suffer a distressing withdrawal illness when they stop using it. Although some patients experience mild discomfort if medication is stopped abruptly, gradually tapering the dose to zero creates no problems. Finally, tolerance does not occur for the antipsychotic effects of the drugs. Clearly, the long-term use of antipsychotic medication can cause problems, tardive dyskinesia being the most serious. Drug addiction, however, is not one of them.[17]

Minimizing Side Effects

Drug Selection

There is no evidence that one antipsychotic drug is more effective than any other. Although antipsychotic drugs vary in potency, less potent drugs can be just as effective as more potent ones, even for the sickest patients. That one drug is more potent than another means only that the more potent drug is effective in smaller doses. For example, trifluoperazine (Stelazine) is a more potent drug than chlorpromazine (Thorazine). About 5 milligrams of trifluoperizine is equivalent in antipsychotic efficacy to about 100 milligrams of chlorpromazine. When the doses are properly adjusted, both are equally effective.

Since there are many antipsychotics with similar therapeutic effectivness on the market, a physician usually selects an antipsychotic for a patient because of its particular side effects rather than its particular therapeutic effects. All antipsychotics cause movement side effects, sedation, and hypotension, but the intensity of each varies from drug to drug. If the psychiatrist wants to minimize the movement disorders—for example, Parkinsonism, dystonia, or akathisia—he is likely to select chlorpromazine. Unfortunately, he can minimize the movement side effects only at the expense of increasing sedation. On the other hand, if he wants to minimize sedation, he will probably select haloperidol or trifluoperizine. However, he will decrease sedation at the expense of increasing the likelihood of movement abnormalities. For each patient, the physician tries to choose the drug that will cause the least annoyance and discomfort. If the side effects are too onerous, the patient will refuse to take the drug.

At one time, psychiatrists supposed that sedating phenothiazines would be the best treatment for patients who were excited or hyperactive, whereas the so-called activating phenothiazines would be best for those who withdrew socially, failed to talk, or moved very little or very slowly. However, there are no controlled observations to substantiate this conjecture. Current medical opinion is that both hyperactive and withdrawn patients are helped by both activating and sedating drugs.

If you fear that a relative is suffering unnecessarily from side effects of antipsychotic drugs, you should consult with the patient's psychiatrist and discuss the possible explanations. Are you sure the symptoms are really side effects? Could they be symptoms of the underlying disease? Has the patient been taking the drug long enough for some of the initial side effects to wear off? Most patients will be disagreeably sedated during the first 10 days or so on medication. This side effect is a necessary evil. Could the situation be improved by lowering the dose? This remedy may be feasible after the acute symptoms have abated. Would it help to change drugs? Each patient will tolerate some drugs better than others, but you cannot expect to find an antipsychotic with no bad side effects. Do not expect the psychiatrist to try the entire pharmacopea. You might reasonably expect her to try two or three drugs, each with a different spectrum of side effects. But when the patient begins taking a different drug, do not be impatient. The effects of the change in drugs may not be immediately apparent because it takes months for all traces of an antipsychotic to leave the body. Changing drugs rapidly would only lead to confusion; if the side effects were to improve, the psychiatrist would have no idea which drug caused the improvement. Finally, remember how sick the patient was without treatment. He may have to tolerate some unpleasant side effects to get the therapeutic benefit, the return to rationality.

If a patient has been taking antipsychotic medication, but his symptoms have not improved, is he likely to respond to a different drug? He might, but then again, he might not. One authority recommended that, if a patient does not respond to one drug in a few weeks, a second drug should be tried, but there is no point in changing drugs every few days.[18] Another authority recommended that, if a patient fails to respond to a second antipsychotic, drug therapy should be discontinued and the diagnosis reevaluated.[19] Unfortunately, about 10 percent of schizophrenia patients fail to respond to any antipsychotic medication.[20] These patients should not continue taking drugs that have, for them, only risks and no benefits.

Dose

The minimum effective dose is often called the threshold dose. If a patient receives less than the threshold dose, he does not benefit from the drug. Doses much higher than the threshold usually do not bring increased benefits. Furthermore, these higher doses may bring increased side effects at first and, perhaps, an increased risk of tardive dyskinesia later. The optimal dose is therefore only slightly more than the threshold dose.[21]

If a patient does not respond to doses that are usually effective, will larger doses, two, three, or ten times the normal amount, be effective? Researchers are not in complete agreement on the answer to this question, but the best summary of their results is, "maybe, but probably not." Occasionally, prescribing a very large dose for a *short* time might be an acceptable procedure for seriously ill patients, but there is no evidence that it is an effective one.[22] Fortunately, the patient will not die from an overdose—doses 10 times the ordinary dose are not lethal. In fact, no one has established the lethal dose of chlorpromazine. Because of the danger of tardive dyskinesia, trials with large doses must be conducted cautiously. The psychiatrist should plan to decrease the dose as soon as the symptoms are under control or to stop the medication entirely if the symptoms have not improved after two or three months.

Determining the correct drug dose for each patient is important but difficult. Drug doses are given by weight, usually specified in milligrams. (A milligram is one one-thousandth of a gram.) The dose will be higher if the patient is receiving a low-potency drug than if he is receiving a high-potency drug. Nevertheless, a higher dose of a low-potency drug may produce the most acceptable combination of therapeutic effects and side effects for some patients. When a patient receives a new antipsychotic drug, you cannot determine that the effective amount of medication has been increased or decreased simply by knowing that the number of milligrams has been increased or decreased. You must also know the relative potencies of the new and old drugs. This seemingly obvious point can be overlooked even by psychiatrists. Some of Sylvia Frumkin's unexplained improvements and relapses may have resulted from irrational changes in medication. She failed to improve on 1800 milligrams of chlorpromazine per day but improved rapidly when switched to 90 milligrams of haloperidol. Haloperidol is not a better drug than chlorpromazine, but 90 milligrams of haloperidol is the equivalent of 4500 milligrams of chlorpromazine. Although a psychiatrist would not intentionally triple a patient's medication, Sylvia Frumkin's physician did just that when he switched her from chlorpromazine to haloperidol.[23]

A proper dose depends on the particular patient as well as the drug because different people metabolize drugs at different rates. Even when two patients of the same sex and weight receive equal doses of chlorpromazine, the levels of the drug in their blood may be very different. Psychiatrists could compensate for these individual differences by adjusting each patient's dose after measuring the amount of chlorpromazine in the blood. But this procedure is expensive and not available everywhere. Therefore, because of these practicalities, blood concentrations of antipsychotic drugs are not commonly measured.

The slow onset of action of antipsychotic drugs impedes the determination of correct doses. Typically, the relief from schizophrenic symptoms may not occur for several weeks after beginning drug therapy. This delay does not mean, however, that the dose is too small. Because of the slow elimination of antipsychotics, a patient who stops taking these drugs may go several weeks without a relapse. This does not mean, however, that she does not need drug therapy. Active metabolic products of the drug may remain in her body for several months. Furthermore, the slow action makes it difficult to determine if any increase in dose has caused improvement or if any decrease has caused a relapse.

After an acute schizophrenic episode has been controlled, the maintenance dose should be as small as possible to minimize the chances of tardive dyskinesia. Unfortunately, the slow action of antipsychotic drugs frustrates attempts to find the optimal dose. Suppose that a patient is taking a drug that is clearly effective, and the psychiatrist decides to reduce the dose slightly to determine whether a lower dose will suffice. How long should the psychiatrist and patient wait for a return of symptoms before trying a second dose reduction? There are no absolute rules. The doctor and patient have to use their own judgment, always balancing the immediate side effects and the risk of tardive dyskinesia against the consequences of another episode of schizophrenia.

9

Diagnosing Affective Disorders

The term *affective disorders* is currently the preferred term for the group of illnesses that includes depression, mania, and manic depression.[1] To oversimplify a bit, these are illnesses in which the afflicted person suffers from extreme and inappropriate changes of mood. The inappropriate mood can be either an energetic, overactive, overconfident, wired high (mania) or a sad, guilt-ridden, discouraged, no-fun, no-energy low (depression). In some patients, mania is an irritable mood; the person is chronically angry, belligerent, and impatient. Other patients are loquacious and feel elated and self-important. But whether irritable or elated, mania is a mood in which the person is psychologically and behaviorally superactivated. Of course many other moods can be extreme or inappropriate. A mother may be so fearful of a bus accident that she refuses to let her child go on a school trip, or a man may physically attack his wife's lover. Although these extreme moods may be unreasonable or damaging, they are not necessarily evidence of an affective disorder. Only extreme depression and elation or irritability figure importantly in the affective disorders.

Affective disorders are usually clearly distinguishable from schizophrenia. In affective disorders, emotions, rather than thoughts, are abnormal. Of course, people who are in a depressed or manic mood can have strange thoughts, but these seem to be set in motion by the disturbance of mood, rather than vice versa. Affective disorders are less debilitating than schizophrenia. Many victims of an affective disorder enjoy extended periods of normality between episodes of mania or depression. During these times, the person is normally productive both socially and occupationally. During periods of mild mania, the person may be more than normally productive due to his high energy level, optimism, and self-confidence. But the mildly manic person sits on a shaky pedestal. He may recklessly quit his job to write the great American novel, squander the family savings on high stakes gambling in Las Vegas, or destroy his good marriage to pursue a new love affair.

Affective disorders are common. They occur in many different societies and are even described in the writings of the ancient Greeks.[2] In the United States and Western Europe, it is estimated that 18 to 23 percent of women and 8 to 11 percent of men suffer from at least one clinically significant episode of an affective disorder, usually depression, at some point during their lives.[3] Few will escape contact with this form of mental illness. Therefore, you should learn to recognize its early signs so that you will know when to seek treatment for yourself or a family member. Too often, affective disorders invade a victim's life insidiously—the victim or the victim's family is not fully aware that a mental health problem has been gradually developing.

In the *Diagnostic and Statistical Manual of Mental Disorders* (called the *DSM-III*, see Chapter 3), severe affective disorders are divided into two categories called bipolar disorder and major depression. Bipolar disorder is an illness that includes at least one manic episode as well as one or more episodes of depression. Major depression is a similar illness but without any manic episodes.

Diagnostic Criteria for a Manic Episode

A manic episode is defined in the *DSM-III* by the following five criteria, labeled A through E. All five criteria must be met before a person can be diagnosed as having such an episode.

Criterion A

One or more distinct periods with a predominantly elevated, expansive, or irritable mood. The elevated or irritable mood must be a prominent part of the illness and relatively persistent, although it may alternate or intermingle with depressive mood.[4]

This criterion establishes two requirements for the diagnosis of a manic episode. The first is that mania is recognizably unusual; the afflicted person's mood is clearly different from her normal moods. The second fact is that the mood change occurs in distinct periods; the mood comes and goes in "episodes." Between the manic episodes, there are usually periods of normality or periods of depression. In some cases, the victim's personality may appear dominated by wide swings of mood from mania to depression. Usually, a patient remains in each phase for weeks or months, but, occasionally, a patient will alternate much more rapidly between mania and depression. Cases have been reported in which the person's mood swings daily from one extreme to the other. Still other patients may experience depressive symptoms mixed with the mania. The switching between two abnormal moods that superficially seem to be polar opposites is the origin of the *DSM-III* term *bipolar disorder*. It is also the origin of the older term *manic depression*, the term that Emil Kraepelin applied to the illness when he first described it in the medical literature near the end of the nineteenth century. Another descriptive name for bipolar disorder is *moodswing*, as it has been called by Dr. Ronald R. Fieve in his popular book of the same name.[5] The *DSM-III* definition of bipolar disorder differs from earlier definitions of manic depression, however, in that a manic episode alone is sufficient to make the diagnosis. The earlier definitions required both episodes of mania and depression. The authors of the *DSM-III* omitted reference to depression in the criteria for bipolar disorder because they believed that all or almost all patients who suffer a manic episode will also suffer from depression at some time. Thus, the occurrence of mania, but not depression, diagnostically distinguishes between major depression and bipolar disorder.

When irritability predominates, the person may make frequent hostile remarks, become enraged at the most minor frustrations, or launch into unprovoked angry tirades. For example, a woman may stamp her foot and angrily announce, "I'm just furious," when she sees that her visiting mother, who is trying to be helpful, has used a piece of steel wool to scour a pan. The angry daughter claims, "It's perfectly obvious that steel wool will shed filthy rust particles all over the kitchen." With that declaration, she marches to her bedroom and slams the door so hard the wood trim is knocked loose from the door frame. Irritability is also expressed as low tolerance to frustration and impatience. Thus, a woman may come home from work expecting to begin making dinner immediately, but she finds that the kids have left a pot with burned refried beans stuck to the bottom in the sink. She flies into an angry tirade, demanding that the negligent children be punished. She then announces her categorical refusal to have anything more to do with cooking—ever.

When expansiveness predominates, the person is grandiose, overconfident, gregarious, loquacious, and probably a bit too loud. For instance, a man may announce that he has just talked the bank loan officer into lending him $200,000 to start a new company to manufacture his invention, a microcircuit for home computers. He also gives a friend a golden opportunity to become one of the original stockholders. He claims, "There's no way you can make less than a million!" This garrulous man may even succeed in persuading his friend to invest in the business.

Dr. Ronald Fieve recounted an expansive manic episode of psychotic proportions experienced by one of his patients, William Smythe. Mr. Smythe was a highly successful businessman. One day, feeling absolutely on top of the world, Mr. Smythe hired a young man in a white uniform driving a white horse and carriage to parade him down Fifth Avenue. Along the way, Mr. Smythe picked up a young couple just engaged to be married. When they politely refused his offer to take them out to dinner, he went to his bank and obtained $50,000 in silver dollars and in twenty, fifty, and one hundred dollar bills. As the three rode down the avenue, they threw money to the people on the street, creating quite a commotion. Everyone, from hippies to well-dressed matrons, ran from every direction to grab as much as they could. The adventure finally ended at a fancy restaurant where Mr. Smythe gave his new friend $500 to buy a tie and jacket to satisfy the restaurant's dress code. He gave another young man $1000 to buy a new guitar. The meal ended with a circle of reporters around Mr. Smythe's table and all the money gone. He had to pay the restaurant bill with a check.[6]

Criterion B

Duration of at least one week (or any duration if hospitalization is necessary), during which, for most of the time, at least three of the following symptoms have persisted (four if the mood is only irritable) and have been present to a significant degree:

1. increase in activity (either socially, at work, or sexually) or physical restlessness

2. more talkative than usual or pressure to keep talking

3. flight of ideas or subjective experience that thoughts are racing

4. inflated self-esteem (grandiosity, which may be delusional)

5. decreased need for sleep

6. distractibility, i.e., attention is too easily drawn to unimportant or irrelevant external stimuli

7. excessive involvement in activities that have a high potential for painful consequences which is not recognized, e.g., buying sprees, sexual indiscretions, foolish business investments, reckless driving.[7]

This criterion helps distinguish the manic mood from other emotional states. The increased activity (symptom 1) may show up in numerous ways. The patient may take on more work than she can handle. She may make grandiose plans and begin multiple projects that she cannot possibly complete. She may be restless and constantly in motion—wiggling, walking, moving in quick-step. The increase in activity is often expressed sexually. For example, a man may exhibit a change in his typical sexual behavior, demanding that his wife have intercourse with him several times a day; a woman may have an affair when it is not her usual style to be promiscuous.

It is easy to spot overactivity in speech (symptom 2). In the manic mood, the patient talks too much, too loud, and too fast. His verbal output can be so rapid, intense, and insistent that others never get a chance to speak. Nonstop, noninterruptible talking is such a striking and frequent symptom of mania that it has been given its own name, pressure of speech. When the symptom is severe, the person may talk so fast that he cannot be understood.

Thinking, like speaking, is speeded up during a manic episode. The patient's ideas seem to come in swarms. She cannot complete one line of thought before it is replaced by another. This symptom is called flight of ideas (symptom 3). When the ideas fly too fast, they become disorganized and worthless, but when the symptom is only mild, the quick flow of ideas may be productive. Dr. Fieve described the work habits of a number of artists whom he believed experienced intermittent mildly manic episodes. Among these artists are Honoré de Balzac, Vincent Van Gogh, and Ernest Hemingway. These men experienced periods of frenetic productivity when their ideas seemed to come with unusual ease and rapidity. Robert Schumann, the great romantic composer and psychiatric invalid, experienced periods when his musical ideas came profusely and without effort. At other times, however, he could compose nothing.[8]

Almost invariably, a person in a manic mood is overconfident and has an exaggerated opinion of her importance and power (symptom 4). A woman may think she is ravishingly beautiful and sexually irresistible. She may try to use her sexual powers to influence her boss, minister, or psychiatrist. A man may believe he can succeed in any undertaking, whether it be in business, in politics, at the dice table, or with women. Grandiosity can take on delusional intensity. A patient may believe that she has been anointed by God to accomplish His mission on earth by giving her body sexually to all who need it. This mission may have been revealed to her by hallucinatory voices. Another patient may believe that he has discovered a new form of energy that can be harnessed to accelerate spaceships to velocities exceeding that of light. He thinks that his discovery has not been accepted at NASA only because the agency has a vested interest in the entrenched military–industrial complex.

When a psychiatrist sees a patient with delusions and hallucinations, the physician's first inclination may be to diagnose schizophrenia. Indeed, manic delusions and schizophrenic delusions are sometimes similar. In mania, however, the delusions are thought to be caused by an abnormal mood and are present only during episodes of manic excitement. In schizophrenia, the delusions can exist when the patient is calm and even when, under the influence of drug treatment, the patient pays no attention to them because he realizes they are just delusions or meaningless hallucinations. The manic patient is always responsive to external stimuli and can be distracted from his own train of thought. By contrast, the patient with schizophrenia can become totally preoccupied with his inner fantasies. He can become withdrawn from the outside world; sights and sounds do not distract him. Nonetheless, the similarity between schizophrenic and manic delusions probably has led to the overdiagnosis of schizophrenia, especially during the period when American psychiatrists were influenced by the dictum, "even a trace of schizophrenia is schizophrenia" (see Chapter 4).

When manic self-confidence and grandiosity are not too severe, they can be infectious, even inspiring. Some people believe that certain influential political figures suffered from mania. Manic episodes may have been responsible for Hitler's ability to mesmerize a crowd. He had an exalted view of himself, believing that he was the greatest German in history. Often he was irritable. An angry tirade, complete with pressure of speech, against the alleged enemies of the Reich was often used as a technique of persuasion. Hitler's grandiosity invaded other spheres. He believed, completely erroneously, that he had great talent as a painter. Hitler also suffered periods of depression. He ended his life in a joint suicide with his mistress, Eva Braun.[9] Dr. Ronald Fieve argued that Abraham Lincoln, Theodore Roosevelt, and Winston Churchill all experienced mania to some extent.[10] High-powered businesspeople, too, often show symptoms of mania in their energetic entrepreneurial wheeling and dealing.

A person experiencing a manic episode may have a decreased need for sleep (symptom 5). He may toss and turn in bed, becoming furious with frustration because he is unable to sleep. He may work or play indefatigably for days, scarcely sleeping at all. Balzac, Van Gogh, and Hemingway all worked furiously for weeks without seeming to get tired. During one excited period lasting 42 days, Hemingway slept only two-and-a-half hours a night.[11]

Distractibility (symptom 6) is another sign of mania. The rushing stream of thought is easily diverted. The seriously manic patient cannot keep his attention on a single subject for an effective length of time. Minor stimuli in the environment, even the sound of his own words, may distract him. He forgets what he is trying to say and does not complete one statement before going on to the next. A patient might be ranting about what should be done to punish the school board for hiring a fourth assistant superintendent, but when he hears the sound of a barking dog, he changes the subject to the scandal in the county over the animal control program. Before this indictment is complete, however, the sound of his own voice saying "dog" may make him begin lecturing about the problem of "log" exports to Japan that is causing the loss of sawmill jobs in his home state of Oregon. While the patient believes that he is brilliant and in control of his life, his distractibility significantly impairs his ability to manage his business and social affairs.

During a manic episode, the patient may seem to be totally oblivious to the possibility that any of his endeavors have negative consequences (symptom 7). Careless gambling sprees, irresponsible sexual affairs, and squandering of money are common symptoms of mania. Hitler, for instance, often seemed incapable of grasping the possibility of military failure. And Mr. Smythe, who enthusiastically and confidently squandered over $50,000 in a few hours by throwing money to people on the street and thrusting expensive gifts on strangers, seemed totally insensitive to his own recklessness.

Criterion C

Neither of the following dominate the clinical picture when an affective syndrome (i.e., criteria A and B above) is not present, that is, before it developed or after it has remitted:

1. preoccupation with a mood-incongruent [inconsistent with the prevailing mood] delusion or hallucination . . .
2. bizarre behavior[12]

The purpose of this criterion is to help distinguish between a manic episode and schizophrenia. In schizophrenia, the patient may be preoccupied with delusional thoughts and hallucinations even when he is not in an agitated or excited mood. Bizarre behaviors such as catatonic stupor, grimacing in the mirror, refusing to use the toilet, and dressing aberrantly can also occur when a patient is in a comparatively calm emotional state. This pattern of behavior does not occur in mania. Although the person may act strangely or experience delusions and hallucinations in the heat of manic excitement, these symptoms disappear when the superexcited state passes.

Criterion D

Not superimposed on either Schizophrenia, Schizophreniform Disorder or a Paranoid Disorder.[13]

According to the *DSM-III*, a patient cannot be diagnosed as having both schizophrenia and manic episodes. Some psychiatrists think this restriction is a mistake, but until stronger evidence is accumulated for the possible coexistence of the two disorders, they will be officially regarded as mutually exclusive. Although Criteria C and D may seem to be the same, they make an important distinction. Criterion C aims to prevent the error of calling schizophrenia mania, and Criterion D says that one person cannot have both mania and schizophrenia at the same time.

Criterion E

Not due to any Organic Mental Disorder, such as Substance Intoxication.[14]

We already mentioned in Chapter 4 the problem of misdiagnosing abnormal behavior as a mental disorder when it is actually a symptom of an illness with known cause and treatment. It is especially important to rule out the possibility that the behavior of an excited patient is a response to a drug. Amphetamine, cocaine, hallucinogens, and steroid hormones such as estrogen can cause symptoms similar to mania.

Diagnostic Criteria for a Major Depressive Episode

A certain amount of sadness is a normal part of the human condition and does not indicate a need for psychiatric treatment. Sorrow, disappointment, and discouragement are natural and healthy responses to an important loss or failure, such as a death in the family or a divorce. People recover, as nature takes its course, usually without psychiatric treatment.

The illness of depression resembles normal sadness, but it is enhanced in both duration and intensity, and it may occur in the absence of any severe loss or failure. In its milder forms, the illness can wear the guise of normality. When people are sad, they may believe their mood is a response to failure to be promoted at the office, stock market losses, absence of a daughter who has gone away to college, or some other loss. But these ready justifications may really be rationalizations. In truth, the depression may be a condition of the brain that is imposing itself upon the problems of living. Depressive illness often becomes severely distressing and debilitating before the patient or his family recognize the need for treatment.

The members of the *DSM-III* task force, after much discussion and some field testing, finally agreed on five criteria for detecting a major depressive episode. The illness is called "major" depressive episode rather than just depressive episode to distinguish it from normal depressive emotions and from certain milder depressive conditions that are also defined in the *DSM-III*.

Criterion A

Dysphoric mood or loss of interest or pleasure in all or almost all usual activities and pastimes. The dysphoric mood is characterized by symptoms such as the following: depressed, sad, blue, hopeless, low, down in the dumps, irritable. The mood disturbance must be prominent and relatively persistent, but not necessarily the most dominant symptom, and does not include momentary shifts from one dysphoric mood to another dysphoric mood, e.g., anxiety to depression to anger, such as are seen in states of acute psychotic turmoil. (For children under six, dysphoric mood may have to be inferred from a persistently sad facial expression.)[15]

The word *dysphoric* is of Greek origin and means "unpleasant" or "unwell," the opposite of *euphoric*. This criterion, then, states that depression is unpleasant and deenergizing. It prevents the afflicted person from enjoying herself as she normally does. The patient is aware of her bad mood, and she reports on her emotional state by saying she feels sad, blue, depressed, and so on. Although the bad mood always occurs to some extent, it need not be the dominant symptom of depression. In some cases, the depressed person's inability to concentrate, make decisions, or sleep may concern her more than her bad mood.

Criterion B

At least four of the following symptoms have each been present nearly every day for a period of at least two weeks (in children under six, at least three of the first four).

1. poor appetite or significant weight loss (when not dieting) or increased appetite or significant weight gain (in children under six, consider failure to make expected weight gains)

2. insomnia or hypersomnia

3. psychomotor agitation or retardation (but not merely subjective feelings of restlessness or being slowed down) (in children under six, hypoactivity)

4. loss of interest or pleasure in usual activities, or decrease in sexual drive not limited to a period when delusional or hallucinating (in children under six, signs of apathy)

5. loss of energy; fatigue

6. feelings of worthlessness, self-reproach, or excessive or inappropriate guilt (either may be delusional)

7. complaints or evidence of diminished ability to think or concentrate, such as slowed thinking, or indecisiveness not associated with marked loosening of associations or incoherence

8. recurrent thoughts of death, suicidal ideation, wishes to be dead or suicide attempt[16]

Changes in appetite and sleep pattern (symptoms 1 and 2) are often called biological or vegetative symptoms of depression. Of course, all the symptoms are biological because they originate in the brain. But these first two seem to lack psychological components. It is important to note that the symptoms are specified as changes in the usual eating or sleeping pattern. A person who has always eaten like a bird does not have a depressive symptom just because he customarily does not eat much. Although depression usually causes appetite to diminish, resulting in weight loss, it can cause weight gain. Either too much or too little sleep qualifies as a symptom. A depressed person who sleeps too little usually wakes up too early in the morning, but failure to fall asleep at night or wakening in the middle of the night also qualify. Sometimes the patient may sleep more than usual and may even stay in bed almost around the clock.

Psychomotor agitation or retardation (symptom 3) refers to changes in the speed and reactivity of the person's mental processes and overt behavior. The word *psychomotor* can be divided into two parts, *psycho*, meaning "mind" or "mental", and *motor*, meaning "movement" or "behavior." *Agitation* means "a speeding up" and *retardation* means "a slowing down."

In psychomotor agitation, the depressed person is visibly nervous and overactive in his speech, behavior, and emotional responses. He may complain and worry much too much or generally display attitudes of anxious, antagonistic, pessimistic, or self-deprecating overactivity. He may pace the floor, wring his hands, or twiddle his hair while wailing desperately about unhappy themes. A woman we know with agitated depression scratched her head continuously while worrying about spending too much money; she actually wore all the hair off her scalp in two spots, each one about an inch in diameter.

Thinking, speech, and movement are slower than normal in psychomotor retardation. Behavior associated with retardation is the opposite of verbosity and energy. People may become impatient trying to converse with a person who has retardation because he speaks with the speed of the proverbial "molasses in January." Listeners do not want to interrupt, but sometimes they get so tired of waiting that they just break in. Most of the patient's words are monosyllables, and in severe cases, he may be completely mute. Perhaps the retarded speech of depression is the antithesis of manic pressure of speech.

Bob exemplifies a person who suffered from recurrent depression with retardation. He and his wife, Jane, both worked for a hospital, he as an accountant, she as a nurse. Jane could always tell when Bob was entering another active phase of his illness because he became uncommunicative. For example, when she tried to discuss plans about how they each would get to work the next day (they had only one car, worked different shifts, and had to go grocery shopping), Bob seemed unable to talk. He tried to speak up and would say "Well...," but then no ideas came to him. He seemed confused and disconnected. His mind was stuck while Jane waited for a response. Sometimes Jane just gave up on joint planning and made arrangements herself.

Activities other than speech are affected, too. The patient performs less work and participates in fewer activities; in fact, his whole body moves more slowly. Retardation can become so severe that the depressed person does not want to move at all. Sometimes Bob developed this symptom. When he and Jane both worked the day shift, they often rode their bicycles to work. Ordinarily, Bob was a strong bike rider and often pressured Jane to ride a little faster than she really wanted to. But when Bob got depressed, he rode so slowly that Jane became impatient. When they came to a hill, the depressed Bob got off his bike and walked with it. On several occasions, he stopped moving entirely and just sat down, remaining motionless, staring at the street for several minutes.

Psychiatrists use the Greek word *anhedonia* as a name for symptom 4, loss of interest or pleasure in usual activities. *Anhedonia* means "an inability to experience pleasure." For example, a woman who normally works hard and enjoys her job may lose interest in it and may even have difficulty going to work. A man who usually loves to take a female companion to a fancy restaurant and the theater afterward may find himself "too tired for it now" or claim, "I don't like it as much as I used to." A man who has always loved to ski and who customarily spends more than his recreation budget allows on ski trips may decide that it is "too expensive." A woman who is normally sociable and enjoys conversation may become withdrawn and uncommunicative with her friends and relatives.

A reduction in the desire for and joy of sex is especially common in a major depressive episode. Bob experienced this symptom. He and Jane were often quite exuberant sexually. But when Bob got depressed, he became sexually passive. Sometimes he even felt resentful at the prospect of having intercourse. He would become a bit hostile toward Jane near bedtime when he sensed that she was feeling sexy. During one of his sexually apathetic periods, he actually found himself thinking how much he would like it if sex just did not exist. He felt he would then be free of the conflict his lack of enthusiasm always created.

Symptom 5, loss of energy and fatigue, fits into the concept of depression as a deactivation or slowing down of mental and behavioral processes. Loss of energy does not quite mean what retardation means, although the two may have a common cause originating in the brain. A person with agitated depression, without retardation, is nonetheless capable of feeling "just exhausted" and may proclaim, in an agitated way, her imperative need for sleep. Loss of energy can also be combined with retardation, of course. Bob, whose retardation often interfered with his bicycle riding, sometimes spent the better part of entire weekends in bed. He did not have the energy to wash the car and mow the lawn. Jane would eventually do these chores for him. It took all the discipline Bob could muster just to get to work on weekdays.

Bob also exhibited feelings of worthlessness, self-reproach, and guilt (symptom 6). Bob's colleagues regarded him as competent. But when he was depressed, he became obsessed with the idea that he was not doing a good job anymore and that his colleagues had no respect for him. Sometimes, when he thought no one would hear, he exclaimed aloud, with hateful self-reproach, "You're stupid!" Inevitably, Jane overheard him berating himself and tried to stop him. She wondered if he was angry at her or if there was something she could do to help him relax. But her concern was of no avail, for it only caused Bob to be overcome with guilt about damaging their marriage and diminishing Jane's happiness by being such an albatross around her neck.

In a small minority of depressed patients (about 10 percent), the feelings of worthlessness, self-reproach, and guilt can become so intense that they activate delusions or even hallucinations. A hallucinating depressed person may hear a voice that berates him and calls him names because of his past errors and shortcomings. In depression, however, the voice usually does not speak as prolifically as it does in schizophrenia.

Depressive delusions differ in several ways from schizophrenic delusions. The delusions of depression typically concern poverty, medical illness, or punishment for imaginary sins. They seldom have the bizarre, magical quality that is almost the trademark of schizophrenic delusions. Depressive delusions are not systematized as schizophrenic delusions are. A patient with systematized delusions believes that all his experiences are caused by a single delusional entity; for example, the content of television programs, the pronouncements of the Pope, the flight patterns of insects, the machinations of international politics, and the patient's own mind are all controlled by one pervasive force. In nonsystematized delusions, unreal beliefs do not necessarily have the same cause. A depressed woman may erroneously believe that she is suffering abject poverty and has also contracted cancer.

Diminished ability to think or concentrate (symptom 7) is one of the most common complaints of people with depression, especially if their occupation calls for much listening, reading, writing, or complex decision making. A depressed college professor, despite heroic efforts to exercise will power, may find it impossible to keep his attention fixed on the doctoral thesis he is supposed to be evaluating. A competent lawyer, when depressed, may find herself unable to listen attentively to her clients and unable to assimilate the details of a case. A depressed author may stare at the typewriter for weeks without typing a word. Bob, who was an accountant, worked more slowly and made more computational mistakes when he was depressed.

Thoughts of death and suicide and suicide attempts (symptom 8) is perhaps the symptom that impresses us most with the clinical significance of depression. Approximately 15 percent of the people who suffer from depressive episodes die by suicide, and suicide is the second most frequent cause of death in people between the ages of fifteen and twenty-four. (The most frequent cause is automobile accidents.) Suicide, however, is not always a symptom of depression. On the contrary, suicidal thinking and behavior also frequently occur in schizophrenia. Suicide may even occur in the absence of mental illness. Sometimes soldiers in battle commit suicide as an act of heroism.

An overt suicide attempt is a severe symptom. Having morbid thoughts of one's own death also qualifies as a depressive symptom. Bob frequently had suicidal thoughts when he was depressed. While driving home from the hospital, he would suddenly imagine that he was going to get killed by steering his little car into a bridge abutment or under the rolling wheels of a log truck. When sitting at home or at work, he would brood gloomily on the fact that he still had to live through another thirty years, a prospect that seemed to be a grinding ordeal. "Another thirty years of this?" he would think. "How will I make it to the end? Why can't the race be shorter?" He would ask himself these questions as he ruminated about his imagined professional failures, his sexual inadequacy, and the burden he placed on Jane.

Criterion C

Neither of the following dominate the clinical picture when an affective syndrome (i.e., criteria A and B above) is not present, that is, before it developed or after it has remitted:

1. preoccupation with a mood-incongruent delusion or hallucination. . .
2. bizarre behavior[17]

This criterion is a repeat of Criterion C for manic episode. Its purpose is also the same—to distinguish depression from schizophrenia. The source of confusion is the occurrence of delusions, hallucinations, and bizarre behavior in both schizophrenia and a minority of cases of depression. In depression, delusions and hallucinations occur only while the person is depressed. After the acute episode of mood disturbance has passed or before it starts, the patient is not troubled with hallucinated voices and untrue beliefs. As we mentioned, schizophrenic delusions often develop gradually during the prodromal phase of the illness and persist during the residual phase. During these times, the schizophrenia patient may be aware of the delusions and voices and may know that they are symptoms of illness. In fact, he may undertake active measures to play them down or ignore them. Nonetheless, they are present, and he knows they are. Bizarre behaviors, such as failure to talk or move, also do not occur in depression except during the acute episode of altered mood.

Criterion D

Not superimposed on either Schizophrenia, Schizophreniform Disorder, or a Paranoid Disorder.[18]

This criterion is a repeat of Criterion D for a manic episode. It specifies that the psychiatrist is not allowed to diagnose a major depressive episode and a schizophrenic disorder in the same patient at the same time. Again, some authoritative psychiatrists think this prohibition is unjustified by the facts. We will be watching for revisions of this criterion in future editions of the *DSM-III*.

Criterion E

Not due to any Organic Mental Disorder or Uncomplicated Bereavement.[19]

As usual, the psychiatrist must rule out the possibility that the depressed mood is a result of some illness other than depression or that it is a reaction to the death of a close friend or family member. There is always some degree of depression accompanying the pain and suffering of a nonpsychiatric illness. This type of depression is described as *secondary* to the illness, and it is excluded by Criterion E. According to the *DSM-III*, the depression that is secondary to the flu, for example, is a different condition than the primary mental illness of depression.

Certain drugs given for high blood pressure often produce psychological depression. Alcohol is another surreptitious culprit. A person who is abusing alcohol may be seriously depressed due to his overuse of the drug as well as his knowledge that he has a destructive and debilitating addiction. Sometimes cause and effect are reversed. A person who suffers from depression may be using alcohol as a self-administered drug treatment for the mental illness.

Criteria for Depression with Melancholia

The *DSM-III* describes one special subtype of depression called depression with melancholia. This Elizabethan-sounding phrase designates a particular form of depression that must meet an additional set of diagnostic criteria. We describe depression with melancholia here because some psychiatrists believe that it should be treated differently from major depression that does not satisfy the criteria for melancholia.

Depression with melancholia requires that the patient feel "loss of pleasure in all or almost all activities, lack of reactivity to usually pleasurable stimuli (doesn't feel much better, even temporarily, when something good happens), and at least three of the following:

a. distinct quality of depressed mood, i.e., the depressed mood is perceived as distinctly different from the kind of feeling experienced following the death of a loved one

b. the depression is regularly worse in the morning

c. early morning awakening (at least two hours before usual time of awakening)

d. marked psychomotor retardation or agitation

e. significant anorexia or weight loss

f. excessive or inappropriate guilt[20]

These symptoms defining melancholia overlap with the symptoms of major depressive episode defined in Criterion B. To have melancholia, the patient must be particularly apathetic and incapable of feeling pleasure. This symptom is similar to the fourth symptom of depression listed in Criterion B, except that with melancholia, the anhedonia must be severe. In addition to anhedonia, the patient must have three of the six symptoms that define melancholia.

Some symptoms from Criterion B for major depressive episode are not included in the six symptoms of melancholia. For example, the inability to concentrate and recurrent thoughts of death contribute to a diagnosis of major depressive episode but not to the additional diagnosis of melancholia. Of course, a patient who has depression with melancholia may suffer from an inability to concentrate in addition to his melancholic symptoms.

Some other symptoms are more narrowly defined for diagnosing melancholia than for diagnosing the broader affective disorder, major depression. For example, several kinds of sleep disturbance are symptoms of depression, but only awakening at least two hours earlier than usual is symptomatic of melancholia. Either weight gain or weight loss is a symptom of major depression, but only weight loss is a symptom of melancholia.

The first two symptoms on the list for melancholia—distinct quality of depressed mood and feeling more depressed in the morning—are not included in Criterion B for major depressive episode. Perhaps some amplification of these would be helpful.

The patient may describe the distinct mood as a pervasive sense of despair and hopelessness. She may assume that her feelings are justified by external events and so can give reasons for her unhappiness. But these reasons are probably unconvincing, as arbitrary as using the little fork for salad. If asked, she says that her mood is quite different from how she would feel if she lost her job or if a close relative died. Indeed, melancholia seems to have a life of its own. Its intensity and longevity appear to be out of proportion to any loss, failure, or disappointment. The patient's desperation stems, perhaps, from her certain conviction that she is suffering from a permanent and incurable condition. Love, money, achievement, and amusement cannot help. If asked what might make her well, her response may be, "not having to be me": Melancholia is as much a part of her as the color of her eyes. No tears and no language can express the depths of her despair.

But I have that within which passeth show—
These are but the trappings and the suits of woe.

Hamlet, Act I, Scene ii, line 85)

A patient with symptom b usually feels most depressed early in the morning. Even though he may have been awake for hours before he gets out of bed, he does not feel alert. Some patients are extremely confused in the morning. John, a graduate student who had depression with melancholia, regularly studied at home in the evening. Almost as regularly, he left for school in the morning without the books and papers he had brought home the previous evening. Each day when the phone rang at 10:00 A.M., his frustrated and annoyed wife knew it was John asking her to bring him the materials he had forgotten.

Other patients are agitated and fearful in the morning. Jennifer, a dressmaker, feared that a cutting error would ruin a customer's expensive fabric. Just anticipating the day's work made her nauseated; about once a week she actually vomited before going to work. Still other patients have such retardation that they cannot get out of bed; some are chronically late to work. Many patients with severe morning symptoms function somewhat better in the afternoon and evening, but there is no time of day when their melancholic mood is completely absent.

10

Depression

Many symptoms of schizophrenia, like the devils that danced in Sylvia Frumkin's pillowcase[1], are so bizarre that one easily sees that the patient is ill. When a person has depression, however, the existence of an illness is less obvious. Usually, a depressed person's thoughts are neither bizarre nor patently incorrect. The reasons he gives for feeling depressed make sense in comparison to the reasons a schizophrenia patient gives to explain her strange behaviors. When a person suffers from depression, both the afflicted person and his family are often unsure whether problems of living are causing the feelings of depression or whether the feelings of depression are causing the problems of living. If problems of living are primary, perhaps the depression will clear up when the problems are solved. In this case, psychotherapy, rather than pharmacotherapy, would be the appropriate first line of treatment. In depression, unlike schizophrenia, psychotherapy is usually possible. Most depressed people use language normally and can communicate with a therapist. On the other hand, if the patient had no major problems of living before he became depressed, it might be surmised that he has a biochemical problem that did not originate from environmental stress. Psychotherapy alone may not be a sufficient treatment for this patient.

When we first encounter a friend or relative who has become depressed, we may try to help. It seems so obvious that he is not as worthless as he thinks, that his life is not an unrelenting shower of failures. A logical examination of his situation should persuade him that his life is actually quite successful and enjoyable. We may try to improve his mood by providing some pleasurable experiences. Then we expect him to "snap out of it." When our efforts to help do not work, we feel dismayed. As our friend continues spending his days in tears, berating himself for nonexistent sins, and refusing pleasure because he believes that he does not deserve it, we begin to realize that he has something more than the sadness that all people experience from time to time. A suicide attempt may convince us that he has a serious illness. Our friend's depressed mood is not as easy to cure as we first expected it to be. Common-sense treatments do not help because his extreme and inappropriate emotions are caused by illness.

Depression is a serious mental health problem both because it is prevalent and because it can have serious consequences. The most obvious consequences of depression are deterioration of work performance, marital unhappiness, and personal misery. Fortunately, both pharmacological and psychotherapeutic treatment of depression have improved greatly over the last thirty to forty years. In 1940, only about 40 percent of hospitalized patients recovered within one year. This statistic shows that available treatments were virtually ineffective because about 40 percent of all depressed patients recover without treatment. Now, however, the rate of recovery within one year approaches 85 percent. This does not mean that 85 percent of depressed people are permanently cured. About half of them will suffer at least one relapse. Nevertheless, modern treatment has made it possible for people who have recovered to spend months or years without episodes of depression.[2]

Prevalence of Depression

Depression is so prevalent that it has been called the common cold of mental illness. Its exact prevalence is not known because reliable measurements require consistent diagnostic criteria. Until the publication of the *DSM-III*, different researchers used widely different criteria to diagnose depression. The *DSM-III* has provided generally accepted diagnostic criteria, but no studies on the prevalence of depression based on the *DSM-III* criteria are yet available. The best estimates indicate that between 10 and 20 percent of the U.S. population experiences at least one episode of a major affective disorder. About one in five victims receives treatment and about one in fifty is hospitalized.[3] The probability that you or someone close to you will suffer from depression is high.

Depression is not related to socioeconomic class. Low status in society does not cause the illness and high status does not prevent it. These facts have been determined by survey research in which persons representing all social strata were asked if they had ever had symptoms of depression at any point during their lives. The wealthy, however, may suffer less when they do become depressed because they can afford treatment. Perhaps for this reason, a survey in which a person is asked about depressive symptoms he is currently suffering will reveal that people in the lower social classes have more symptoms. Members of racial minorities suffer no more depression than members of the white majority. In fact, depression is slightly more prevalent among whites than among nonwhites.[4]

Depression can occur at any age. It is uncommon in children but strikes with equal probability at all times during adult life.[5] Sex is one demographic feature that can be used to predict who will become depressed. Depressed females outnumber depressed males by about two to one.[6] This sex difference cannot be explained by the fact that women visit doctors more often and so are more likely to be diagnosed as having the illness. Myrna Weissman and Jerome K. Myers of the National Institute of Mental Health attempted to find the prevalence of depression in each sex by administering a structured psychiatric interview to about one thousand people randomly selected in New Haven, Connecticut. They found that about 26 percent of the females but only 12 percent of the males had suffered from a major depression.[7]

In our opinion, feminists need not search to find excuses for this sex difference. Such a search implies that depression is shameful; it implies that admitting a greater incidence of depression among women is tantamount to admitting inferiority. Yet no one treats the greater incidence of heart disease in men as evidence of inferiority. We do not know whether the traditional role of women in society contributes to the greater prevalence of depression among women. We do not think, however, that this prevalence can be fully explained by an oppression theory because many of the disadvantages often experienced by women—for example, unemployment and low family income—do not predict depression and because depression is not prevalent among other disadvantaged groups.[8]

Like schizophrenia, depression is thought to occur in all cultures.[9] Its prevalence is similar in Western Europe, South Korea, Japan, and Indonesia. Like the specific symptoms of schizophrenia, the specific symptoms of depression are culturally determined. The Indonesians rarely commit suicide, but the Dutch and Japanese living in Indonesia have about the same suicide rate in Indonesia as in their homeland. In the West, the depressed patient is likely to talk about guilt and self-reproach: "If only I hadn't yelled at him, he wouldn't have left." "If only I had studied harder in school, I would be able to properly provide for my family." The Western patient may be reticent about mentioning that he lost 10 pounds last month or that he wakes up between 4:00 and 5:00 A.M. even though he does not have to be at work until 8:00 A.M. In non-Western countries, patients are more likely to describe physical symptoms such as sleep disturbance, loss of appetite, dry mouth, and headaches. They rarely express feelings of guilt.

If the constellation of symptoms is different in Indonesia and in the United States, how do scientists and physicians know that the depression of the Indonesians is the same disease as the depression of the North Americans? The answer is that they do not know, at least not with great certainty. Psychiatrists who have examined patients in several cultures have expressed their clinical judgment that depression among Africans is the same disease as depression among New Yorkers. No one will know whether this opinion is correct until patients in many cultures have been diagnosed using the rigorously validated criteria or until laboratory tests that are specific for depression are perfected. Perhaps the dexamethasone suppression test (Chapter 3) will be helpful for this purpose.

Occasionally, depression is a fatal illness. The overall mortality rate in depressed patients is substantially higher than in the general population. Accidents and suicides account for most of these additional deaths.[10] Depression dramatically increases the risk of suicide. Accurate figures are difficult to find, but the best estimates indicate that 7–15 percent of people suffering from depression commit suicide.[11] In the total population, only 1.0–1.4 percent dies by suicide.[12] About half of all suicides in the entire population occur in people suffering from depression.[13] Therefore, only 0.5–0.7 percent of the nondepressed population commits suicide. Thus, depression increases the risk of suicide about twenty-fold.

Causes

The hypothesis that stress and misfortune cause depression is intuitively reasonable, but the demographic data do not support it. As we just discussed, depression is not related to socioeconomic status or to race. Because depression probably occurs in all cultures, it probably does not result from the stress of living in an industrialized society.

Studies of stress in the lives of depressed patients suggest that, while stressful events may precipitate depression, many depressions are unrelated to life's problems and disappointments. Depression is, however, associated with environmental stress much more often than is schizophrenia. Children who have experienced the death of a loved one are about two to three times more likely to suffer from depression in adulthood than are children who did not experience bereavement. But only about 30 percent of depressed adults suffered bereavement as children.[14] If the remainder of the depressed adults suffered a different form of childhood deprivation, it has not been identified.

Depressed people report more recent stress in their lives than normal people do.[15] About 25 percent of depressed people say that they recently experienced one or more severe stresses such as death in the family, divorce, birth of child, or change of job. Only about 5 percent of nondepressed people report similar stress.[16] These reports are, however, difficult to interpret. Perhaps depressed people are more sensitive to stressful events and report them more often than normal people even when the actual circumstances of those who are depressed are not unusually stressful. In some cases, depression may be the cause rather than the result of a stressful life event. Depression certainly creates marriage problems. It can cause job performance to deteriorate, perhaps resulting in loss of the job. It can alienate friends. In a recent objective study, a cause and effect relation between stressful events and depression was not found. For a two-year period, depressed patients and healthy volunteers filled out weekly or bimonthly questionnaires about stressful events in their lives and about depressive symptoms. There was no evidence that stressful events preceded symptoms of depression.[17]

We conclude that the relation between stress and depression is, at most, weak. Stress, especially stress in personal relationships, might cause depression in susceptible people, but it does not precipitate the illness in everyone. Only about 20 percent of the people experiencing a severely stressful event become depressed, and furthermore, depression often occurs in the absence of any obvious stressful circumstance.[18]

Because depression is only weakly related to achievement or failure, to good fortune or misfortune, we suspect that susceptibility to depression might be genetic. Unfortunately, adoption studies of depression have not been done. The best evidence for genetic susceptibility comes from twin studies. Identical twins have a 40 percent concordance rate for depression while fraternal twins have only an 11 percent concordance rate.[19] This difference can be interpreted in two ways. If you see the genetics glass as half full, you might conclude that the difference in the concordance rates between identical and fraternal twins suggests a genetic component in depression. But if you view the glass as half empty, you will focus on the fact that the concordance rate for identical twins is not 100 percent. Therefore, you will conclude that the environment makes a significant contribution to major depression. As we have emphasized throughout our discussion, both heredity and environment can influence the development of a mental illness. Therefore, both conclusions are probably valid.

Many papers have been published showing that depression tends to run in families, implying that this tendency provides evidence for the genetic hypothesis. The roles of heredity and environment are hopelessly entangled in family studies. We do not think these studies can demonstrate the role of either heredity or the environment.

The evidence for a genetic component in bipolar illness is much stronger than the evidence for a genetic component in major depression. The concordance rate for identical twins is high (72 percent) for bipolar illness.[20] In addition, the concordance rate is virtually the same for identical twins reared apart and those reared together.[21] The likelihood that close relatives will be affected is also greater for bipolar illness than for major depression.[22] Most important, however, is an adoption study done in Belgium by Julien

Mendlewicz and John D. Ranier which was modeled after Seymour Kety's adoption studies of schizophrenia.[23] Mendlewicz and Ranier looked for affective illness (bipolar disorder or major depression) in the biological and adoptive parents of adopted children with bipolar illness. They also examined the biological and adoptive parents of healthy adopted children. Eighteen percent of the biological parents of the bipolar adoptees had an affective illness while only 1–4 percent of the parents in the other groups were afflicted. Bipolar illness clearly has a genetic component. Again, we stress that the existence of a genetic component does not rule out environmental causes. Stress may indeed be a precipitating factor.

11

Treating Depression with Drugs and Psychotherapy

Patients suffering from depression often respond to drugs. But, in contrast to schizophrenia, in which drug treatment is required, depression often can be effectively treated without drugs. In recent years, several psychotherapeutic techniques have been developed specifically to treat depressed patients. However, in some severe cases neither drugs nor psychotherapy work and electroconvulsive shock may be required.

In the scholarly literature and at cocktail parties, proponents of drug therapy argue with proponents of psychotherapy. For many years, argument was the only method available for comparing drug treatment with psythotherapy. More recently, psychotherapists have begun to design scientific tests to measure the effectiveness of psychotherapeutic methods. These tests are modeled on the tests used to measure drug effectiveness. Medical insurance companies have encouraged this research because they do not want to reimburse for a treatment without having proof of its effectiveness. As a result of this work, there is now good information on three different psychotherapeutic treatments for depression.

We focus our discussion of drug treatment for depression on a group of drugs called tricyclic antidepressants because these are the most commonly used and the most thoroughly studied. In the next chapter, we discuss other drug treatments as well as electro-convulsive shock. When we cover mania in Chapter 14, we discuss lithium therapy for both mania and depression.

Tricyclic Antidepressants

Tricyclic antidepressants are not stimulants. Unlike caffeine and amphetamine, they do not keep the patient awake. They do not produce euphoria in either depressed or healthy people. In fact, if a healthy person takes these drugs, he feels sleepy, tired, clumsy, and perhaps a bit unsteady on his feet. He may also experience an increase in anxiety. If he takes the drugs for several days, these symptoms will increase. He may then begin to experience difficulties in concentrating and thinking.[1]

The response of a depressed person to the antidepressants is quite different. For the first week after beginning treatment with a tricyclic antidepressant, the patient probably does not notice much change in her symptoms. But sometime during the second or third week, the depression starts to lift. Sleep disturbance and appetite improve; guilt and suicidal thinking disappear.[2] As the depressed mood lightens, the patient may say that she feels "normal" for the first time in many months. She begins to enjoy life again.

Of course, all patients do not receive such miraculous relief. All symptoms do not improve at the same time. Sleep disturbance may improve within a few days while the depressed mood continues for three to four weeks. Clearly, antidepressants are not an ideal treatment. Sometimes one or more symptoms persist. One patient, for example, may continue to have occasional suicidal thoughts whereas another may have occasional bouts of guilt. Still another may appear symptom free to family and friends; however, the patient remains aware of some remnants of his depression. Clearly, some patients are helped more than others. Some people, unfortunately, are not helped at all.

Even when treatment is successful, the patient may relapse occasionally. He may have episodes of sadness, irritability, or early morning awakening. These relapses should not be surprising. The effects of antidepressants, like the effects of antipsychotics, do not outlive the presence of the drug in the brain. The drug does not cause a permanent change in the state of the depressed brain and, hence, the drug is not a permanent cure for depression.

Case Studies

Beatrice and Derek both suffered from depression, but their symptoms were quite different. We tell their stories to illustrate the effectiveness of drug treatment on two people who had quite different patterns of symptoms.

Beatrice: Depression with Agitation

For several years, Beatrice had been irritable, but then for a six-month period, her irritability bordered on the irrational. She screamed in anger or sobbed in despair at every dirty dish left on the coffee table or on the bedroom floor. Each day the need to plan the dinner menu provoked agonizing indecision. How could all the virtues or, more likely, vices of hamburgers be accurately compared to those of spaghetti? A glass of spilled milk was an occasion for panic. Beatrice would bolt from her chair and run from the dining room. Ten minutes later, she would realize that the spilled milk was insignificant. She had her whole family walking on eggs. She thought they would be better off if she were dead.

Beatrice could not cope with her job. As a branch manager of a large chain store, she had many decisions to make. Unable to make them herself, she would ask employees who were much less competent for advice, but then she could not decide whose advice to take. Each morning before going to work, she complained of nausea. In public, she was usually able to control her feelings of panic and felt a little better when she actually arrived at work and was away from the wary eyes of her family.

Beatrice's husband loved her, but he did not understand what was wrong. He thought that she would improve if he made her life easier by taking over more housework, cooking, and child care. His attempt to help only made Beatrice feel more guilty and worthless. She wanted to make a contribution to her family. She wanted to do the chores "like normal people" did but broke down crying at the smallest impediment to a perfect job. Because Beatrice's volatility put a stress on her marriage, the couple went to a psychiatrist for marriage counseling. The psychiatrist failed to diagnose Beatrice's depression. He provided marriage counseling that was designed for healthy people. Consequently, the counseling failed. Months passed, and Beatrice's problem became more serious. Some days she was too upset to go to work. She stopped seeing her friends. She spent most of her time at home either yelling or crying. Finally, Beatrice's husband called the psychiatrist and insisted that something was seriously wrong.

After a diagnostic interview, the psychiatrist suggested that she enter the hospital. According to her hospital records, her diagnosis was pseudoneurotic schizophrenia, a category that had always been poorly defined and is no longer used. The psychiatrist prescribed phenothiazines and group therapy. During the three weeks in the hospital, Beatrice relaxed, and her husband had a needed rest. When released, Beatrice continued to take phenothiazines as an outpatient. The drugs decreased her agitation but did not stop the crying or lift the depressed mood. Continued psychotherapy also failed to help. Two years and several thousand dollars later, Beatrice decided to look elsewhere. She asked her psychiatrist to recommend a colleague. That was not easy for a woman who could not decide between hamburgers and spaghetti!

The second psychiatrist did not change Beatrice's medication immediately, but she did continue psychotherapy, trying to teach Beatrice to respond more rationally to other people's behavior. Beatrice agreed with this approach in principle, but it did not keep her from yelling at her husband and children and feeling worthless and guilty afterward. Finally, after a few tearful months, the psychiatrist began to question her colleague's diagnosis and prescribed antidepressant medication for Beatrice. Ten days later, Beatrice told her psychiatrist that a 100-pound weight had suddenly been lifted from her shoulders. For Beatrice, it was not "a beautiful day, but . . ." anymore; it was simply "a beautiful day." No qualifications were necessary. Either hamburgers or spaghetti was fine for dinner. The psychiatrist was almost as delighted as Beatrice.

Beatrice has been taking antidepressants for three years. She tried drug holidays twice, but each time she became depressed and agitated within about ten days after stopping the medication. She may need drug treatment indefinitely.

Beatrice's response to antidepressants sounds almost too good to be true. But Beatrice's story is not fictional. We know Beatrice and are familiar with her psychiatric history. But her story does not end here because antidepressants did not solve all of Beatrice's problems. She remained a bit irritable, and she occasionally panicked at the inevitable small disasters of family life—the dent in the car and the leak in the washing machine. These remaining symptoms suggested that antidepressants alone were not adequate medication. Therefore, a few months after prescribing antidepressants, the psychiatrist added lithium (Chapter 14), and Beatrice became less irritable and less agitated. Now Beatrice rarely panics. When she does, she recovers quickly. When the house is more cluttered than she can tolerate, she gets annoyed, but she no longer screams at the children. Beatrice's husband has a mate again. Her children see their mother laugh.

Beatrice, like Jill in Chapter 3, had difficulty getting the correct diagnosis. Because effective treatment depends on correct diagnosis, both women suffered needlessly for several years. Because Beatrice did not have schizophrenia, antipsychotics did not help her very much, in spite of the fact that phenothiazines do have weak antidepressant effects. Beatrice suffered from a major depression; antidepressants changed her life. Although Beatrice did not satisfy all the *DSM-III* criteria for bipolar disorder, she had almost enough symptoms to satisfy them. And lithium helped. Accurate diagnosis is not just an academic nicety; the patient's health and sometimes her life depend on it.

Beatrice's story illustrates the progress that psychiatry has made during the last ten to fifteen years. No one should be too critical of Beatrice's first psychiatrist. When Beatrice first became ill in 1969, diagnosis was much more difficult than it is now. The *DSM-III* had not yet been published. The criteria for the diagnosis of affective disorder had not been as well established. Different psychiatrists used different criteria, and many had no explicit criteria at all. They relied purely on clinical judgment. If Beatrice had walked into the office of her first psychiatrist in 1982 instead of 1969, he might well have provided the correct diagnosis.

Derek: Depression with Retardation

Derek's condition was less serious than Beatrice's. His depression was not incapacitating; yet treatment greatly improved his life. Derek had probably suffered from depression all of his adult life but was unaware of it for many years. Derek called himself a night person, claiming that he could not think clearly until after noon even though he was often awake by 4:00 A.M. He tried to schedule his work as editorial writer for a small town newspaper so that it was compatible with his depressed mood at the beginning of the day. Therefore, he scheduled meetings for the mornings; talking with people got him moving. He saved writing and decision making for later in the day.

Derek had always been a thoughtful person and was often preoccupied. His family and colleagues grew used to his apparent inattention and absentmindedness. He often failed to answer people when they spoke to him. Sometimes they were surprised to hear his slow, soft-spoken reply 20 or 30 seconds later. His wife tried to be patient when it took him 20 seconds to respond to, "Do you want coffee or tea tonight?" Derek's private thoughts were rarely cheerful and self-confident. He felt that his marriage was a mere business partnership. He provided the money, and she provided a home and children. Derek and his wife rarely expressed affection for each other. Occasionally, he had images of his own violent death in a bicycle crash, in a plane crash, or in a murder by an unidentified assailant.

Derek felt that he was constantly on the edge of job failure. He was disappointed that his editorials had not attracted the attention of larger papers. He was certain that several of the younger people on the paper had better ideas and wrote more skillfully than he did. He scolded himself for a bad editorial that he had written ten years earlier. Although that particular piece had not been up to his usual standards, everyone else on the paper had forgotten it a week after it appeared. But ten years later, Derek was still ruminating over that one editorial.

Although Derek was distressed much of the time, the possibility that he had a psychiatric illness never occurred to him. First of all, he did not know anything about mental illness. Second, he certainly was not incapacitated. He did his job. He and his wife did not fight; they merely failed to love each other. He took care of his family. He participated in sports, playing basketball and softball for his newspaper's team in the city league. Occasionally, he took his family on overnight bicycle trips that required much initiative, organization, and energy. He was supportive of his children and interested in their schoolwork and friends.

Derek could be cheerful when the social situation required him to be. His colleagues found him pleasant and easy to get along with. But, when by himself or alone with his wife, Derek could not keep up the illusion. His thoughts and talk reflected hopelessness and self-deprecation. Life was not much fun. Even Derek's recreational activities originated in a sense of duty to family or community. He would never be offered a job on a big city paper. Most important, he could not make his wife love him.

Derek attributed his inability to enjoy himself and his methodical, passionless marriage to his severe Anglo-Saxon protestant upbringing. He had been taught that open expressions of affection were ill-mannered. He had never seen his own parents embrace in their fifty years of marriage. In his family, humility was valued more than self-confidence. He had been brought up to do the "right thing," not to enjoy himself. Raucous merrymaking was only for the irresponsible. Even a game of Go Fish had to be played in secret when he was a child.

Derek brushed off his morning confusion as a lack of quick intelligence. He had no way to know that it was a symptom of depression. He never realized that his death images might be suicidal thinking. People do not talk about such things. For all Derek knew, everyone had similar thoughts.

Derek might have continued living his battleship-gray life had it not been for the local college. One winter Derek signed up for an evening course called "The Use and Abuse of Psychoactive Drugs" because he wanted to be able to provide accurate background information in future newspaper articles on drug use among high school and college students. The course covered psychiatric as well as recreational drugs. When the professor listed the symptoms of affective disorders on the blackboard, Derek had a flash of recognition. Perhaps he suffered from depression with melancholia.

Derek then consulted with a psychiatrist, who confirmed his suspicion and prescribed imipramine. A week later, Derek was sleeping until his alarm went off. Two weeks later, at 9:00 A.M. he was writing his column and making difficult decisions about editorials on sensitive topics. He started writing some feature stories on drugs just because he was interested in the subject. Writing was more fun than it had been in years. His images of his own violent death disappeared. His wife found him more responsive. He conversed with her enthusiastically and answered her questions without the long delays that had so tried her patience.

Antidepressants, however, did not solve all Derek's marital problems. Derek and his wife had gotten so good at doing their duty that they could not devote a day or even an evening to enjoying themselves without feeling guilty. Even the bicycle trips had been justified as good for the children, nonpolluting, and good exercise. Derek and his wife had to learn to enjoy each other.

Derek's marital problems had been the result of his depression, not symptoms of it. His improvement gave both Derek and his wife hope that happiness was possible, that they were not forever controlled by the asceticism of their Puritan ancestors. They also obtained marriage counseling, hoping to solve the problems created by Derek's long-standing depression. The mood of Derek's marriage suggested that his wife might also be depressed. Therefore, the therapist's first task was to examine Derek's wife for symptoms of mental illness.

If you are incapacitated by a psychiatric illness, the need for help will probably be fairly obvious. But you may not be able to find treatment by yourself. A relative may have to help. If, like Derek, you are not incapacitated, you will not get help unless you decide that you have a problem. We are not recommending that you diagnose your own psychiatric condition or decide how it should be treated. Those responsibilities belong to the psychiatrist. But the psychiatrist will not have a chance to help you unless you know enough about psychiatric illness to guess that you may be afflicted and then to seek diagnosis and treatment. Making that guess may prevent you from suffering unnecessary misery. Derek suffered for many years because he knew nothing about mental illness and concluded, "I'm just not an optimistic person."

The Effectiveness of Tricyclics

If you were skeptical that antidepressants really work, you might suspect that Derek's improvement was merely a placebo effect.

After all, Derek was never really sick. You may further claim that all people have periods when they are less moody and when they can concentrate better. Of course, the possibility of a placebo effect can never be ruled out when considering a single case history, but the improvement in Derek's ability to sleep is a phenomenon that can be observed and measured by someone other than the patient. This improvement suggests that the drug effect is real. In the remainder of this chapter, we present more scientific evidence for this conclusion.

Collecting Evidence

Beatrice's and Derek's stories illustrate the changes that anti-depressant drugs can produce in depressed patients, but anecdotes are not evidence. Therefore, we must examine the scientific evidence that antidepressants actually work. The evaluation of anti-depressants has the same problems as the evaluation of antipsy-chotics. First, to distinguish between spontaneous recovery and true drug response, researchers must include a placebo group in their study. The placebo control group is even more important in studies of antidepressants than in studies of antipsychotics because about 35 percent of depressed patients get well spontaneously dur-ing the four to six weeks required to test an antidepressant.[3]

Determining the appropriate dose is a second problem. The effective doses are not as well established for antidepressants as for antipsychotics. In many research studies, as well as in many doctors' offices, patients receive doses that are smaller than optimal.

A third problem is patient compliance with the physician's orders. Antidepressants are frequently given to outpatients. These patients often do not understand that the drug will have no effect for a week or more. When they do not feel better in a few days, they become convinced that the drug is not working and they quit taking it. Other patients continue medication and feel much better after a week or ten days. But, because they do not realize that they are likely to relapse without the antidepressant, they too stop taking the drug. Thus, many are depressed again when they return to the clinic for evaluation. Antidepressants taken according to directions and in adequate amounts may be much more effective than is indi-cated by current research.

Most studies of antidepressant effectiveness proceed somewhat as follows. Patients entering a hospital or outpatient clinic are diagnosed as depressed by the specific procedure used in that particular facility. (Because most of the research on antidepressant effectiveness antedates the *DSM-III*, the patients studied in one facility may have had somewhat different symptoms than the patients studied in another.) After diagnosis, the researchers rate the severity of each patient's depression, using a standardized procedure, for example, the Hamilton Rating Scale.[4] An interviewer using the Hamilton Scale studies the patient's history, observes his behavior during the interview, and listens to his answers to specific interview questions. He gives the patient a score for each of seventeen symptoms. (The Hamilton Scale includes most of the symptoms for a major depressive episode listed in the *DSM-III*.) The higher the score, the more severe is the depression. For example, the patient receives one point for retardation if he delays slightly in answering questions. He receives four points for retardation if he does not speak at all during the entire interview. He receives one point for suicidal thinking if he claims that life is not worth living but four points if he has actually made a serious suicide attempt. The scores for individual symptoms are added to produce an overall measure of severity.

After his depression has been evaluated, the patient is randomly assigned to either the drug group or the placebo group. The experiment must be double blind; that is, neither the patient nor the doctors and nurses who rate his improvement know which group he is in. After the patient has taken the drug for one to four months, the severity of his depression is rated again. Finally, the researchers break the code and find out whether the patients taking tricyclic antidepressants have improved more than the patients taking placebo.

About ninety studies measuring the effectiveness of tricyclic antidepressants were published between 1958 and 1972, and their findings are not all in agreement.[5] About two-thirds of these studies found that antidepressants were more effective than placebo. The rest found that antidepressants and placebo were about equally effective. None found that placebo was more effective than antidepressants. This line score is not, perhaps, very impressive. If antidepressants really work, why do one-third of the studies find that they do not? The three problems previously mentioned—inaccur-

ate diagnosis, inadequate dosage, and poor patient compliance—
may contribute to this lack of effectiveness.

When the data from all the research reports are combined,
there is no doubt that antidepressants are an effective treatment
for depression.[6] Nevertheless, this finding does not mean that they
are a desirable treatment. If they are only slightly effective, the risk
of side effects may not be worth the benefits. Alternatively, other
treatments may be safer and/or more effective.

During a drug trial lasting a few months, a depressed patient
has about a 70 percent chance of improving on antidepressants and
about a 30 percent chance of improving on placebo. Antidepressant
drugs approximately double the chance that he will improve. (In
comparisons to antipsychotics, antidepressants do not seem very
impressive. Very few schizophrenia patients improve on placebo,
but about 90 percent improve on antipsychotics.) If the patient has
been depressed for only a few weeks and is not in severe distress,
patient and physician may decide to wait and hope for spontaneous
remission. But if the patient, like Beatrice or Derek, has been troubled by depression for years, he should probably begin antidepressant therapy.

Relief from Symptoms

Do antidepressants decrease all the symptoms of depression? Or
do they just improve some while leaving others intact? You might
intuitively predict that medication would be effective for the symptoms that people usually think of as involuntary, such as sleep
disturbance and appetite suppression, but would not work as well
on guilt and depressed mood. In fact, antidepressants improve virtually every symptom of major depression as described in the *DSM-
III*, but the changes in involuntary, or vegetative, symptoms are
most pronounced.[7] Antidepressants decrease sleep disturbance,
especially early morning awakening. Like Derek, most patients stop
waking up several hours before the alarm goes off. They begin to
eat more and to gain weight. Antidepressants improve mood and
change hopelessness to hope. For example, Beatrice felt that the
weight of the world had been lifted from her shoulders. Antidepressants also relieve guilt. Suddenly, Beatrice could accept the

love her family had been giving her for so long. Derek stopped scolding himself for the bad editorial he had written ten years earlier. In addition, antidepressants can change apathy to activity. Beatrice began to share responsibilities for making dinner, helping the children with their homework, and cleaning the house, and she felt proud of herself—almost like a small child discovering that, like grownups, she can tie her shoes. Antidepressants also relieve anxiety. Before treatment, Beatrice constantly anticipated failure. She was certain that a glass of milk would spill at dinner and that she would scream at the offender, spoiling the meal for the entire family. Now she has confidence that she can accept minor accidents.

With the help of antidepressants, patients not only move faster, they also think faster. Because *mood disorder* is a catchword for depression and because the depressed mood is the most pervasive symptom to an observer, the patients' complaints of cognitive confusion and an inability to make decisions tend to be neglected. Recall that Derek claimed that he was too confused to make decisions in the morning. He felt that antidepressants decreased his morning confusion and so enabled him to work effectively and make decisions throughout the day.

Derek's subjective evaluation of his improvement was probably valid. In several experiments on depressed patients, researchers measured cognitive difficulties before treatment and cognitive improvement during antidepressant therapy. In one experiment, people were asked to press one button in response to one stimulus and to press a different button in response to a second stimulus.[8] Depressed people performed this task much more slowly than healthy people, but the patients increased their speed within a week of beginning treatment with antidepressants. In fact, their speed increased before other symptoms of depression were relieved. In another experiment, depressed patients performed more poorly than healthy people in a short-term memory task. The patients' memory became more accurate during antidepressant therapy. Memory often improved before the depressed mood lifted.[9]

Limitations of Antidepressants

Antidepressants are not, however, a cure for whatever ails you. These drugs help patients with a major affective disorder. They are not useful in treating schizophrenia and hypochondriacal or hysterical illnesses.[10] Because they do not prevent bizarre thoughts, they often fail to help patients with delusional depression.[11] Patients with delusional depression believe things that are contrary to fact. For example, they may imagine that they have committed crimes or that someone is trying to murder them because they do not deserve to live. Simply believing that one's life has been worthless does not, however, qualify as a delusion. Perhaps antidepressants do not help delusional patients because such patients have a thought disorder in addition to their mood disorder. Fortunately, patients with delusional depressions often respond well to a combination of tricyclics and antipsychotics.[12]

Antidepressants do more harm than good for some patients with bipolar illness: the drugs can evoke episodes of mania. But for other bipolar patients, the combination of a tricyclic for depression and lithium for mania is very successful.[13] Therefore, a psychiatrist prescribing a tricyclic antidepressant for a patient with such symptoms of bipolar illness as agitation or hostility must watch carefully for manic or hypomanic behavior. Finally, antidepressants will not cure the consequences of depression. If depression has impaired work performance or damaged personal relationships, relieving the depression does not solve these problems. The patient does, however, become capable of working on them, perhaps with the help of psychotherapy.

If antidepressants were used optimally, they might help more than 70 percent of depressed patients. Improved diagnosis and improved selection of patients for antidepressant therapy should increase the percentage of people helped. Patients who do not have an affective disorder and delusional patients treated with an antidepressant alone swell the ranks of drug treatment failures.

A patient may also fail to improve with antidepressants because she is not getting the correct dose; a larger or smaller dose might have worked. When the same dose (adjusted for body weight) of an antidepressant is given to many different people, it produces a wide range of drug concentrations in the blood because some patients metabolize antidepressants much faster than others. In a two-part study, the blood concentration of the antidepressant, imipramine, and its active metabolites was first measured in patients who were separated into three groups: those with low, medium, and high plasma levels.[14] Only 29 percent of those with low levels responded to the drug; 64 percent of those with medium plasma levels responded; and 93 percent of those with high plasma levels responded. Overall, 60 percent of the patients were drug responders. This 60 percent figure is close to the 70 percent success rate that is usually reported when blood levels are not monitored.

In the second stage of the experiment, the nonresponders with low plasma levels were given higher doses so that their plasma levels entered the therapeutic range. This procedure turned many nonresponders into responders and increased the overall percentage of responders to 84 percent.

The initial dose used in this experiment was at the upper end of the range usually prescribed by physicians. Yet 40 percent of all the patients in this study did not obtain a therapeutic plasma level. If, in a large population, half the nonresponders with inadequate plasma levels became responders when their plasma levels were raised, the effectiveness of antidepressants would increase from 65–70 percent to 85–90 percent, a substantial improvement. Other antidepressants may have different requirements. For example, nortriptyline has a "therapeutic window"—plasma levels that are either too high or too low are ineffective.[15] Very few clinical studies of antidepressant effectiveness have measured plasma levels. Therefore, we can only surmise that many of the nonresponders did not obtain a plasma level within the therapeutic range.

Preventing Relapses

After a depressed patient has obtained relief from antidepressant medication, can he expect to remain symptom free or will he suffer a relapse? Unfortunately, without continued treatment, about 40–50 percent of the patients relapse within 6 to 12 months. If the patient continues to take antidepressant medication, the likelihood of relapsing decreases from 40–50 percent to 15–25 percent.[16] We do not know how to interpret the relapses that occur during maintenance therapy. Perhaps antidepressants cannot prevent relapse in some patients. On the other hand, relapses might be due to failure to take medication or to lowering of the dose.

The patient is less likely to relapse if treatment is not stopped as soon as the symptoms of depression are relieved.[17] G. L. Klerman's group at the National Institute of Mental Health (NIMH) treated a group of depressed patients with a tricyclic antidepressant for six weeks and selected only those who responded favorably to participate in the maintenance phase of the project. During the maintenance phase, one group of patients received a tricyclic for the next eight months while two control groups received either a placebo or no treatment. Only 12 percent of the tricyclic group but about 33 percent of the control groups relapsed during the maintenance period.

Psychiatrists do not know precisely how long a patient should continue to take antidepressants once his depression is in remission. Probably, he should stay on medication for six to eight months and then try taking doses that are decreased gradually until he is completely off the drug. The results of the NIMH study suggested that six to eight months of maintenance therapy can prevent a first episode patient from becoming a chronic patient.[18] Perhaps longer treatment permits a more complete recovery and forestalls the development of a lifelong problem. But depression is sometimes a chronic disease. It is for Beatrice. Antidepressants worked for her, but she relapsed when she and her psychiatrist experimented with a drug free period. About 10–15 percent of depressed patients have multiple relapses, and thus appear to have a chronic illness.[19] Even after several years of successful treatment with psychotherapy and antidepressants, some patients relapse within a few months when the antidepressant is replaced with placebo.[20] These patients need indefinite medication. The only way to determine whether a patient needs continuing medication is to withdraw it and observe the consequences.

Many of the patients whom physicians in family practice and internal medicine label "crocks" are patients with chronic depression. These patients visit primary care physicians frequently, usually with vague complaints.[21] Often their depressions go undiagnosed and, hence, untreated. The doctor cannot find a nonpsychiatric illness and because he is not skilled at psychiatric diagnosis, he does not recognize depression. Under pressure from the patient to "do something," he may prescribe Valium. (Valium is an antianxiety drug described in detail in Chapter 15.) It is not very effective in the treatment of major depressive disorder. When Valium is prescribed for a person suffering from depression, that person is not getting proper medical care.

Comparative Benefits of Psychotherapy and Drug Therapy

Effective Psychotherapeutic Treatments

We did not give psychotherapy very high marks as a treatment for schizophrenia. We pointed out that the effectiveness of traditional psychotherapy greatly depends on the skill and personality of the therapist. Because neither the treatment procedures nor the treatment goals are well specified, the technique is almost immune to evaluation. Nevertheless, the evaluations that have been done showed that psychotherapy could not cure schizophrenia or even relieve its symptoms. The situation is quite different for depression. Several psychotherapeutic treatments for depression have been developed in such detail that essentially the same treatment can be given by anyone who is properly trained. In addition, the development of rating scales for the severity of depression has made it possible to specify what success means and to measure that success. As Myrna M. Weissman, a scientist at the National Institute of Mental Health, said, comparisons of psychotherapy and drug therapy can now progress "from ideology to evidence."[22]

Several psychotherapeutic treatments have come through such evaluations with very high marks. Not only do these new treatments work, they are an affordable choice for a large number of patients. In many of these treatments, a therapist meets with a group of patients. In this format, cost is decreased and the number of patients who can be treated is increased. A patient entering one of these newly developed psychotherapy programs as an outpatient will probably spend a few months and a few hundred dollars. In contrast, if he enters psychoanalysis, the cost is measured in years and thousands of dollars.

Three well defined psychotherapies have been tested on depressed patients, and all three appear to be effective. Because we are focusing primarily on drug treatments, we discuss these psychotherapeutic treatments only briefly. Weissman, Klerman, and their colleagues used a treatment that dealt with the patient's day-to-day interactions. The therapists described their psychotherapeutic techniques as follows: "The therapy was primarily supportive in nature with emphasis on the 'here and now,' and oriented around the patients' current problems and interpersonal relations. Patients were assisted in identifying maladaptive patterns and attaining better levels of adaptive response, particularly in family or social interactions. Therefore, no attempt was made to uncover unconscious material, modify infantile drives or induce a strongly regressive transference."[23]

Cognitive therapists used a second approach that is based on the belief that depression results when a person views his experience so that he is pessimistic about his future.[24] His depressed thoughts develop from certain attitudes and assumptions. For example, he may think, "Unless I do everything perfectly, I am a failure." Therefore, these therapists assign tasks designed to counteract this assumption. Success at each task gives the patient confidence to approach the next one and shows him that his self-reproaches are incorrect.

The third technique, used by behavior therapists, stemmed from the concept that a person becomes depressed when he does not receive sufficient positive reinforcement for his efforts.[25] A positive reinforcement is any pleasant event that is contingent upon the person's behavior. A smile in return for a compliment is a positive reinforcement, but a new car spontaneously delivered by a wealthy parent is not. Behavior therapists try to teach depressed people skills that will increase the number of positive reinforcements they receive. Learning social skills increases the reinforcements received from other people. Participating in pleasant events increases the reinforcements from the environment. Learning self-control increases feelings of self-worth.

Drug therapy and psychotherapy are both effective treatments for depression, but we cannot give you a simple answer to the obvious question "Which is more effective?" In some studies, psychotherapy has been found to be as effective as drug therapy.[26] Some studies show that it is less effective than drug therapy.[27] Still other research shows that it is more effective than drug therapy.[28]

Simply stating that both treatments work does not provide an adequate description of their effects. The NIMH group attempted to analyze the effects of each in some detail. These researchers' findings are interesting, but because many of them have not yet been replicated by other researchers, these findings must be considered tentative.

Combining the Two Treatments

If both psychotherapy and drug therapy are effective, is the combination better than using either one alone? Some studies suggest that the answer is yes, but others disagree.[29] The idea that the two treatments work well together is a relatively new one and is an anathema to many who support just one method. Some psychiatrists who rely on drug therapy believe that psychotherapy is, at best, a waste of time. At worst, it stirs up the patient and increases the neurochemical abnormalities that were initially responsible for the illness. Some psychotherapists, particularly those trained in the Freudian tradition, believe that drugs will prevent a patient from facing and solving complex problems. They believe that patients must have a certain amount of discomfort to motivate them to seek psychotherapy and delve into the origins of their depression. If antidepressant drugs are too successful, they may remove that motivation. Some therapists fear that drug therapy will persuade the patient that the illness is beyond his control and thus discourage him from working hard in psychotherapy.

The NIMH group has done the most extensive research showing that a combination of drug therapy and psychotherapy was more effective than either treatment alone. The two therapies tended to affect different symptoms so that each treatment was effective precisely where the other was weak. Drugs had a greater and more immediate effect on sleep disturbance and appetite. Drugs also improved depressed mood and apathy, but only, after several months of use. On the other hand, psychotherapy improved mood and apathy within one month, but had little effect on sleep disturbance. Although poor social adjustment does not contribute to a diagnosis of depression, it is worth noting that psychotherapy, but not pharmacotherapy, improved social adjustment as an additional benefit. Social adjustment was measured by work performance, communication with others, and friction in relationships.[30]

Other investigators disagree with the conclusions of the NIMH group. Beck and his colleagues, the major proponents of cognitive therapy, found no clear differences between the symptoms affected by the two types of therapy, although the patient's view of himself and his future were the first symptoms to be affected by cognitive therapy.[31] We are partial to the conclusion that different treatments influence different symptoms because it explains why the

NIMH researchers and others found that a combination of drugs and psychotherapy worked so well. (Beck's group did not use a combination treatment.) Perhaps psychotherapy can help the patient solve the interpersonal problems caused by depression only after antidepressants have relieved the most severe symptoms. Until then, a patient is likely to be the victim of the vicious and depressing beast known as the "yeahbut." This patient responds to every suggestion of the therapist with, "Yeah, but I am too depressed to . . ." (do whatever the therapist has suggested).

One reason that psychotherapy increases treatment effectiveness is that it keeps the patient in a treatment program. A treatment cannot help patients who do not participate. Patients are more likely to complete a psychotherapy program than a drug therapy program and are still more likely to complete a program in which the two treatments are combined.[32] The NIMH group found that only 30–50 percent of the patients receiving drug therapy alone completed the program. The reasons for this high dropout rate are not completely clear. Treatment failure and worsening depression were not responsible for this high dropout rate among the drug patients because about the same number of psychotherapy and drug therapy patients dropped out for these two reasons. Furthermore, the drug patients did not drop out because they recovered and felt no further need for treatment. Most were still depressed when they left. But many of the drug patients failed to complete treatment for such reasons as missed appointments, failure to take medication, and drug side effects. These reasons for dropout suggest that the psychotherapist plays an important role in keeping the patient in the program. He reminds the patient to keep appointments, encourages him to take his medications, and makes certain that he understands what to expect from the medication.

Is the combination treatment best for all patients, or do some patients do just as well with only psychotherapy or only pharmacotherapy? The questions are obviously important if each patient is to receive the most effective treatment without receiving unnecessary treatments. Several research groups tried to find out whether patients with melancholia respond differently to treatment than do those without melancholia. The NIMH group found that melancholic patients required antidepressants; they did not respond to psychotherapy alone.[33] Optimal treatment was a combination of antidepressants and psychotherapy. Blackburn and his colleagues came to a different conclusion. The most severely ill patients, who were not necessarily the melancholic ones, did best with a combination therapy but cognitive therapy alone was the treatment of choice for the others.[34] The presence or absence of melancholia did not help these researchers predict which treatment would be more effective. Beck's group, like Blackburn's, found no relation between melancholic symptoms and response to cognitive therapy or drug therapy.[35] Brown and Lewinsohn found that neither initial severity nor the pattern of symptoms could be used to predict which patients would respond best to behavior therapy.[36] However, they selected their patients from those who answered an advertisement for depression treatment, and thus their patients may not have been as ill as the patients requesting treatment at hospital clinics.

The disagreements resulting from different studies make it difficult to draw definite conclusions at present, but we will hazard a guess about what future research will show. Patients with severe depression accompanied by melancholia will probably respond best to a combination of antidepressants and psychotherapy. An antidepressant drug without psychotherapy will help, but is not the optimal treatment. Less severe depressions should first be treated by psychotherapy alone. Drugs should be added if the patient fails to respond to psychotherapy. If the symptoms suggest that the depression is one aspect of a bipolar illness, medication will almost certainly be necessary. Lithium is the drug of choice for bipolar patients, but sometimes an antidepressant is also necessary to combat depressive episodes.

Long-Term Benefits

Suppose a patient can be treated successfully by drugs and/or psychotherapy. Are the long-term benefits greater for one type of treatment than for the others? To ask the question another way, does one treatment have only temporary effects while another has long-term benefits? The answer seems to be no.[37] One year after the end of treatment, the NIMH group interviewed patients who were successfully treated with drugs and/or psychotherapy. They found that about 80 percent of them had no symptoms or only mild symptoms. If a patient responded to his original treatment, his likelihood of staying well was not affected by the type of treatment he received.

Beck's group obtained similar results. This finding shows that treatments are best evaluated by their immediate results. This conclusion is somewhat surprising, especially to those espousing insight-oriented psychotherapy. If psychotherapy really restructures the personality, its effects ought to last longer than the effects of a drug that leaves the body in a few weeks. Apparently, all that really matters is alleviating the depression that exists when treatment begins.

If treatment were not terminated at the end of a few months, but continued for an entire year, would more patients remain symptom free? For drug treatment, we have already answered this question in the affirmative. But does continuing psychotherapy prevent relapses? The NIMH relapse data showed that drug treatment had a statistically significant effect on relapse rate, but psychotherapy did not.[38] The difference between the rates in the two treatments was small, however, and did not demonstrate that drug treatment is consistently superior to psychotherapy in preventing relapse. In our view, psychiatrists do not yet know whether antidepressant drug therapy prevents relapse more effectively than psychotherapy.

Choosing a Treatment

The treatment chosen by a patient with chronic depression is often influenced by philosophical and emotional as well as medical considerations. Some depressed patients choose to live with depression indefinitely rather than to take antidepressants. These patients are opposed to a drug dependent life. We suspect that they would not have this objection if the drug were not a psychoactive one. They would probably not object to a drug dependent life if they were diabetic and dependent on insulin. Many women who refuse antidepressants probably do not mind being "dependent" on birth control pills. They may feel that chronic consumption of a drug that controls the ovaries is acceptable, but chronic consumption of a drug that controls the brain is not. (People are often unaware that birth control pills work because they affect the brain.) Some patients feel that if a drug does not effect a permanent cure, it is merely a "cover-up" and a "cop out" and, as such, is morally reprehensible. We do not agree. To put treatment of depression in a medical context, keep in mind that the only medical diseases that can actually be cured by drugs are those caused by bacteria. Most other illnesses, such as heart disease, arthritis, and ulcers, are chronic conditions. Like depression and schizophrenia, they can be controlled but cannot be cured by drugs.

Although we have no ethical or philosophical objection to long-term maintenance treatment with antidepressants, we think that these drugs, like any others, should be used only when the benefits outweigh the risks. The risks and benefits must be assessed for each patient individually. Chronic use of antidepressants is probably quite safe for medically healthy young and middle-aged adults. The older antidepressants may pose a danger to people with certain medical conditions, particularly cardiovascular disease, but some of the newer antidepressants are much safer to use when these conditions exist.[39] People with cardiovascular disease are not prohibited from using antidepressants, but their medical condition must be closely monitored.

No one can know with certainty what treatment will work best for a particular patient, but treatment cannot begin until the psychiatrist makes the best decision she can. Beatrice clearly had severe melancholic symptoms and probably needed drug therapy. If antidepressants had posed a slight medical risk, Beatrice might have decided to take them anyway. A person with milder symptoms might elect not to take that risk. For Beatrice, depression was serious and was ruining her life. Her husband was running out of patience. Her children were losing respect for her. She was in danger of losing her job. Psychotherapy was not sufficient to help Beatrice overcome her morning attacks of nausea, her inability to make decisions, or her irritability. Beatrice improved so dramatically with drugs that she did not continue psychotherapy. But continued therapy probably would have helped. Once she was well enough to make decisions, psychotherapy could have taught her how to enforce them without provoking hostility. Once she managed to remain at the table when the milk spilled, psychotherapy could have taught her how to ask for help with the cleanup.

Like Beatrice, Derek had melancholic symptoms and improved, as predicted, with antidepressants. However, his condition was not as serious. Even though Derek was depressed, his job performance remained adequate. Because his schedule was flexible, he could work around his morning confusion. He could still enjoy his children. He could tolerate occasional bouts of inefficiency and guilt. If antidepressants had posed a serious medical risk, perhaps Derek should have rejected drug therapy. With or without drugs, Derek could probably have benefited from psychotherapy. Antidepressants would not alleviate his marital difficulties. Perhaps psychotherapy would help him improve his marriage, especially if his wife joined him in treatment.

It is hard to guess how long Beatrice or Derek or any other patient will need drug therapy or psychotherapy. In the absence of hard data, each patient and his psychiatrist must be guided by their subjective impressions of the effectiveness of antidepressants and/or psychotherapy. Some patients will need continual treatment throughout their lives. Because there is no drug without risk, most patients should periodically discontinue antidepressants to find out whether drug therapy is still needed.

Misuse of Antidepressants

Like any drug, antidepressants can be misused by physicians. Physicians may prescribe them without paying adequate attention to the diagnosis. An incorrect diagnosis can have consequences far more serious than suffering a few unnecessary side effects and wasting money. On rare occasions, antidepressants have provoked a psychotic episode in patients with schizophrenia. Careful discrimination between unipolar and bipolar illness is important because antidepressants used alone can provoke an episode of mania in a bipolar patient.[40] Depressed bipolar patients should receive lithium along with the antidepressant.

An inadequate assessment of the patient creates a danger of suicide by overdose. Unfortunately, unlike an overdose of phenothiazines, an overdose of antidepressants can be lethal. The fatal dose is usually 10–15 times the prescribed daily dose.[41] According to a suggestion in the standard medical textbook on pharmacology, no more than a week's supply of antidepressant should be dispensed to an acutely depressed patient.[42] Hospitalizing severely depressed patients is safer yet.

The first symptoms of acute poisoning are usually excitement and seizures. The patient then lapses into a coma. At this point, he should be treated in an intensive care unit because of the danger of death due to heart failure. In one to three days, the coma passes into a second phase of excitement and delerium.The patient must be monitored closely for several days after the delerium has passed because the danger of heart failure is still present.

Antidepressants are misused when they are prescribed without careful consideration of the side effects (see Chapter 13). For some patients, these side effects are potentially dangerous.

Antidepressants are misused if the physician does not carefully explain the treatment to the patient. Because hopelessness is a symptom of depression, the patient who expects rapid relief and does not find it may despair quietly and conclude, "Nothing works for me." She may then stop taking her antidepressants. D. A. W. Johnson in Manchester, England, examined the compliance of patients receiving antidepressants prescribed by primary care physicians.[43] Five weeks after their first visit to the doctor, 57 percent of the patients who still felt depressed had stopped taking their medication. Most of these patients stopped because they did not feel better in a few days and concluded that the drug was not working. Others stopped because of side effects, because they did not believe that medication was the correct approach to their problems, or because of fear of dependence or addiction. The physicians had little chance to correct misconceptions because the patients ignored the doctors' requests to return for follow-up care.

Johnson's study emphasized the point made earlier that a treatment program using antidepressant drugs alone is ineffective for the simple reason that about half the patients do not complete it. Combining pharmacotherapy with psychotherapy keeps the patients in treatment and helps them solve some of the problems created by depression. Using pharmacotherapy as the only treatment for depression may not, strictly speaking, be misuse, but it is depriving the patient of optimal treatment.

Antidepressants are frequently underused; that is, they are not prescribed for patients who might benefit from them. The underuse of antidepressants often results in the overuse of addictive and less effective drugs, such as barbiturates and antianxiety drugs (see Chapter 15). Myrna Weissman and her colleagues were interested in whether most patients suffering from depression received adequate treatment. They gave psychiatric interviews with questions about drug treatment to over five hundred adults from a random sample of the population of New Haven, Connecticut.[44] Fifty-five percent of the people suffering from depression had taken psychoactive drugs within the past year, but only 17 percent had taken antidepressants. Thirty-five percent had taken antianxiety drugs, and 17 percent had taken barbiturates. (Some had taken more than one kind of drug.) Failure to diagnose depression and prescribe antidepressants not only deprives patients of adequate treatment. Inaccurate diagnosis and improper treatment may actually create a drug abuse problem if the patients self-medicate with alcohol or obtain multiple prescriptions of barbiturates or antianxiety drugs.

The failure of nonpsychiatric physicians to diagnose and prescribe adequately for patients with affective disorder is illustrated by a study conducted by J. H. Barbar in Glascow, Scotland.[45] Researchers examined 101 patients diagnosed as depressed by physicians in general practice. The physicians spent an average of six minutes with each patient before diagnosing and prescribing. They referred only 2 percent of the patients to psychiatrists and prescribed drugs for about 90 percent of them. Although the physicians had diagnosed all of these patients as suffering from depression, they prescribed antidepressants for only about 75 percent of them. They prescribed sedatives, antianxiety drugs, and antipsychotics for the remainder. Not only was the diagnosis perfunctory, but the medication prescribed was frequently inconsistent with the diagnosis. Furthermore, when antidepressants were prescribed, the dose was often too small to be effective.

Similar results were obtained in the study conducted in Manchester, England.[46] In this study, as in the Glascow one, researchers found that many depressed patients received an antianxiety drug rather than an antidepressant. Thirty-five percent of those receiving an antidepressant drug received a dose so small that it probably had little or no effect. Similar prescribing practices prevail in the United States. Most physicians practicing in general hospitals prescribe antidepressants, but the average daily doses are far too small to be effective. Not surprisingly, the doctors who complained that the drugs were ineffective were those who prescribed very small doses.[47]

An interesting sidelight to the Manchester study is that the researchers asked the physicians where they got their information about the drugs they prescribed. Their answer was always, "from the drug companies." Apparently, even this information never reached the patients. Patients claimed to receive their information from the mass media, not from their physicians.

It should not be surprising that nonpsychiatric physicians frequently fail to diagnose and treat adequately patients with affective disorders. Effective treatments for depression have been available in this country only since 1957. Physicians who graduated from medical school earlier did not learn about these treatments in school. Modern diagnostic methods are even newer, and they are time consuming. Diagnosing depression with a structured interview takes about one and a half hours. It is not realistic to expect a physician to administer such a lengthy diagnostic test when he must see 15–30 patients per day. Perhaps through improved continuing education, the physician can be trained to detect psychiatric problems. But detection is not diagnosis. We think that the only practical hope for widely available accurate diagnosis is the computerized diagnostic questionnaire (see Chapter 3).

Addiction and Tolerance

Like antipsychotics, antidepressants do not produce addiction in the usual sense of the term. They do not produce euphoria and hence do not tempt patients to take more than is medically justified. Furthermore, these drugs have no recreational value for non-patients.[48] Usually, the drugs do not bring harm to the user or to others. The benefits of the drugs far exceed their harmful side effects. In addition, antidepressants do not cause tolerance; that is, the patient does not need to increase his dose to maintain the antidepressant effect.

In a sense, antidepressants do produce physiological dependence. If a patient suddenly stops taking antidepressants, he may experience a withdrawal syndrome that includes muscle aches, gastrointestinal distress, and anxiety.[49] These symptoms sound alarmingly similar to the symptoms of opiate withdrawal. But the two syndromes are not the same. If the antidepressant patient tapers off his withdrawal of antidepressant over a two-week period, he usually has no discomfort. But even gradual opiate withdrawal over 10–15 weeks causes withdrawal symptoms. The antidepressant patient will not crave antidepressants once withdrawn. Of course, if he becomes depressed again, he may want to resume his medication. But this is rational, not addictive, behavior. In contrast, detoxification usually does not terminate the craving of the opiate addict. She continues to crave the drug for months or years, or as some addicts say, forever.

12

Other Treatments for Depression

Monoamine Oxidase Inhibitors

Monoamine oxidase inhibitors (MAOIs) are the second most common chemical treatment for depression. These drugs are named for their biochemical function. They inhibit the enzyme, monoamine oxidase, that breaks down monoamines by oxidation. (The transmitters norepinephrine, dopamine, and serotonin are all monoamines.) These drugs are clearly effective in the treatment of depression; that is, they work more effectively than placebos.[1] According to most controlled studies of effectiveness, monamine oxidase inhibitors do not work as well as tricyclics, but there is some disagreement. Some studies showed that the two treatments were equally effective. However, no one claimed that MAOIs were more effective than tricyclics.[2]

Most psychiatrists in the United States use MAOIs less frequently than tricyclics.[3] Their standard dogma is that tricyclics are better for patients with melancholic symptoms, such as sleep disturbance and appetite depression.[4] MAOIs are most likely to be prescribed after tricyclics have failed. Psychiatrists believe that some of the patients who do not respond to tricyclics respond to MAOIs, but there have been no studies that tell how many.[5] If the patient cannot tolerate tricyclic side effects but still needs antidepressant medication, the psychiatrist may decide to try an MAOI. For example, a physician who prescribed tricyclics for an elderly male suffering from depression might find that each drug caused urinary retention as a side effect. This physician might then prescribe an MAOI for his patient before deciding that pharmacologic treatment was not possible.

Many British and some American psychiatrists think that patients with certain specific symptoms, such as anxiety, hypochondria, fear, and fatigue, are particularly good candidates for MAOI treatment.[6] Using symptomatology to decide on a tricyclic versus an MAOI may be an accurate basis for prescribing a drug or it may be pure superstition. The data are scanty and do not justify a firm conclusion. Thus, psychiatrists are still uncertain about how to select the patients for whom MAOIs are the preferred treatment.

No one is certain of the optimal dose of either class of drug. This uncertainty makes studies purporting to compare them difficult to interpret. Studies showing that tricyclics are superior may have used inadequate doses of MAOIs, and the reverse may be true for studies showing that MAOIs and tricyclics are equally effective.[7] The effective dose of MAOIs, like the effective dose of tricyclics, is not the same for all patients. To find out if a patient is receiving an adequate dose, it is necessary to do a blood test that measures the actual inhibition of monoamine oxidase. Consequently, all that can be said now is that, with adequate doses, MAOIs are an effective treatment for depression.

Electroconvulsive Therapy

Effectiveness of Treatment

Passing large amounts of electric current through the brain seems more like a punishment than a treatment. *One Flew Over the Cuckoo's Nest* has fed public disapproval of electroconvulsive therapy (ECT), just as it has fed public disapproval of antipsychotic drugs.[8] The shock treatment described in Kesey's book inspired sheer terror. When shock hit Kesey's hero, McMurphy, his convulsing muscles jammed him against the straps that held his wrists and ankles.

The shock "bridges him up off the table till nothing is down but his wrists and ankles. . . ."[9] Chief, one of McMurphy's fellow patients, described the aftermath of shock treatment as "that gray zone between light and dark, or between sleeping and waking, or between living and dying, where you know you're not unconscious anymore, but don't know yet what day it is or who you are or what's the use of coming back at all—for two weeks."[10] Every reader and movie patron felt the terror with McMurphy and Chief. ECT as depicted by Kesey is all risk and no benefit: no one ever improves as a result of shock treatment. Indeed, ECT was not an appropriate treatment for McMurphy. He had no diagnosable condition that justified the treatment.

In fact, modern ECT is a very effective treatment for depression and is not the harrowing experience described by Kesey.[11] Many depressed patients who do not respond to antidepressants will respond to ECT. ECT is most often required for patients suffering from delusional depression. Only 40 percent of these patients improve on drugs, but 80–90 percent of the drug failures improve with ECT. Patients who have depression with melancholia and do not improve with drugs have an 80–90 percent chance of improving with ECT.[12] On the other hand, ECT is not particularly successful with patients whose depression is clearly a response to stress. Among these patients, only 26 percent of the drug failures respond to ECT.[13]

For many patients, a treatment that relieves depression rapidly is more than desirable—it is lifesaving. As we mentioned earlier, victims of depression have much higher death rates than do healthy people. Although the exact figures vary, a survey of studies on death rates in depression indicates that during the three to five years following treatment, the death rate of patients treated with ECT is less than one-third that for untreated patients.[14]

Like the other treatments we have discussed, ECT is not a permanent cure for depression. Without maintenance treatment, about half the patients relapse within a year. If, however, ECT is followed up by prophylactic treatment with tricyclics or lithium, the rate of relapse decreases to about 20 percent.[15] In one study, patients receiving no maintenance therapy were ill about eight weeks during the first year following ECT; those receiving lithium treatment were ill less than two weeks.[16] Clearly, patients whose depression is severe enough to warrant ECT should receive careful follow-up care.

Risks of Treatment

Just how dangerous is ECT? ECT today is less dangerous and less frightening than depicted in Ken Kesey's novel. The convulsions and resulting bone fractures have been eliminated by the use of anesthesia and muscle relaxants. The administration of oxygen and artificial respiration ensures that the patient's brain and other organs will not be deprived of oxygen if breathing stops temporarily. Patients are now instructed not to eat or drink for four to eight hours before each treatment so that vomiting is eliminated.[17]

In spite of these precautions, ECT is not entirely safe. Occasional deaths are reported, usually due to cardiac arrest. It is difficult to compare the number of deaths caused by ECT to the number of lives it prolongs because data on mortality from depression are scanty and vary from study to study. However, David Avery and George Winokur at the University of Iowa compiled mortality data from many different studies of depressed patients. Their summary suggested that about 10 percent of untreated depressed patients die during the three years after they become ill. Only about 3 percent of the patients receiving ECT die during the same period.[18] According to these data, ECT saves the lives of about 7 percent of the people receiving it. On the other hand, ECT kills only between 0.01 and 0.8 percent of the patients who receive it.[19] These statistics indicate that ECT prolongs between 10 and 100 times as many lives as it takes. The number of lives saved is probably underestimated by this calculation because a patient who receives ECT is usually seriously ill and, therefore, is probably more prone to suicide and accidental death than are other depressed patients.

One might suppose that passing large amounts of current through the brain must cause permanent damage. Indeed, ECT has caused brain damage in animal experiments, but more shocks, more prolonged shocks, or more intense shocks were used than are used in ECT treatment of depressed patients.[20] Some autopsy reports describe brain damage in patients who had received ECT, but there is no way to know whether ECT caused the damage. Many of these patients were severely disturbed. Their psychiatric symptoms might have been the result of brain damage that occurred long before they received ECT.

Only when the patient with brain damage dies shortly after receiving ECT can doctors find out whether ECT is the culprit. If the pathologist believes that the brain damage is recent, ECT might well be to blame. If the damage is several years old, ECT is not the cause. But because patients rarely die soon after receiving ECT, there is not enough information to draw any firm conclusions. The few autopsy reports describing recent brain damage in ECT patients predated the use of anesthesia and oxygen. Thus, inadequate oxygenation during ECT delivery might have caused the brain damage.[21] In the modern literature, we found only one case describing brain damage in a patient who died two months after ECT. In this patient clearly, the damage had been present for more than two months.[22] Another kind of observation also suggests that ECT does not cause gross brain damage. One patient's brain was inspected with computerized tomography (see Chapter 1) before and after ECT; no changes were found.[23] Of course, none of this rules out the possibility of microscopic changes in the brain cells and synapses, changes that could be just as devastating to brain function as gross damage visible at autopsy or with computerized tomography.

The only convincing way to find out whether ECT causes permanent, significant brain damage is to ask the patients how they feel and watch how they behave. Although most patients are confused and disoriented immediately after ECT, they recover quickly. According to the patients, memory loss is the only problem that outlasts this immediate confusion. Dr. Larry Squire at the University of California at San Diego devised elaborate tests to find out whether this complaint was justified. To some extent, it was. Patients clearly had memory deficits for the first few weeks after ECT. They had difficulty in reading and recalling a short story or in drawing a geometric design from memory. They could not remember current events, television shows, or past events in their own lives. Fortunately, Dr. Squire found that memory recovered virtually completely. The only clear deficit that remained was amnesia for the few days before the ECT treatments.[24] Though memory loss can be avoided almost completely if only one side of the brain is shocked, some psychiatrists continue to give ECT bilaterally because they believe that it is more effective. Others disagree.[25]

In spite of the results of memory tests, many patients insisted that they had permanent deficits. They were certain that their memory was not as good as it used to be. They felt that something subtle was wrong that the psychologist's memory tests did not detect. Perhaps they were right. Dr. Squire's tests hinted, but did not con-

they learned that it causes catecholamines to leak out of the synaptic vesicles into the interior of the synaptic terminal where the transmitter is destroyed by enzymes. Because nerve impulses can release only transmitter that is inside vesicles, reserpine treatment depletes the transmitter available for release.

The discovery of iproniazid, the original monoamine oxidase inhibitor (MAOI), further bolstered the catecholamine/indoleamine theory of depression. Iproniazid was first used to treat tuberculosis. Doctors noticed that it often improved the depressed mood that is so common in patients with chronic illness. MAOIs increase the amount of catecholamines or indoleamines in the synaptic cleft by inhibiting the enzyme (monoamine oxidase) in the presynaptic terminals that destroy these transmitters. When the transmitters are not destroyed, the amount in the vesicles increases. Consequently, more is released in response to a nerve impulse. According to the transmitter deficiency theory of depression, the increased transmitter release is the basis of the antidepressant action of MAOIs. Thus, the cellular actions of reserpine and MAOIs both fit the theory: reserpine decreases transmitter release and causes depression while MAOIs increase transmitter release and relieve depression.

Experiments on the effects of imipramine on the brain provide additional evidence that a deficiency of norepinephrine is important in depression. Because the chemical structure of imipramine is similar to that of the phenothiazines, imipramine was examined during a search for improved antipsychotic drugs. Although imipramine did not have antipsychotic properties, it did lighten the mood of some patients who had depressive symptoms in addition to schizophrenia.[2] The Nobel Prize-winning biochemist Julius Axelrod and his colleague Jacques Glowinski showed that imipramine increased transmission at norepinephrine synapses by blocking the reuptake of norepinephrine into presynaptic endings. As a consequence, the transmitter was available for binding to postsynaptic receptors for a longer time.[3] To demonstrate the effect of the drug, they first determined how much norepinephrine was taken up by presynaptic endings in the absence of drug treatment. They injected radioactive norepinephrine into the ventricles (fluid filled spaces) of a rat brain. Next, they removed portions of the rat's brain and washed it to remove any radioactive norepinephrine that was not bound to the nerve cells. Finally, they measured the amount of radioactivity in the washed brain to discover how much radioactive norepinephrine had been taken up by the presynaptic endings. In their next experiment, Glowinski and Axelrod measured the effect of imipramine on norepinephrine uptake. They repeated the initial experiment, but one hour before injecting the radioactive norepinephrine, they treated the rat with imipramine. The imipramine decreased the amount of radioactive norepinephrine taken up by the presynaptic endings. This finding indicated that imipramine increased the amount of time that norepinephrine is available to the postsynaptic receptor before it is taken up by the presynaptic ending.

Later experiments in which a variety of tricyclic antidepressants were used showed that these drugs inhibited the reuptake of norepinephrine and serotonin but not dopamine.[4] Antidepressants differ from each other in their relative abilities to block norepinephrine and serotonin reuptake. Some, like amitriptyline, have their greatest effect on serotonin reuptake. Others, like desipramine, have their greatest effect on norepinephrine reuptake. Still others, like imipramine, effectively block the reuptake of both transmitters.[5]

The antidepressant effect of reuptake blockers and monoamine oxidase inhibitors and the depressant effects of reserpine provide the major evidence for the catecholamine/indoleamine theory of depression.[6] Of course, the mere fact that tricyclic antidepressants block reuptake does not prove that the catecholamine/indoleamine theory is correct. Some entirely different and unknown effect of these drugs might be responsible for their clinical effectiveness. One argument for the importance of reuptake blockade parallels one of the arguments that dopamine-receptor blockade is responsible for the clinical action of antipsychotics. As we pointed out in our discussion of schizophrenia, increasing available dopamine with amphetamines causes schizophrenic symptoms. These symptoms can be alleviated by antipsychotic drugs. Similarly, depleting nerve endings of catecholamines and indoleamines with reserpine can cause depression. This depression can be alleviated by antidepressant drugs.

The most powerful argument connecting dopamine-receptor blockade with the effectiveness of antipsychotics is that the clinical potency of an antipsychotic is well correlated with its ability to block dopamine receptors. Unfortunately, we cannot make a similar argument for the tricyclic antidepressants because antidepressants are not very different from each other in potency. Therefore, the evidence that blockade of reuptake is the basis of antidepressant action is not nearly as strong as is the evidence that blockade of dopamine receptors is responsible for the clinical actions of antipsychotics.

If the transmitter deficiency theory were correct, then depressed people should be deficient in norepinephrine and/or serotonin. This predication is difficult to test because scientists cannot directly measure transmitters in the human brain. However, they think that they can identify low or high transmitter levels by measuring breakdown products of some transmitters in urine or cerebrospinal fluid. The assumption behind taking these measurements is that more transmitter produces more breakdown product. The major breakdown product of brain norepinephrine, 3-methoxy-4-hydroxyphenylglycol (MHPG), is most conveniently measured in the urine. Unfortunately, the amount of MHPG in the urine is not a perfectly accurate measure of norepinephrine in the brain because only about half the urinary MHPG originates in the brain.[7] Nevertheless, some depressed patients have low urinary MHPG levels. Presumably, these patients are deficient in norepinephrine.

How can the depression of the patients who do not have an abnormally low amount of MHPG in their urine be explained? Perhaps these patients are deficient in serotonin. Measuring the major breakdown product of serotonin, 5-hydroxyindoleacetic acid (5-HIAA), is more difficult than measuring MHPG because 5-HIAA must be measured in the cerebrospinal fluid. Nevertheless, the measurement has been made on a substantial number of depressed patients; about 25 percent of them have low levels of 5-HIAA.[8] Presumably, these patients are deficient in serotonin.

The catecholamine/indoleamine theory would be convincing if every depressed patient had low 5-HIAA or low MHPG but not both. These findings would imply that there are two biochemical groups of depressed patients—those in one group are deficient in serotonin and those in the other are deficient in norepinephrine. Some research psychiatrists think that these two groups exist.[9] Others disagree.[10] The dissenters find that depressed patient's MHPG levels do not fall neatly into a high MHPG group and a low MHPG group. In fact, the range of levels of urinary MHPG is similar in depressed patients and healthy people. They find that many depressed patients have neither low MHPG nor low 5-HIAA and that a few have both. Unfortunately, we have to summarize the results of this type of research by saying that we do not have any firm evidence for transmitter deficiencies in depressed people.

The catecholamine/indoleamine deficiency theory fails to account for all the actions of tricyclics.[11] The long interval between beginning medication and relief of symptoms is difficult to explain for antidepressants, just as it was for antipsychotics. Reuptake inhibition begins as soon as the drug is absorbed into the blood, but relief from depression takes from seven to fourteen days. This time lag reveals that increasing norepinephrine or serotonin cannot, by itself, cure depression. At most, it is only the first step. In addition, some new and very effective antidepressants such as iprindole and mianserin have little effect on reuptake.

Because an increase in the amount of transmitter in the cleft is not an explanation for all the actions of antidepressants, scientists have recently begun searching for other changes in nerve cells caused by these drugs. One of their hypotheses is that antidepressants would alter the rate of transmitter synthesis and breakdown. If so, the drugs might increase the amount of transmitter released even if they did not affect the total amount present in the nerve cells at any one time. But the results of these investigations have been disappointing. Some experiments have shown increases while others have shown decreases. The results seem to vary with the investigators, the particular antidepressant used, and the transmitter measured.[12]

At about the time that antidepressants begin to work, certain types of postsynaptic norepinephrine receptors become less sensitive to transmitter.[13] Some scientists think that the effectiveness of antidepressant drugs depends, at least in part, on this decrease in receptor sensitivity. We speculate that the biochemical events causing depression progress as follows. In some patients, the initial malfunction is a deficiency of transmitter. This deficiency causes receptors to become supersensitive. In other patients, there is no transmitter deficiency. Receptor supersensitivity may be the primary defect. Perhaps, to alleviate depression, all functions of the norepinephrine synapses must be normalized. If so, an antidepressant must be able to increase the available transmitter and normalize receptor sensitivity. It appears that most antidepressants can do both. However, an antidepressant that has only one of the effects might still be useful for some patients.

We do not know for certain that a depressed person has super-sensitive catecholamine or indoleamine receptors, but the idea that receptor sensitivity can change in disease states and in response to drugs is not just idle speculation. In neuroscience, there are many well-documented examples.[14] Several types of synaptic receptors, including norepinephrine receptors, become supersensitive when they are deprived of transmitter. In addition, all biological treatments for depression decrease the sensitivity of postsynaptic norepinephrine receptors. These treatments include conventional tricyclics, newer antidepressants that do not inhibit reuptake, MAOIs, and electroconvulsive therapy. In addition, the supersensitivity theory accounts for the time lag that exists between the beginning of drug therapy and the relief of symptoms. The decrease in depressive symptoms and the decrease in receptor sensitivity begin at the same time.[15] In summary, supersensitivity of the norepinephrine receptor may be an important part of the cellular explanation of depression, but we do not think it is the complete explanation. That we do not yet have.

Side Effects of Antidepressants

Antidepressants are no exception to the dictum that all drugs have unwanted side effects.[16] Fortunately, most side effects are transient; they are the worst during the first one to two weeks of therapy and tend to decrease thereafter. Here we discuss some of the most common ones. However, we do not provide a complete list of side effects and contraindications in this chapter.

Modifying norepinephrine-receptor sensitivity and inhibiting norepinephrine and serotonin reuptake are not the only ways that antidepressants alter synaptic function. Blockade of certain acetylcholine synapses is responsible for the anticholinergic side effects: dry mouth, blurred vision, urinary retention, impotence, and constipation. These side effects are both more common and more severe in patients taking antidepressants than in patients taking antipsychotics, and tricyclics are worse offenders than are MAOIs. Most anticholinergic side effects are not serious, but urinary retention and severe constipation can be. Should either of these occur, the patient should alert his physician immediately. Anticholinergic side effects are particularly likely to occur with a sudden increase in dose. For this reason, most physicians start the patient on a small dose and increase it gradually.

Unfortunately, many patients with schizophrenic symptoms also have depressive symptoms. But many of these patients should not receive both antipsychotics and antidepressants. The two types of drug should be used together only with extreme caution because the anticholinergic effects of one can add to the anticholinergic effects of the other. Occasionally, the summed effects of the two drugs cause a severe anticholinergic crisis, with such symptoms as delerium, seizures, and heart irregularities.

Fortunately, tricyclics do seem to distinguish between norepinephrine and dopamine synapses. Because these drugs do not block dopamine synapses, they do not cause the motor side effects that are so often troublesome to patients taking antipsychotics. In particular, tricyclics do not cause tardive dyskinesia. In high doses, tricyclic antidepressants can block norepinephrine receptors. Scientists do not know whether this action is significant in humans, but it may contribute to some of the side effects of antidepressants.

Because tricyclics affect norepinephrine and acetylcholine synapses, they affect the cardiovascular system. Synapses using these transmitters control heart rate and blood pressure. These synapses are in the brain, in the heart, and on the muscles controlling the size of the blood vessels. Because control of heart rate and blood pressure is so complex, the precise effect of antidepressants varies from patient to patient. Usually, heart rate increases and blood pressure drops, but the opposite effects can also occur. The most serious effect of tricyclics on the heart is that its rhythm may become abnormal. Orthostatic hypotension, dizziness due to low blood pressure in the brain (see Chapter 8), is common in patients taking tricyclics. Occasionally, there is a decrease in the ability of the heart to pump blood, leading to cardiac failure. Because of these cardiovascular side effects, tricyclics must be prescribed with extreme caution for patients with cardiovascular disease and for elderly persons.

Tinnitus, ringing in the ears, has recently been reported by a few patients taking tricyclics.[17] Its cause is unknown. Although we have found only one published study on this side effect and although the study did not use placebo controls, we find the report credible for two reasons. First, tinnitus is a rather specific symptom, and the patients had no reason to expect it. Second, the tinnitus disappeared when tricyclics were discontinued or reduced. In some cases, dose reduction eliminated the tinnitus without causing a relapse of depression.

In the last few years, scientists have developed several new antidepressants with chemical structures that are quite different from the conventional tricyclics. Some are unusual variations of the tricyclic structure; others have varying numbers and configurations of carbon rings. Some of these compounds have very different side effects from the conventional tricyclics. In particular, the new antidepressants may not cause adverse effects on the cardiovascular system and may produce fewer anticholinergic side effects.[18] These antidepressants are, however, not as well studied as the conventional ones. Thus, the full spectrum of their side effects may not be known.

MAOIs have some of the same side effects as tricyclics—for example, mild anticholinergic side effects and orthostatic hypotension. But MAOIs pose some serious dangers that tricyclics do not. Because inhibition of monoamine oxidase prevents the normal metabolism of many foods and drugs, MAOIs can cause toxic chemicals to accumulate in the blood. For example, a patient taking MAOIs must avoid foods containing the amino acid, tyramine. In a healthy person, tyramine is metabolized by monoamine oxidases in the liver and never affects other organs. But the liver of a patient taking an MAOI cannot efficiently metabolize tyramine; hence, it enters the circulation. Tyramine releases catecholamine from the nerve terminals that regulate blood pressure, causing a sudden increase in blood pressure and, occasionally, even a stroke. Smaller amounts of tyramine cause milder increases in blood pressure and a variety of unpleasant symptoms such as a throbbing headache, nausea, and vomiting. Unfortunately, a wide variety of foods contain enough tyramine to be dangerous. Aged cheese is the main culprit, but many other foods such as beer, wine, chocolate, and liver are also hazardous.[19]

Likewise, patients taking MAOIs probably should not use nose drops or cold remedies that shrink mucous membranes. These drugs are chemically similar to catecholamines and are normally metabolized by monoamine oxidases. When MAOIs prevent the metabolism of these drugs, their concentration in the blood may become sufficient to cause dangerous increases in blood pressure.

Patients taking MAOIs must use other drugs very cautiously

and must take smaller doses than typically prescribed.[20] These drugs include alcohol, barbiturates, opiates, and tricyclic antidepressants. Because of the inhibition of monoamine oxidase, drugs metabolized in the liver remain in the blood and in the brain for much longer than they normally would. If a second dose is taken at the usual interval, drug concentration may become dangerously high. In addition, the combination of MAOIs and tricyclics poses a special risk. It can cause high fever, convulsions, and death. Some psychiatrists, however, believe that the combination can be used safely if the patient is monitored carefully so that any problem can be treated before it becomes serious.

Even a clear-thinking and conscientious person who is not depressed might have difficulty remembering all the prohibitions—from cheese to nose drops—that accompany MAOIs. Following complex instructions becomes more difficult when depression causes cognitive problems. The patient may eat dangerous foods inadvertently in a restaurant or when visiting family or friends. Furthermore, the suicidal patient can use the prohibited foods to serve his suicidal intentions.

Although the dangers are real dangers, they should not preclude the prescription of MAOIs. For many patients, their benefits outweigh their risks. Fatalities are rare, about 0.4 per 100,000 patients.

The physician may be uncertain about how to respond when a patient reports side effects from antidepressants. These side effects, like those of antipsychotics, are often similar to symptoms of the original disease. Common symptoms of untreated depression and anxiety, such as fatigue, constipation, sweating, dry mouth, and palpitations, can also be side effects of antidepressant drugs. When a patient complains about side effects and the symptoms are merely annoying, the physician might: (1) decrease the medication if he thinks the symptoms are due to overdose, (2) increase the medication if he thinks the symptoms are due to depression, or (3) keep the dose the same if he thinks the symptoms are normal side effects that will decrease with time. Of course, if the side effects are medically dangerous (for example, severe constipation or inability to urinate), the psychiatrist cannot take any chances. The patient must cease taking the drug and be treated for the side effect.

There is no convincing evidence that one antidepressant is more effective than any other. Physicians frequently choose an antidepressant based on the patient's symptoms. It is a common belief that the sedating antidepressants are the best choice for agitated patients while the nonsedating drugs are best for those with psychomotor retardation. This method of selection is a commonsense approach, but research has not supported it. The antidepressant effect of a drug is unrelated to its sedative properties. Often, the choice of a particular antidepressant, like the choice of a particular antipsychotic, is dictated by its side effects. A person who must be alert on the job (for instance, someone operating heavy machinery) is usually given a nonsedating antidepressant. A person who has trouble falling asleep may be given a sedating antidepressant with instructions to take the entire daily dose at bedtime.

14

Lithium, Mania, and Depression

Bipolar disorder is much less common than major depression, but it is not a rare disease.[1] In fact, it is about as common as schizophrenia. One's lifetime expectancy for bipolar disease is between 0.5 and 2.0 percent. Because major depression is about ten times as prevalent, this percentage indicates that about one out of every ten patients with an affective disorder has at least one episode of mania. Bipolar illness is about equally common in men and women.[2] It usually begins in young adulthood, typically in the late twenties or early thirties. It is no respecter of social class or upbringing. Stress and loss, whether occurring in childhood or near the time of illness, cannot account for it.[3] The adoption study previously described suggests that genes play a major role.[4] Some studies found that the families of bipolar patients tend to be unstable, but this finding does not demonstrate that unstable families cause bipolar illness.[5] More likely, the genes that afflict the children with bipolar disorder are also present in the parents, thus producing unstable families.

Acceptance of Lithium in Psychiatry

Lithium carbonate is a very effective treatment for affective illness, particularly bipolar disorder. Unlike antipsychotics and antidepressants, lithium carbonate is not a complex organic molecule; it is a simple salt. Lithium was introduced into psychiatry in 1949 by John Cade, an Australian psychiatrist and researcher who was testing the hypothesis that uric acid caused excited behavior. When he injected the lithium salt of uric acid, lithium urate, into guinea pigs, they became calm and unresponsive instead of excited. When he put them on their backs, they lay quietly instead of trying to scramble to their feet. When he poked or prodded them, they did not scamper away. Cade concluded that lithium was a calming drug. In another of those leaps of faith that are possible only outside the jurisdiction of a strict drug regulatory agency, he tried lithium carbonate on ten patients with mania, on six with schizophrenia, and on three with depression. Only the manic patients were helped, but these patients improved dramatically.[6]

Although Cade's clinical trial was successful, his report generated very little interest among psychiatrists, perhaps for a number of reasons.[7] Maybe the psychiatrists just could not believe that a simple salt could treat a disease as complex as manic-depressive psychosis, now called bipolar disorder. Or perhaps they could not believe that a single drug could protect against both mania and depression. If so, they were espousing the fallacy that causes many a layman to reject all psychiatric drugs: drugs can only suppress; they cannot normalize. Or perhaps the psychiatrists were not excited because the drug companies had no interest in promoting a drug on which they could not make huge profits. Because the chemical itself is plentiful and cheap, it could not be patented and given a fancy name like "Normavil" and an accompanying fancy price.

Until the middle 1960s, lithium treatment and research were kept alive primarily by the Danish psychiatrist, Mogens Schou, who firmly established the effectiveness of lithium. Schou's research persuaded most psychiatrists that lithium was an effective treatment for mania, but it was not approved by the U.S. Food and Drug Administration (FDA) until 1970.[8] The FDA held back out of concern that lithium was dangerous. In the 1940s, lithium had been widely used as a salt substitute for cardiac patients. Dosage was not monitored, and consumption of toxic quantities led to coma and death in a few patients. The FDA scientists insisted on extensive testing before they were persuaded that, properly monitored, lithium treatment was safe. Finally, it was approved for the treatment of bipolar disorder, but not for any other diagnoses.[9]

Lithium Treatment for Mania

Lithium calms manic patients. Continued lithium therapy protects them against future manic episodes and against future depressive episodes. Lithium's effects can be astounding. When the drug removes the wraps of mania, it often reveals a healthy person, a person very different from the bipolar patient.

Anna's story, which follows, illustrates the change lithium can bring about in the life of a bipolar patient. (Anna's story is elaborated from a case described by a team of well-known psychiatrists at the National Institute of Mental Health [NIMH] and the Illinois State Psychiatric Unit).[10] Anna was a 21-year-old college student. Before she became ill, Anna was sedate and polite, perhaps even a bit prim. During the fall of her sophomore year at college, she had an episode of mild depression that began when she received a C on a history paper she had worked quite hard on. The same day she received a sanctimonious letter from her father reminding her of the financial hardships he was undergoing to send her to college. He warned her to stick to her books and not to play around with men. Anna became discouraged. She doubted that she deserved her parents' sacrifice. Anna's depression did not seem unusual to her roommate, to her other friends, or even to Anna herself. It seemed a natural reaction to her father's unreasonable letter and her fear that she could not live up to the standards he set. In retrospect, this mild depression was the first episode of her bipolar illness.

Several months later, Anna became restless, angry, and obnoxious. She talked continuously and rapidly, jumping from one idea to another. Her speech was filled with rhymes, puns, and sexual innuendoes. During Christmas vacation, she made frequent and unwelcome sexual overtures to her brother's friend in the presence of her entire family. When Anna's mother asked her to behave more politely, Anna began to cry and then slapped her mother across the mouth. Anna did not sleep that night. She sobbed. Between sobs she screamed that no one understood her problems, and no one would even try. The next day, Anna's family took her to the hospital. She was given chlorpromazine, which calmed her. When she was discharged two weeks later, she was less angry and no longer assaultive. But she was not well and did not go back to school. Her thought and speech were still hypomanic (slightly manic). She had an exaggerated idea of her attractiveness and expected men to fall for her at the first smile. She was irritated when they ignored her attentions. Depressive symptoms were still mixed with the manic ones. She often cried when her bids for attention were not successful or when her parents criticized her dress or behavior.

Anna returned to school the following fall but suffered another depressive episode, followed by another attack of mania within seven months. She had to withdraw from school and enter the hospital. This time, Anna was fortunate to enter a research unit that was authorized to use lithium. The psychiatrists diagnosed her illness as bipolar disorder. Because she was so agitated, they began treatment with chlorpromazine as well as lithium. The initial sedative action of the chlorpromazine rapidly calmed her agitation, and this drug was discontinued after only a few days. As the effects of the chlorpromazine subsided, the lithium began to take effect. After seventeen days on lithium, Anna's behavior was quite normal. She was attractively and modestly dressed for her psychiatric interviews. Earlier, she had been sloppily seductive: hair in disarray, half-open blouse, smeared lipstick, bright pink rouge on her cheeks, and bright green make-up on her eyelids. With the help of lithium, she gained some ability to tolerate frustration. During the first week of her hospital stay, she had screamed at a nurse who would not permit her to read late into the night in violation of the ward's 11:00 P.M. "lights out" policy. On lithium, Anna was still annoyed by this "juvenile" rule, but she controlled her anger. She gained some insight into her illness, recognizing that her manic behavior was destructive to herself and others. She also recognized the depression that was often mixed with the mania. She speculated that the mania was an attempt to cover up depression. She admitted, "Actually, when I'm high, I'm really feeling low. I need to exaggerate in order to feel more important."

Because Anna was on a research ward, the effectiveness of lithium had to be verified by removal of the drug. When she had been off lithium for four to five days, Anna began to show symptoms of both mania and depression. She threatened her psychiatrist, and as before, the threats were grandiose with sexual overtones. In a slinky voice, she warned, "I have ways to put the director of this hospital in my debt. He crawled for me before and he'll do it again. When I snap my fingers, he'll come down to this ward and squash you under his foot." Soon afterward, she threatened suicide. She later explained, "I felt so low last night that if someone had given me a knife or gun, POW." By the ninth day off lithium, Anna's speech was almost incomprehensible: "It's sad to be so putty, pretty, so much like water dripping from a faucet. . . ." (Is it surprising that distinguishing a hostile manic patient from a schizophrenia patient is so difficult—that mistakes are often made?) Lithium therapy was reinstituted, and within about sixteen days, Anna again recovered and was discharged on lithium.

Anna's recovery is typical. Within one to two weeks of beginning lithium therapy, most manic patients are well on their way to recovery. Because lithium produces no enduring sedative effects, it does not slow down patients' thoughts or subdue their feelings. Thus, college students can return to school and work normally. Managers, executives, and writers can perform as well as they did before they became ill. Lithium patients feel the normal range of human emotions. Mania is prevented, but happiness is not. These patients experience love, sexuality, pride, friendship, and compassion just as normal people do. Likewise, the depression that may have been mixed with the mania is gone, but the ability to feel sadness is not. Lithium patients are disappointed by failure, and they grieve at the loss of a loved one. Indeed, normal people who take lithium for a few days or weeks experience its side effects but do not detect any dramatic psychological changes. Some experience a slight feeling of detachment, as if they were viewing the world from behind a glass wall. Most notice no change in mood or alertness.[11] The normalizing effects of lithium on mood have been likened to the normalizing effects of aspirin on temperature. Aspirin brings down a fever but does not change the temperature of a healthy person.

Lithium does not work for everyone who needs it. Although the results of research studies vary, it is fair to say that about 80 percent of all manic patients respond to lithium.[12] Psychiatrists do not know how to explain the failures. Improper diagnosis is always a possible explanation, but we have no direct evidence to support it. Another possible explanation is that there are several biologically different categories of bipolar patients—one category includes those who are responsive to lithium and one includes those who are nonresponsive. This hypothesis is supported by the fact that lithium responders are more likely than nonresponders to have bipolar patients in their immediate families.[13] Still another possibility is that the nonresponders have not received an adequate dose of lithium. Some might respond to a higher dose. Lithium is effective only if its concentration in the blood is maintained within narrow limits. Too little is ineffective. Too much is toxic.

Lithium's ability to protect patients against relapse is so dramatic that the effect of placebo is inconsequential by comparison. One of the pioneers in lithium therapy, Mogens Schou, compared the relapse rate when patients and doctors knew that placebo had been substituted for lithium with the relapse rate when patients and doctors were blind to placebo substitution. The two relapse rates were not different.[14]

Is lithium a specific treatment for mania or might other treatments be equally effective? The other obvious candidates are antipsychotics. Researchers have done a number of studies to find out which treatment is more effective, but they have not managed to resolve the issue.[15] Antipsychotics, because of their initial sedative effect, act more promptly than lithium to slow speech, inhibit aggressiveness, and decrease rapid-fire activity. Lithium works only gradually and does not decrease manic symptoms for seven to fourteen days. Some psychiatrists, like Anna's, recommend a few days of antipsychotic treatment along with lithium treatment until the lithium begins to work. Manic patients receiving only antipsychotics and those receiving only lithium score very closely on psychiatric rating scales that measure mania; yet more lithium patients become well enough to leave the hospital. Some psychiatrists suggest that this discrepancy between the measurements on rating scales and hospital release rates exists because the rating scales are insensitive to the different effects of the two drugs. They believe that antipsychotics subdue manic patients while lithium normalizes them. Obviously, this hypothesis cannot be substantiated until improved rating scales are developed.

Like other psychiatric drugs, lithium is not a permanent cure. If the patient stops taking it, he is likely to relapse into mania or depression. Double-blind studies prove unequivocally that lithium protects bipolar patients against both mania and depression. Without lithium, the typical bipolar patient has about one manic episode every fourteen months and about one depressive episode every seventeen months. With lithium maintenance, his manic episodes occur only once every nine years and his depressive episodes only once every four years. Without lithium, he spends an average of eight to thirteen weeks per year in the hospital. If he takes lithium, he is hospitalized for less than two weeks per year.[16]

One group of psychiatrists tried to estimate the economic benefits of lithium treatment.[17] Lithium capsules, accompanied by a monthly or bimonthly blood test and a brief psychiatric interview, are obviously much cheaper than intensive psychotherapy and eight weeks of hospitalization per year. Lithium has cut in half the cost of treating bipolar disorder. In the United States, this savings represents approximately 270 million dollars per year. The patients and their families are not the only people to benefit from these savings. Anyone who buys medical insurance benefits, too. Lithium also permits bipolar patients to be economically productive. Before lithium, bipolar illness caused a loss in work productivity equaling about 152 million dollars per year. Lithium has decreased this yearly loss to about 40 million dollars. Again, this savings benefits everyone, not just the patients and their relatives.

The Role of Psychotherapy

We were unable to find a single controlled study on the effectiveness of psychotherapy in treating mania. However, Ronald R. Fieve discussed psychotherapy for bipolar patients in his book *Moodswing*. Fieve is one of the foremost authorities on lithium in the United States but was trained in the psychoanalytic tradition. He described the frustrations of the early years of his career, which he devoted to treating depressed and manic patients with psychotherapy. He did not think he accomplished very much. When a manic patient improved after months of therapy, he was never certain that psychotherapy had played a role. The improvement was usually a spontaneous mood swing and did not last very long. When he began to treat patients with antidepressants and lithium, he saw dramatic improvement in just a few weeks. With lithium maintenance therapy, the improvement was permanent.[18]

Fieve's observations are, of course, only anecdotal; they are not scientific evidence. Yet there seems to be no experimental evidence for or against the effectiveness of psychotherapy for mania. We surmise that research psychiatrists do not want to waste their time proving what seems obvious from clinical experience—that psychotherapy is not an effective treatment for mania.

Fieve's view of the appropriate uses of psychotherapy is similar to that of Gerald Klerman and Myrna Weissman at the NIMH.

Fieve recognized that problems in living often result from prolonged affective illness. Psychotherapy is often helpful in solving
these problems once the underlying mania and depression have
been relieved.

Should Hypomania Be Treated?

When a depressed person refuses maintenance drug treatment, she
is expressing an opinion about antidepressant drugs and making
inferences about long-term drug use. For instance, she may not like
the idea that her mental health depends on a drug. She may not
want to admit that she has a chronic illness. She may not be willing
to tolerate the side effects. In spite of these objections, she is not
choosing illness in preference to health. Some bipolar patients may
refuse lithium maintenance for these same reasons. But others refuse
lithium for a different reason: they do not want to be cured. They
enjoy their hypomanic periods and are loath to give them up.
Artists may feel that they are most creative when hypomanic; businesspeople may feel most enterprising; homemakers may feel most
efficient.

In *Moodswing*, Ronald R. Fieve told the story of a well-known
modern painter who suffered from a bipolar illness that threatened
to destroy his life.[19] During his hypomanic periods, the artist was
enormously productive. His canvases were bright and showed a
creative use of color. Thus, he gained considerable critical acclaim.
Unfortunately, his moods and hence his work were not consistent.
Hypomania inevitably gave way to depression. During his depressed
periods, the artists not only refused to paint, but refused to eat. He
would not see his friends. He slept 16 hours out of 24.

In spite of the debilitating depressions, the artist was reluctant
to take lithium. He feared that, without hypomania, he would lose
his creativity. Without his hypomanic passions and generosity, his
family and friends might cease to love him. The risks were too
great. He would not give up hypomania merely to escape the
depression that inexorably followed. Fieve commented that as long
as a patient is merely hypomanic, he should not be pressured into
taking lithium.

But when the hypomania becomes mania, some treatment must
be initiated. Late one night, a 747 from New York to San Francisco

made an unscheduled stop in Chicago so that the artist could be taken off the airplane and hospitalized. He had adamantly insisted on holding a prayer meeting in the aisles, and the flight attendants could not control him. During another manic period, he squandered all his family's resources on a trip to Hawaii that he was certain would put him in contact with influential art dealers. In fact, the artist could not negotiate with art dealers while in a manic state. His demanding and arrogant tone antagonized them. The manic artist nonetheless painted energetically, convinced that his work was inspired. In reality, it was merely disorganized. After his manic high receded, he realized that his "inspiration was ridiculous."

After the manic episode on the 747, Ronald Fieve felt that the artist needed continuous lithium therapy. Fieve persuaded him to examine the havoc left in the wake of mania. The artist realized that another episode might destroy his family. In spite of his fears, he decided to take lithium. His fears were unfounded. He did not need hypomania to paint: his paintings continued to be well received. Fieve did not describe the effect of lithium on the artist's family, but we suspect that he did not need hypomania to be lovable. Normal hugs and thoughtful small gifts probably made his family happier than did explosive bear hugs and extravagant purchases he could ill afford.

Lithium Treatment for Depression

Once a bipolar patient has responded to treatment, lithium prevents relapses of both depression and mania, just as it did for Anna. Might lithium also be an effective treatment for depressive episodes in bipolar patients or patients suffering from major depression? The research data on lithium as a treatment for depression are not very encouraging. Some depressed patients respond to lithium, and the drug is more likely to succeed with bipolar patients than with unipolar patients. But a tricyclic is more apt to produce results if a person begins treatment in a depressed episode.[20] Unfortunately, some bipolar patients do not respond well to tricyclics. Instead of restoring the normal mood, a tricyclic may precipitate a switch from depression to mania. When a psychiatrist prescribes an antidepressant for a bipolar patient, he should observe the patient very carefully. If manic symptoms develop, the patient must cease taking the tricyclic. Some recent evidence indicates that maintaining an adequate lithium level may prevent the switch to mania that is occasionally caused by tricyclics.[21] If this finding proves to be correct, tricyclics will become more useful to bipolar patients.

Although lithium is not an effective drug for terminating an episode of depression that is already in progress, it does prevent depressive relapses both in patients who have major depression without mania and in those who have bipolar disorder.[22] Twenty to 30 percent of depressed patients taking lithium relapse in a year, about the same percentage that relapses on tricyclics. The fact that 70 percent would relapse on placebo shows that both treatments are effective.

When a patient suffers from recurrent depression, the psychiatrist, in consultation with the patient, must decide whether the patient should take preventive medicine and, if so, whether it should be lithium, an antidepressant, or both. If the symptoms are primarily depressive, but there are also hints of mania (for example, irritability or restlessness), lithium may be the best choice. If the patient suffers frequent depressive episodes on lithium, a combination of lithium and a tricyclic is likely to be the best treatment.[23] However, if adding the tricyclic provokes mania, lithium alone may be the only practical approach. At present, psychiatrists have no a priori way of predicting precisely what treatment will work best for a particular patient. Of course, side effects are also a major consideration in drug selection. If the patient cannot tolerate anticholinergic side effects, perhaps lithium is the better choice. If the patient's work requires delicate coordination, he may not tolerate the lithium tremor. (We discuss lithium side effects later in this chapter.)

The Biology of Lithium

As we might have expected from our study of antidepressants, lithium affects both norepinephrine and serotonin synapses. During the first few days of lithium treatment, transmitter synthesis and breakdown increase. This increased metabolism of transmitter would increase the amount of transmitter in the cleft. On the other hand, lithium decreases release of transmitter and enhances its reuptake.

These effects would decrease the amount of transmitter in the cleft.[24] Lithium also decreases the effectiveness of catecholamine synapses by inhibiting the synthesis of camp that is normally activated by norepinephrine.[25] But these effects on synapses cannot be the basis of lithium's therapeutic effects because the synaptic changes begin almost simultaneously with lithium treatment while symptoms of mania are not relieved for one to two weeks. Furthermore, the effectiveness of lithium often increases over several months. Therefore, a correct explanation of lithium's therapeutic effects must be based on cellular changes that build up slowly over weeks or months after lithium therapy has begun.

The major unanswered question about the biological effects of lithium is how lithium can protect against both mania and depression. Some investigators have suggested that depression is caused by supersensitive receptors (Chapter 12) and mania, by subsensitive receptors. The cause of the supersensitivity is unknown, but researchers think that the subsensitivity might result from an excess of norepinephrine. The scientists hypothesized that lithium stabilizes the membrane, preventing both supersensitivity and subsensitivity.[26] There is some evidence for this hypothesis, but it is not overwhelming. Lithium can prevent drug-induced supersensitivity at catecholamine synapses, but it fails to prevent drug-induced subsensitivity.[27] The only evidence for the receptor subsensitivity explanation of mania is a single report that manic patients have an abnormally high level of norepinephrine in their cerebrospinal fluid.[28]

The following explanation might resolve the paradox of how lithium protects against both mania and depression. However, we emphasize that our explanation is only speculative. We present it as a framework on which to hang the experimental facts, not as a proven theory. Assume, as we did in Chapter 12, that depression is always associated with a supersensitivity of norepinephrine receptors that may or may not be accompanied by a catecholamine deficiency. Also assume that excessive stimulation of catecholamine receptors can provoke mania. In the bipolar patient, perhaps the release of norepinephrine intermittently becomes much greater than normal. We do not know what causes these norepinephrine surges, but they might be a response to environmental events. During a norepinephrine surge, the patient has both an excess of norepinephrine and supersensitive norepinephrine receptors. His norepinephrine response becomes excessive, and he switches into mania. Lithium can prevent the switch into mania by preventing supersensitivity and, hence, the excessive response to a burst of norepinephrine production. At the same time, preventing supersensitivity protects against depression because supersensitive receptors cause depression in the absence of excess norepinephrine.

Side Effects

When we discussed antipsychotics and antidepressants, we preceded our discussions of their side effects with a description of how these drugs act on the brain. We then tried to explain the side effects in terms of the biology. For lithium, we can only describe the side effects. Neuroscientists do not yet understand their biological basis.

Lithium can produce many unpleasant side effects, but fortunately, most patients experience only a few. Even these usually disappear in one to four weeks. The most common side effects are weakness, tremor, fatigue, nausea, vomiting, abdominal cramps, diarrhea, weight gain, sleeplessness, and lethargy.[29] The psychiatrist should warn the patient of these temporary side effects and encourage her to persist with lithium therapy until she has had a chance to reap its benefits. A fine tremor is the only neurological effect that is likely to remain beyond the first month of therapy.[30] The tremor will not bother most patients but may disturb those whose livelihoods depend on precise coordination. For instance, surgeons, dancers, jewelers, violinists, and athletes may be unwilling to tolerate the lithium tremor. Fortunately, it can frequently be alleviated by propanalol, a drug that blocks certain norepinephrine receptors.[31]

The major danger in lithium therapy is that the prescribed dose will be too high, resulting in lithium poisoning. The psychiatrist cannot know the correct dose in advance because each patient's body eliminates lithium at a different rate. Determination of the correct dose requires measurement of lithium concentration in the blood. At the beginning of treatment, the amount of lithium in the patient's blood changes rapidly. Therefore, lithium concentration must be measured frequently. After the proper dose is established and the lithium concentration stabilized, blood concentration needs to be measured only three to twelve times per year. Reasonably frequent measurements are important because changes in diet, health, and activity can cause marked changes in lithium concentration even though the patient is taking his lithium precisely as directed. Failure to adjust lithium intake can cause relapse when the lithium level is too low. Toxicity can result when the lithium level is too high.[32]

Lithium toxicity primarily affects the brain. Its symptoms are confusion, slurred speech, drowsiness, loss of balance, tremor, vomiting, diarrhea, and eventually, coma and death.[33] Some of these symptoms, such as drowsiness and diarrhea, are similar to those occurring at the beginning of lithium therapy. Therefore, during the early stages of drug treatment, frequent measurement of blood levels may be needed to distinguish normal side effects from incipient toxicity. If these symptoms occur in a patient who has been taking lithium for some time, the drug should be stopped and the patient should receive immediate medical attention.

Lithium sometimes affects the kidneys.[34] The kidney concentrates waste molecules so that they can be excreted in the urine with minimal loss of water. In about 7–13 percent of lithium patients, the kidney's ability to concentrate urine is decreased. Thus, these patients drink large quantities of water and excrete large quantities of dilute urine. Although frequent urination is a nuisance, it is not known whether the water loss indicates any significant kidney damage. Reports that the microscopic anatomy of the kidney is not quite normal in some lithium patients cause additional concern. Again, no one knows whether this slight abnormality is a sign of significant damage. However, there are no documented cases of kidney failure associated with lithium therapy.[35] In several studies that compared kidney function in lithium patients with kidney function in psychiatric patients taking other drugs, no evidence was found that lithium causes kidney damage.[36] The proper control group is important in studies of the effects of the drug on the kidneys because there is evidence that patients about to start lithium therapy have more kidney damage than healthy volunteers.[37]

In summary, we are uncertain whether lithium causes significant kidney damage. We think that for people with a severe affective disorder, the benefits of lithium maintenance are greater than the risks, but the risk cannot be ignored. If you or a relative take lithium, we suggest that you ask the prescribing doctor to keep you informed about current research on the effects of lithium on the kidney. Once or twice a year, ask him to reassess with you the risks and benefits of continued treatment.

15

Anxiety

Anxiety is fearful anticipation. No one likes it, but it serves useful purposes. It prevents procrastination. Without anxiety, people would play the third little pig, lazing the time away. Anxiety helps the student study instead of partying all night and sleeping all day. It prevents recklessness. Without anxiety, people would drive too fast or climb mountains without extra clothing. Anxiety subdues agressiveness. It forces the breadwinner to remain polite in the face of her boss's rudeness. Anxiety has to be unpleasant. It forces people to perform unpleasant tasks in order to avoid even greater evils.

Anxiety, however, can be excessive. It can be so intense, pervasive and persistent that it is an obstacle rather than a warning or an aid. It can be a source of constant pain with little utility. For example: Jane Able was an intelligent, hardworking college freshman. Her grades were good, although they could have been better had she been less anxious. Before her first math exam, she broke out in cold sweat and vomited. During the exam itself, her mind was so overwhelmed with anxiety that she could not see the solutions to problems that were just like the ones that she had easily solved in homework assignments. In a situation where some anxiety was justified, Jane's anxiety was excessive.

Anxiety can intrude in situations where there is much less justification. The character Annie Hall in the movie of the same name was afraid of bugs. Once she became so frightened by a spider in her bathtub that she called her ex-boyfriend to come over and kill it at 3 a.m. Mrs. Angst is an example of another type of irrational anxiety. She peered through the windows of her house but refused to go out for fear that she would be stricken helpless by panic. Her sister had to bring her groceries and other necessities.

John Traurig suffered from depression and the anxiety that usually goes with it. His small reserves of energy were wasted in self-deprecation and worry about his hopeless inadequacy. His anxiety gave him stomachaches and diarrhea. He always had a lump in his throat and had horrible headaches. For many years, his wife tried to cheer him up. She cooked his favorite food and put on pretty dresses. But nothing worked. Finally, she began getting frustrated and impatient. She started to wonder whether marriage was worth such a price, and she told John so. Yet his anxiety remained.

Mr. Mann, the building contractor, had genuinely serious problems. His wife, Mary, found a lump in her breast that the pathologist said was malignant. She had to have her breast removed. To make matters worse, the recent high interest rates had hurt Mr. Mann's business badly. He worried about how he was going to pay the medical bills and what would happen to him and his ten-year-old adopted son if Mary died. He felt he could not carry the entire load alone. Because of this stress, Mr. Mann was having trouble paying attention to his work. He forgot about a meeting he had with a city planning commissioner. Also, he was going to lose money on a remodeling project because he had forgotten to include the cost of the painter's wages when he prepared his bid. Mr. Mann had not been sleeping well, either. Sometimes he realized that the muscles in his face were aching with tension. His blood pressure was up; he felt his heart pound when he went up the steps from the carport. Mr. Mann's brother had died of a heart attack at the age of 47, and Mr. Mann himself already was 46 years old.

For Jane, Annie, and the others, anxiety itself is a major problem. Their anxiety is so intense that it is incapacitating. How should they try to control it? Should they take antianxiety drugs? Drugs would relax muscles, ease headaches, calm the mind, permit a good night's sleep. Mrs. Angst might be able to walk on the street and go shopping like other people; Jane Able could get the excellent grades that she is capable of achieving and that her hard work deserves. We discuss treatment recommendations for Jane, Mrs. Angst, and the three others in the last section of Chapter 16 after we have completed a description of the benefits and risks (especially the risk of addiction) of antianxiety drugs.

Most people are uneasy about using antianxiety drugs, at least those drugs that come in pill form. While people usually understand that too much anxiety causes serious distress and disability, they are nonetheless reluctant to treat it chemically. Psychiatric Calvinism is a more common response to anxiety than it is to schizophrenia or affective disorders. The psychiatric Calvinist believes that proper treatment requires hard work. Taking a pill is not proper treatment but just an easy way out. Despite such reservations, most people understand that some cases of excessive anxiety are nearly impossible to control with known psychological methods and that in these cases anxiety-relieving pills may be justified.

In evaluating antianxiety pills, it is important to reflect on the fact that drugs for relieving anxiety have been in use since before the beginning of written history. Mostly, people have been taking them without giving the issue serious thought and without the advice of a physician. Alcohol is one such antianxiety drug, an exceedingly effective one. Approximately two-thirds of the adult population of the United States, about 140 million people, use alcoholic beverages, and the percentage is much higher in many other countries. Unfortunately, some people use alcohol, and other antianxiety drugs as well, with so little concern about side effects that they harm themselves and their families. Despite the problems associated with antianxiety drugs, insistence on abstinence is not a solution. Alcohol's sustained popularity over thousands of years and the failure of prohibition in the United States make this point well.

Some people may object that alcohol is not really for anxiety relief but rather for recreation and relaxation. But this argument overlooks the fact that the reason alcohol is so good for recreation and relaxation is precisely because it is so effective for anxiety relief. With a little alcohol in the blood, and hence in the brain, people are not so anxious in social situations. Their fear of being embarrassed is decreased, and they are less shy. Indeed, alcohol is a genuine antianxiety drug that pharmacologically falls into the same class as all the drugs prescribed by physicians to treat anxiety. In the medical literature, these drugs are usually referred to as the sedative–hypnotics, and we use this class name in our discussion. (The most common prescription sedative–hypnotics are listed in the Appendix.)

History of Sedative–Hypnotic Drugs

In contrast to alcohol, the prescription sedative–hypnotics are new, and we have had comparatively little cultural experience with them. Barbital, the first sedative–hypnotic barbiturate, was introduced into medicine in 1903.[1] A year later, it was reported in the medical literature that some people were becoming addicted to the drug.[2] Nonetheless, organic chemists working for the drug companies continued to develop the barbiturate family of drugs by making minor chemical modifications of the barbiturate molecule. Twenty-five hundred different barbiturate drugs were synthesized and tested. Most of these were never marketed as medicine, but the fifty or so that were marketed became the dominant pills for anxiety and insomnia until the mid 1950s.

The threat of addiction with prolonged use and the possibility of death from overdose were constant sources of dissatisfaction with the barbiturates. Accordingly, the drug companies were on the lookout for new drugs that would be as relaxing as the barbiturates but less toxic and less addictive. The people at Wallace Laboratories thought they had found such a drug when they introduced Miltown (generic name, meprobamate) in 1955.[3] Miltown was the first in a long parade of new drugs that were introduced as "improvements" over the barbiturates.[4] The drug companies perceived that the people in North America and Western Europe were ready to consume billions of pills for the relief of anxiety, and they started racing with each other to capture a share of an exploding market. Doriden (glutethimide) was introduced by the USV Pharmaceutical Corporation, Quaalude (methaqualone) by William H. Rorer, Inc., Noludar (methyprylon) by Roche Laboratories, and Placidyl (ethchlorvynol) by Abbott Laboratories.[5] The newness of these drugs and their chemical distinctness from the older barbiturates were emphasized not only by their proprietary names but also by particular words selected to describe their effects. Instead of sedative–hypnotics, the new drugs were called minor tranquilizers. They became very popular with both physicians and patients. Miltown was the most popular of all.

The label "minor tranquilizers" was of greater significance in advertising than in pharmacology—the action of the minor tranquilizers was not greatly different from the action of the barbiturates. But because the minor tranquilizers were new, they could be patented, given proprietary names, and exploited for much higher profits than the familiar barbiturates. As the number of users grew from thousands to tens of thousands to millions, reports of overuse and addiction to minor tranquilizers began to appear.[6] Indeed, the drugs introduced in the 1950s were just as lethal and were just as addictive as the barbiturates.[7] Thus, these new minor tranquilizers of the 1950s were a triumph of drug marketing in the absence of any new medical benefit.

The drug companies continued to introduce new sedative–hypnotics throughout the 1960s, and the winner of the race to produce the most popular minor tranquilizer was finally Roche Laboratories, with Librium (chlordiazepoxide, 1960) and Valium (diazepam, 1962).[8] These two drugs are members of the chemical family called benzodiazepines. Thousands of benzodiazepines have been synthesized; over a hundred have been tested for medical use; and six are available in the United States as prescription drugs for the treatment of anxiety.[9] (Benzodiazepines available in the United States are listed in the Appendix.)

By the early 1970s, the benzodiazepines had nearly replaced meprobamate, barbiturates, and the other contenders as drug treatments for anxiety and insomnia. The physicians' and the public's enthusiastic acceptance of the benzodiazepines caused the use of prescription sedative–hypnotics to become much more widespread than it had ever been. The benzodiazepines became the Western world's most frequently prescribed drugs. Of individual drugs prescribed most often, Valium ranked first and Librium, third.[10] In the mid 1970s, the number of prescriptions written for benzodiazepines in the United States approached 100 million, at a cost of about 500 million dollars.[11] The pattern of consumption indicated that 10 to 20 percent of adults in the various countries of the Western world took benzodiazepines on a fairly regular basis. Women were twice as likely to use benzodiazepines as men, and older people were more likely to use them than young people.[12] Dr. D. J. Greenblatt and Dr. R. I. Shader, two prominent researchers on the effects and effectiveness of benzodiazepines, remarked that there was a "benzodiazepine bandwagon."[13]

The reasons for the enormous popularity of Valium and Librium are not fully known. Some people think that the sophisticated advertising of Roche Laboratories was a major factor.[14] Advertisements claimed that Valium and Librium relieved anxiety, tension, and insomnia at doses that seldom produced impairment of intellectual function and without significant threat of addiction when used at the recommended doses. Also, the lethal dose was said to be so high that the pills were ineffective as suicide weapons in the hands of depressed patients. In short, the pitch was that Librium and Valium relieved anxiety with fewer side effects and with greater safety than any of the drugs used previously. Most physicians apparently have been persuaded that these claims are correct. Furthermore, most patients who have taken benzodiazepines seem to be pleased with the results.[15] According to a survey conducted in Europe and published in 1974, people who had used benzodiazepines were only one-half to one-third as likely as people who had never taken these drugs to believe that the drugs "do more harm than good."[16]

The first report of benzodiazepine addiction in the medical literature appeared in 1963, three years after the introduction of Librium. Additional reports trickled in thereafter.[17] The drug ads and established medical opinion discounted these reports as cases of multiple drug overuse in which the original addiction had developed in association with some nonbenzodiazepine drug such as alcohol. Nonetheless, there was a great deal of unfavorable publicity in the mass media about addiction to "tranquilizers," and a wave of concern about benzodiazepine overprescribing began to sweep through the medical community in the early 1970s.[18] In 1975, the United States Food and Drug Administration placed the benzodiazepines on the list of controlled substances, as it had done earlier for the barbiturates and other sedative–hypnotics that were potentially addictive.[19] At about this time, physicians began to be more cautious about prescribing benzodiazepines, and the annual number of prescriptions started to decline. While there had been nearly 100 million prescriptions for benzodiazepines in 1975, there were only about 70 million in 1979.[20] The recent conservative trend in benzodiazepine prescribing has prompted some knowledgeable psychiatrists to express concern that excessive fear of addiction is preventing proper medication for many patients who could safely benefit from benzodiazepines.[21]

Appropriate Use of Benzodiazepines

The vast majority of prescriptions for benzodiazepines are not written by psychiatrists but by physicians in family practice, internal medicine, and gynecology. This pattern has developed not because psychiatrists scorn benzodiazepines but because the patients for whom the drugs are appropriate most frequently go to family practitioners or internists—for example, patients suffering from cancer, painful arthritis, back problems, and other chronic diseases. Physicians often give benzodiazepines to these patients to relieve the anxiety, uneasiness, and dread that accompany their stressful illnesses. Family practitioners also see many patients who have vague complaints of aches and pains that do not lead to a diagnosis of an organic or mental illness. These people can greatly benefit from anxiety relief. The doctor's office is also a frequent stop for those whose main problem is excessive anxiety. These patients have a pounding heart, trouble sleeping and relaxing, headaches, or difficulty catching their breath. These bodily symptoms of anxiety suggest medical treatment, and the family physician can provide welcome relief with benzodiazepines. People who have anxiety-provoking somatic illnesses rarely consult psychiatrists. Those who do consult psychiatrists are more likely to have mental illnesses with bizarre symptoms that are not effectively treated with benzodiazepines. Consequently, psychiatrists are not the leading prescribers.[22]

Numerous symptoms suggest treatment with benzodiazepines. For example, the anxious person typically has a conscious sense of dread and fear. She may worry and ruminate that something terrible is going to happen. She is distractible, irritable, unable to concentrate, and unable to sleep. In addition, her muscles are affected by the anxiety. She feels shaky and jittery. She trembles and her eyelid may twitch. Relaxation is impossible. Her muscles may stay so tense that they ache. Her head aches, too. The strain is visible on her face. Her internal organs are also affected.

She may experience sweating, a pounding and racing heart, cold, clammy hands, a dry mouth, dizziness, light-headedness, tingling of the hands and feet, hot and cold spells, an upset stomach, frequent urination, diarrhea, a lump in the throat, butterflies in the stomach, belching, sighing, and difficulty in breathing.[23]

Excessive anxiety is seldom a disease in itself. More commonly, it springs from some other distinct illness or stress.[24] For most patients, therefore, benzodiazepine treatment should be seen as an effort to relieve suffering but not as a sufficient treatment for the overall condition. Again, a benzodiazepine's effect on anxiety is similar to aspirin's effect on a fever. It makes you feel better, but it is seldom appropriate as a *total* treatment for the illness.

This principle is obvious in patients whose anxiety is secondary to an easily diagnosed nonbrain disease such as appendicitis. The best treatment would be surgery to remove the infected appendix and a benzodiazepine to relieve the patient's worry and fear preceding the operation. If, however, the anxiety is a symptom of an underlying mental illness, such as depression, the appropriate treatment is not so clear-cut. Of course, mental illnesses are more difficult to diagnose conclusively than appendicitis. So the physician may be tempted to treat the visible anxiety with benzodiazepines and forget about the problems that are harder to understand. Treating only the anxiety with a prescription antianxiety drug is only a little wiser than self-medication with alcohol. If you take a benzodiazepine for anxiety, you should probably try to treat the cause of the anxiety with some form of organic or psychological therapy.

Anxiety and insomnia are prominent features of depression. Depression has additional symptoms such as retardation, loss of pleasure, feelings of worthlessness, and suicidal thoughts. If the depression were to be treated only with a benzodiazepine, the anxiety and insomnia might be relieved, but the other symptoms would be relatively unaffected. Several studies have shown that the benzodiazepines are inferior to the tricyclic antidepressants for the treatment of depression.[25] Because depression is common and yet easily overlooked, it is important to check carefully for it before adopting the expedient of benzodiazepine treatment.

Excessive and inappropriate anxiety is the major symptom in some mental illnesses. In the *DSM-III*, these are called the anxiety disorders. Some of the disorders in this group are generalized anxiety disorder, simple phobia, social phobia, obsessive-compulsive disorder, posttraumatic stress disorder, agoraphobia, and panic disorder.[26] The benzodiazepines are not very effective as treatments for obsessive-compulsive disorder and simple phobia.[27] These drugs are probably most effective in relieving generalized anxiety disorder.[28] However, patients with these disorders are thought to have a propensity for overuse and addiction to sedative–hypnotic drugs.[29] This propensity, unfortunately, complicates the treatment. The vast majority of patients for whom benzodiazepines work successfully have short-term anxiety reactions to stress or are in other anxiety states that cannot be clearly diagnosed by criteria in the *DSM-III*.

Agoraphobia, one of the anxiety disorders, is a fear of being alone in public places and is often accompanied by panic attacks in which the victim feels terrified of losing control and behaving in an unspecified bizarre manner. During a panic attack, the victim also suffers somatic symptoms of fear such as shortness of breath and heart palpitations. Although these are symptoms of anxiety rather than depression, the best treatment for panic attacks is a tricyclic antidepressant or an MAOI.[30] But these are not a complete treatment because often the panic attacks create generalized anxiety—the patient becomes anxious that he will have a panic attack. The secondary anxiety is often treated with benzodiazepines. Because patients with generalized anxiety are prone to addiction, they should try to give up regular use of benzodiazepines when the panic attacks are under control. (Again, see the end of Chapter 16 for a more detailed discussion of indications for benzodiazepine treatment.)

Effectiveness of Benzodiazepines

There are few patients or physicians who doubt that the benzodiazepines are effective in relieving anxiety and encouraging sleep, at least during the first month or two of drug therapy. There is less certainty about their effectiveness if therapy is extended.

The effects of benzodiazepines on anxiety can be demonstrated on laboratory animals, such as white rats. In experiments, benzodiazepines make rats less fearful and more willing to perform behaviors for which they are punished. A standard test for the efficacy of an antianxiety drug is to train a rat to press a bar with their feet to obtain a small pellet of food. When this behavior is well learned, the researcher throws a switch so that every time the rat presses the bar, it receives a mild electric shock (punishment) before it obtains the food. A drug-free rat slows down or stops pressing the bar soon after the first shock. If, however, the experimenter gives the rat a shot of Valium, the rat, as if unencumbered by fear, will press and eat, shock notwithstanding.[31]

The efficacy of benzodiazepines in humans has been widely tested in controlled drug trials in which the anxiety-relieving action of the drug is compared with a placebo or some other active drug. One such drug trial was carried out by Peter Hesbacher, Karl Rickels, and several of their colleagues associated with the Department of Psychiatry at the University of Pennsylvania Medical School.[32] They compared diazepam (Valium) to a placebo and to the barbiturate, phenobarbital. The study involved 472 patients, all of whom sought treatment for excessive anxiety. Some of the patients were treated in a medical clinic that served patients with low incomes. Other patients were treated by private physicians in general practice, and still others were treated by psychiatrists in private practice.

At the beginning of treatment, each patient filled out a data sheet consisting of about sixty common symptoms of anxiety (headache, diarrhea, feeling tense, and so on). The patients were asked to rate on a scale of one to four how much each symptom had bothered them during the past week. The patients then had an interview with one of the participating physicians, and the physician scored the severity of the anxiety symptoms on a scale of one to seven.

The physician next gave each patient some capsules containing either diazepam, phenobarbital, or placebo. He explained that the capsules contained a new drug that had been supplied free by a drug company and that it would be "good for your nerves." One capsule was to be taken with breakfast, lunch, and dinner, and two more were to be taken at bedtime. The physician further explained about possible side effects, such as drowsiness and difficulty keeping one's balance, and warned about the hazard of driving a car or operating dangerous machinery while taking the drug. The capsules had been coded by the participating pharmacist, but neither the physician nor the patient knew whether the capsules contained placebo, diazepam, or phenobarbital. The drug that a particular patient received was determined at random. Patients receiving an active drug took 10 milligrams per day of diazepam or 150 milligrams per day of phenobarbital.

The patients returned for evaluation after two weeks and again after four weeks. During these follow-up visits, physicians evaluated the improvement of symptoms and the occurrence of side effects. The physicians also counted the remaining capsules to determine whether the patients had used the drug as directed.

When the data were analyzed, it was clear that both active drugs were superior to placebo in reducing the severity of anxiety symptoms, but neither of the active drugs was consistently superior to the other. Diazepam was associated with fewer reported side effects than phenobarbital, and the number of side effects reported with diazepam was no greater than with placebo. Diazepam was a better drug than phenobarbital from the standpoint of patient acceptability. More diazepam patients than phenobarbital patients took their capsules as prescribed, and fewer diazepam patients dropped out of the study. Also, there were fewer diazepam dropouts than placebo dropouts. Presumably, the phenobarbital patients who dropped out were dissatisfied with the side effects while the placebo patients who dropped out were dissatisfied with their lack of improvement.

Numerous studies similar to the one by Hesbacher and his colleagues have been done by many different investigators. In most of these studies, the benzodiazepine proved to be more effective than placebo. When a benzodiazepine was compared with a barbiturate, the benzodiazepine was almost always equal or superior to the barbiturate in relieving the anxiety symptoms; the barbiturate was almost never superior to the benzodiazepine. The barbiturates rather uniformly produced more side effects than did the benzodiazepines.[33] We conclude, therefore, that the benzodiazepines are indeed an effective treatment for the symptoms of anxiety and that they are as good or better than the barbiturates for this purpose.

How Antianxiety Drugs Act on Neurons

Before about 1975, neuropharmacologists knew almost nothing about how the benzodiazepines and barbiturates acted on neurons to produce relief from anxiety. Recently, however, there has been a leap of progress in understanding this process. As we mentioned in Chapter 2, recent research indicates that sedative–hypnotic drugs probably enhance synaptic inhibition that is mediated by the transmitter called gamma-aminobutyric acid, or GABA. Most likely, GABA is used at more synapses in the brain and spinal cord than any other transmitter. Furthermore, it is used in many different regions of the brain. A drug that modifies the functioning of GABA synapses would be expected to have wide repercussions on brain activity and to cause many observable effects on behavior.

At every GABA synapse thus far investigated, researchers found that GABA was inhibitory; that is, when the axon terminal of a GABA-secreting nerve cell releases GABA at a synapse, the postsynaptic nerve cell responds by reducing its output of nerve impulses. At GABA synapses, as at all others (see Chapter 2), the transmitter molecules must attach (or bind) to postsynaptic receptor molecules to cause a change in the nerve impulse activity of the postsynaptic cell. The receptor molecules are embedded in the membrane of the postsynaptic cell. For each type of transmitter, there is a corresponding postsynaptic receptor that readily binds to the particular transmitter; this receptor does not bind readily to other chemicals or other transmitters. At GABA synapses, GABA must bind to postsynaptic GABA receptors to have its inhibitory effect. This inhibitory effect stops promptly when GABA detaches from its receptors. Because the attachment is not exceedingly tight, GABA does detach fairly readily under normal circumstances. When GABA becomes detached, it may be removed from the synaptic cleft by being taken up into the presynaptic terminal, thus removing the transmitter entirely from the vicinity of the receptor.[34]

During the past five years, scientists in a number of laboratories have obtained good evidence that at many GABA synapses the GABA receptor is closely associated with several other distinct protein molecules in the postsynaptic membrane. One of these associated molecules has been named the benzodiazepine receptor. As its name indicates, this molecule has a specific affinity for binding to benzodiazepine molecules. Another protein associated with the GABA receptor has a specific affinity for binding to barbiturates (and to certain other classes of neurally active drugs). There is no consensus yet about the best name for this molecule, but we call it the barbiturate-binding protein. The GABA receptor, the benzodiazepine receptor, and the barbiturate-binding protein all seem to be mechanically linked to each other so that they form a single complex molecular mechanism. We call this molecular mechanism the GABA receptor complex. When a barbiturate or benzodiazepine molecule binds to its specific binding site on the GABA-receptor complex, the result is an enhancement of inhibition of nerve impulses in the postsynaptic cell.[35]

The mechanisms for enhancement of inhibition are somewhat different depending on whether a benzodiazepine or a barbiturate binds to the GABA receptor complex. When a benzodiazepine binds to the benzodiazepine receptor, the inhibitory response to GABA is enhanced. A benzodiazepine acting alone does not cause inhibition. The details of how benzodiazepine binding enhances the effectiveness of GABA are not understood, but an interaction between the benzodiazepine receptor and other molecules in the GABA-receptor complex must certainly be involved. Many neuropharmacologists hypothesize that there is some natural chemical in the brain that binds to benzodiazepine receptors and that, like Valium, enhances the inhibitory response to GABA. As yet, however, no such Valium-like compound has been conclusively identified.[36]

Barbiturates may have as many as three separate actions at GABA synapses, and all three result in more inhibition of activity in the postsynaptic cell. First, when a barbiturate binds to the barbiturate-binding protein, the protein interacts with the neighboring GABA receptor, causing the receptor to have greater affinity for GABA; that is, it binds GABA more tightly. The increased affinity increases the amount of time that GABA remains attached to its receptor, resulting in a prolonged inhibitory response to GABA. Second, barbiturate binding increases the affinity of the benzodiazepine receptor for benzodiazepines and, presumably, for the hypothetical natural substance that binds to the benzodiazepine receptor. Third, barbiturate binding may mimic the action of GABA itself, directly inhibiting the postsynaptic neuron. This third action means that a barbiturate, by itself, can inhibit neural activity even in the absence of natural GABA or a natural benzodiazepinelike compound. Scientists suspect, but are not certain, that barbiturates can suppress neural activity in still other ways at locations other than GABA synapses.[37]

In summary, a barbiturate can (1) enhance natural GABA inhibition, (2) enhance benzodiazepine action, and (3) directly inhibit nerve impulses in neurons with GABA receptors. By contrast, a benzodiazepine produces only one of these effects: it enhances natural GABA inhibition. Because a barbiturate can enhance inhibition in three ways, whereas a benzodiazepine does so in only a single way, one might guess that the maximum effect of a high dose of barbiturate is more devastating to normal brain function than the maximum effect of a high dose of benzodiazepine. This prediction is generally verified in the clinical data, as we discuss later in this chapter.

An interesting issue is whether low doses of alcohol also enhance inhibition at GABA synapses. Because the effects of low doses of alcohol are similar to the effects of low doses of barbiturates and benzodiazepines, it would be reasonable to expect their cellular mechanisms to be similar. However, there is currently little definitive information about how alcohol produces its observed behavioral effects. Because alcohol has a large number of different actions on cells, it is very difficult to determine which or how many of these actions are important for producing anxiety relief and for promoting sleep.

Side Effects of Antianxiety Drugs

One can think of excessive anxiety as excessive nerve impulse traffic in the brain circuits serving fear and vigilance. There is no experimental proof of this hypothesis, though it is a reasonable one. If it were valid, one could logically believe that the sedative–hypnotic drugs relieve anxiety by helping to inhibit this excessively high level of nervous activity. Unfortunately, though, the drug enhancement of inhibition will also create some unwanted effects. GABA synapses and GABA-receptor complexes are distributed widely throughout the brain and spinal cord and they are involved in circuits underlying many kinds of behavior. Therefore the action of the drugs cannot be confined to just those circuits that serve fear and vigilance. Furthermore, the higher the drug dose, the greater the number of unrelated synapses that will be affected. These effects on unrelated synapses cause side effects.

The side effects that people complain about most are drowsiness, loss of mental acuity, and clumsiness. Because of the extra inhibition in the brain, people have difficulty being alert, thinking, making judgments, reading, or carrying on discussions. Reflexes and skilled movements are also impaired. Driving a car or flying a plane is hazardous when taking antianxiety drugs.[38]

Social restraint and judgment are also impaired by sedative-hypnotic drugs. The drugs may permit people to take risks or engage in behaviors they normally would suppress for fear of embarrassment.[39] These effects are predictable from the animal studies showing that the sedative–hypnotic drugs increase behaviors that are ordinarily inhibited by fear of punishment. To be sure, the relief from social fear (anxiety) is one of the main benefits of a sedative–hypnotic drug. But this benefit is a two-edged sword. Living harmoniously with others requires social restraint. The association of alcoholic drunkenness with impulsive violent crimes and suicide is well known. Perhaps less publicized are the cases in the psychiatric literature in which prescription sedative–hypnotics appear to have released ill-considered hostility or aggressiveness.

Drug-Released Aggression

Peter exemplifies a patient who became unusually hostile while taking an antianxiety drug. Peter was about forty years old and worked as a tree trimmer. In an accident at work, he injured his back, and his family doctor prescribed Valium at 20 milligrams per day to relieve some of the anxiety associated with the stress of pain. After about three days on Valium, Peter began to be unusually argumentative. He knew arguing with his wife was not normal behavior for him and thought the cause was being cooped up at home all day. So he went back to work. However, he immediately got into an argument with a co-worker that escalated into a fist fight. Peter had not gotten into a fight since high school. His wife then insisted that he see a psychiatrist. The psychiatrist decided that Peter had been harboring resentments and that the Valium was decreasing inhibitions, resulting in the expression of hostility. Peter's Valium was discontinued, and the argumentativeness went away after a couple of days. However, the psychiatrist encouraged Peter to see a counselor in his neighborhood mental health clinic so that he could ventilate some of his resentments.[40]

A few case histories, of course, are not proof that benzodiazepines cause excessive aggressiveness. The aggressive behavior might have occurred anyway, given the particular personality and the particular situation. Everyone loses control from time to time, whether or not he is taking a psychoactive drug. In an effort to rigorously evaluate whether benzodiazepines could release social aggressiveness, Dr. Carl Salzman of the Harvard Medical School and several colleagues from Harvard and New York University performed an experiment in which aggressive behaviors were measured in small groups of young men who were subjected to mild frustration.[41] For a week prior to the critical experimental day, the men in some groups were given a small daily dose of Librium while the men in other groups received a placebo. On the day of the experiment, the experimenter asked the men in each group to spend 10 minutes making up a story about a picture they were shown. At the end of the discussion, the experimenter created a frustrating situation by telling each group that its story was inadequate and that the group had to make up a new one. At this point, one of the men (who had taken Librium) became furious and walked out of the study, but the men remaining controlled themselves sufficiently to finish a second story. Later, the psychologists evaluated videotapes of the group discussions to find out whether hostile or assaultive behavior increased after the men were told that they had to make up new stories. On the average, the frustration caused a greater increase in hostility and assaultiveness in the men who had taken Librium than in the men who had taken placebo. This study was double-blind—neither the observers nor the subjects knew who had taken Librium and who had taken placebo. Thus, it would appear that low doses of benzodiazepine do indeed release aggressiveness in some people.

Effects Caused by Dose Increases

When the dose of sedative-hypnotic drugs is increased beyond the minimum level required for anxiety relief, the side effects due to general neural inhibition become dominant and present a syndrome of gross intoxication. The syndrome is similar to alcoholic drunkenness. The intoxicated person becomes unable to pronounce words distinctly or to walk without staggering. His thinking and judgment are grossly impaired.

The effect of further dose increases varies with the sedative–hypnotic drug being used. With most sedative–hypnotic drugs, the person loses consciousness, falling into a coma in which the only behavior left is breathing. Barbiturate-induced coma is commonly used as an anesthesia during surgical procedures. With higher doses yet, even breathing stops. As is well known, barbiturate sleeping pills are a popular suicide weapon. Barbiturates, methaqualone, glutethimide, or meprobamate should never be placed in the hands of a person who has depression or is otherwise prone to suicide. The lethal dose for all of these drugs, including alcohol, is ten to twenty times the daily dose recommended for anxiety relief.[42]

Among all the drugs in the sedative–hypnotic family, the benzodiazepines are the least likely to result in death by overdose. In the absence of other sedatives, a huge overdose of benzodiazepine, fifty or sixty times the dose recommended for anxiety relief, probably will not interrupt breathing, and it is almost always possible to arouse a person from a benzodiazepine stupor. The benzodiazepines cannot be used to produce a coma that is deep enough to serve as surgical anesthesia. Some authorities doubt that a single death has been reported in the medical literature in which the cause of death was incontestably proven to be an overdose of benzodiazepine *alone*.[43] Furthermore, people who are driven to the doctor by excessive anxiety or tension are more likely to have suicidal impulses than those who do not seek such help. Considering the vast number of people who take benzodiazepines, the rarity of lethal overdose is a remarkable fact which, more than any other, justifies the wide acceptance of benzodiazepines by physicians and patients.

The known actions of the benzodiazepines and barbiturates on nerve cells provide a good basis for speculation about why benzodiazepines are less likely to be lethal than barbiturates. As we already discussed earlier in this chapter, the benzodiazepines enhance postsynaptic inhibition by intensifying the postsynaptic inhibitory response to the transmitter GABA. In contrast, the barbiturates enhance inhibition in several different ways.[44] Therefore, it is not surprising that the maximal effect of a high dose of barbiturate is greater than the maximal effect of a high dose of benzodiazepine.

The actions of sedative–hypnotic drugs on nerve cells account for the dangers of combining sedative–hypnotic drugs. Even though benzodiazepines are relatively safe when taken alone, *they are distinctly unsafe when taken in combination with other sedative– hypnotic drugs.* If the nervous system is operating with mildly enhanced inhibition under the influence of a benzodiazepine, a devastating amount of inhibition may occur with the addition of a normally safe dose of another drug that promotes inhibition in additional ways. All the side effects of sedative–hypnotics are enhanced when the drugs are used in combination. For instance, a small dose of benzodiazepine, along with a small dose of alcohol, can impair driving far more than one would predict by adding the separate effects of the two drugs.[45] Although benzodiazepines used alone are rarely, if ever, lethal, a benzodiazepine combined with alcohol can make a lethal cocktail. The same danger exists when benzodiazepines are taken in combination with other prescription sedative–hypnotic drugs.

Effects on Organs Outside the Nervous System

Many side effects of the sedative–hypnotic drugs are produced directly on organs outside the nervous system. Alcohol probably produces the most serious of these effects. The excessive amount of alcohol consumed by heavy drinkers can directly damage the heart, liver, pancreas, gastrointestinal tract, and bone marrow. Excessive drinking is associated with cancer of the mouth, esophagus, liver, and lung. Heavy drinkers also often suffer from vitamin deficiencies that develop because the alcohol, which provides calories, replaces more wholesome foods in the diet. Consequently, heavy drinkers have a substantially higher risk of death from a large variety of diseases than do moderate drinkers or people who do not drink at all.[46]

Barbiturates also have effects on peripheral organs. In the liver, they induce activity in the enzymes that cleanse the blood of foreign substances, such as the barbiturates themselves and other drugs. This faster cleansing action may result in a reduction in the effectiveness of non-sedative–hypnotic drugs that are being used to treat nonpsychiatric illnesses. In addition, barbiturates can inactivate an important liver enzyme called cytochrome P450, resulting in a decrease in the rate at which the liver metabolizes many compounds, including the steroid hormones from the adrenal gland, the ovaries, and testes. In turn, a hormone imbalance may result.[47]

In contrast to alcohol and barbiturates, benzodiazepines have very little significant action outside the brain and spinal cord. The benzodiazepines do not induce drug-metabolizing enzymes in the liver; so they do not significantly interfere with drug treatment of nonpsychiatric illnesses. The most frequently reported nonneural effect of benzodiazepines is skin rash, and even this effect is rare. It is unclear whether rashes are due to the action of the drug on the skin itself or to an action on the central nervous system that secondarily results in a rash. The freedom from threatening nonneural side effects gives the benzodiazepines a genuine therapeutic advantage over other drugs available for the treatment of anxiety and justifies the benzodiazepines' popularity with physicians and patients. As Dr. Ross J. Baldessarini of the Harvard Medical School stated, the use of other drugs, such as meprobamate, barbiturates, glutethimide, and so on, for the treatment of anxiety is now "virtually obsolete."[48]

16

Sedative–Hypnotic Drugs and Addiction

In this chapter, we examine the problem of addiction to sedative–hypnotic drugs. Writers of popular books and magazine articles have lavished attention on this problem. Under sensational titles like "Danger! Prescription Drug Abuse" and *The Tranquilizing of America*, the dangers of benzodiazepines have been proclaimed.[1] In 1979, social concern found an outlet in the United States Congress. The Senate Subcommittee on Health and Scientific Research held a hearing, known as the Valium Hearing, to consider the "growing and very serious public health problem" of benzodiazepine abuse. At this hearing, Committee Chairman Edward Kennedy said, "If you require a daily dose of Valium to get through each day, you are hooked and you should seek help."[2] Drug scares, of course, have been a staple of popular culture since long before the invention of minor tranquilizers, and on some occasions, the media and the government have been profoundly misleading. In the late 1930s, for instance, numerous popular magazine articles, prepared with the help of the U.S. Federal Bureau of Narcotics, played an important role in convincing the American public that marijuana is an addictive killer drug, a doctrine that has no basis in fact.[3]

Today, the principal limitation on the medical use of sedative–hypnotic drugs is fear of physiological dependence and addiction.

In this chapter, we evaluate the risk and severity of addiction. Our focus is on the benzodiazepines, which are the most commonly prescribed sedative–hypnotics. We compare the benzodiazepines with alcohol, which is the most popular sedative–hypnotic, and with the barbiturates, which are the older prescription sedative–hypnotics. We also try to identify some of the reasons why people are induced to overuse drugs. Then we ask to what extent these inducements are associated with the various kinds of sedative–hypnotics. This approach has the advantage of focusing attention on some of the presumed causes of addictive behavior and provides a basis for judgment about how potentially addictive drugs can be used with minimal risk. Next, we offer recommendations for minimizing the risk of addiction when anxiety is treated with benzodiazepines. In the last part of the chapter, we present a few typical situations in which benzodiazepines are used and ask whether the benefits justify the risk. A word of warning: Our recommendations reflect only our best judgment, formed after having read many opinions in the literature. It appears to us that there are no generally agreed upon rules defining proper medical use of antianxiety drugs. Indeed, the complexity of the issue seems to preclude the formulation of any simple set of rules for deciding whether or not a benzodiazepine is justified for a particular patient.

What Is Drug Addiction?

Before we can evaluate the addiction hazard of the various sedative–hypnotic drugs, we need a working definition of *addiction*. Addiction is more than mere physiological dependence, more than the occurrence of a withdrawal illness when a patient abruptly stops taking a drug. Many people who are physiologically dependent on a drug are by no means drug addicts, for example, those people who take proper doses of morphine for intractable pain. People who are addicted to a drug have problems that go far beyond fear of the withdrawal illness. If addiction were nothing more than physiological dependence, it would be simple to cure. The patient would simply check into the hospital, undergo a medically supervised gradual drug withdrawal, and then walk out cured. But anyone who has had experience with Alcoholics Anonymous or any other addiction treatment program will tell you that drug withdrawal does not cure addiction.

There is probably a continuum of drug-taking habits ranging from justifiable medical use, through overuse, to addiction. No clear line separates medical use from overuse, or overuse from addiction. Nonetheless, we find it useful to define *addiction* by three criteria. First, a person with an addiction uses his drug much more frequently and in larger quantities than is medically justified by illness (excessive use). Second, his excessive use causes the undesirable side effects to outweigh the benefits so that his drug taking causes social, psychological, and/or physiological debilitation (unhealthful use). Third, the addict is unwilling to quit taking his drug; the prospect of running out of his drug arouses anxiety and strenuous efforts to obtain an adequate and continuous supply (compulsive use). Thus, addiction involves (1) excessive use, (2) unhealthful use, and (3) compulsive use. This definition emphasizes that addiction is an illness in the sense that it is distressing, disabling, and difficult to stop. Physiological dependence is only one of the factors that contributes to the illness. In fact, it is possible for people to become harmfully addicted to a drug in the absence of significant physiological dependence. For example, some users of amphetamine, marijuana, and LSD behave like addicts even though these drugs usually do not cause prominent withdrawal symptoms when drug taking is suddenly terminated.[4]

It is easy to avoid unhealthful, compulsive overuse of some drugs because the drugs themselves are not especially pleasant and there are few inducements to use them. Addiction to quinine, for instance, is not a major problem. The sedative–hypnotics, though, are difficult to control because their effects and patterns of use encourage people to increase their drug taking even when good health would require that the dosage be reduced or the drug be discontinued entirely.

Prevalence of Sedative–Hypnotic Addiction

Alcohol, the most popular antianxiety drug, accounts for most of the cases of addiction to seductive-hypnotic drugs. When used in small amounts, at the proper time and place, it can relieve anxiety and help people enjoy themselves. But some people like it too much. These people use excessive amounts, without regard for the impropriety and unhealthfulness of their intoxication. Based on data collected by Louis Harris and Associates, personnel at the United States estimated that approximately 10 percent of all people who drink alcoholic beverages get into some fairly serious trouble as a result.[5] These troubles include serious accidents, disease, occupational failure, addiction, wife beating, child neglect, divorce, violent crime, and suicide. The monetary cost of alcohol related problems in the United States was estimated to have totaled about 43 billion dollars in 1975.[6] Sometimes the problem is of short duration and does little permanent harm to the individual. For example, if a young man is arrested for public intoxication and disturbing the peace on a single occasion but has no further problem with alcohol, little damage is done. But frequently, the trouble is not limited to a single incident; instead, it is a never-ending repetitive pattern of binges. There are probably well over five million alcohol addicts in the United States who consume debilitating doses of alcohol day after day, year after year.[7] The result is human misery which, in total, far exceeds that resulting from any other form of drug addiction.

Addiction to prescription sedative–hypnotics also exists with significant frequency in our society. A favorite subject of writers of popular journalism is the pill addiction of celebrities (for instance, Johnny Cash, Elvis Presley, Betty Ford).[8] The existence of pill addiction in famous people tells us little, however, about its numerical prevalence in the general population, and we have been unable to find estimates of this prevalence based on statistically valid surveys. The publicized cases of addiction also fail to make clear whether pill addictions are brought about through the use of prescription drugs alone or through the use of prescription drugs in combination with alcohol. People who are addicted to pills frequently overuse alcohol as well, but they may be more embarrassed about admitting their alcoholism than admitting their addiction to a drug "the doctor ordered." The physician's orders seem to provide an excuse— "I never dreamed the doctor would give me an addictive drug!" Betty Ford, however, is one person who admitted that her problem involved both prescription drugs and alcohol.[9]

Sometimes, apparent addiction may be misinterpreted, even by the patient herself. Simply using a benzodiazepine over a long period does not constitute addiction, just as using morphine for intractable pain over a comparable amount of time is not addiction. We suspect that Barbara Gordon (no relation to the author of this book) misinterprets her own Valium use in her autobiographical book *I'm Dancing as Fast as I Can*.[10] Barbara Gordon took

Valium regularly. While using it, she was competent both on the job and at home. When she decided to stop taking the drug, she became unable to work and her relationship with the man she loved deteriorated. She developed an unspecified psychiatric illness and spent about five months in the hospital. Upon discharge from the hospital, she was still not well. We do not think that Ms. Gordon's long illness resulted from Valium withdrawal because the research literature indicates that the Valium withdrawal illness lasts only two to three weeks.[11] Perhaps, for Ms. Gordon, Valium was a partially effective treatment for a long-standing psychiatric problem, and withdrawal from the drug unmasked its symptoms.

Some data illustrating the pattern of multiple drug use among people who become addicted to prescription sedative–hypnotics were published by Dr. Christer Allgulander of the Department of Clinical Alcohol and Drug Research of the Karolinska Institute in Stockholm, Sweden. Dr. Allgulander studied the drug-taking habits of patients admitted to the institute's Department of Psychiatry during a two-year period for treatment of addiction to sedative–hypnotic drugs. This group of patients constituted about one-third of the psychiatric admissions for all causes. Of these addicted patients, 68 percent had been overusing alcohol and no other drug. Another 23 percent had been using alcohol in combination with prescription drugs. Only 9 percent (3 percent of total psychiatric admissions) were addicted to prescription drugs alone. Of these prescription addicts, who numbered 55, about one-half had used 10 or more different prescription sedatives; only 4 patients had used fewer than 4 different prescription drugs. Allgulander's data indicated that, under the conditions existing in Stockholm, alcohol is the only sedative–hypnotic that leads to addiction when taken alone. Among the prescription drugs, it was impossible to conclude which had the greatest addiction liability since these drugs were always used in combination.[12]

Addiction Liability of Benzodiazepines

Because there are few data on the extent of addiction to benzodiazepines alone, we tried to evaluate their addiction liability and the addiction liability of other sedative–hypnotics by asking whether each sedative–hypnotic drug has properties that are typical of addictive drugs. There are seven properties that we think best predict the addiction liability of a drug:

1. The drug produces euphoria, a high, or other desirable feelings.
2. The drug takes effect rapidly.
3. The drug can be used freely without medical supervision of dose and dose schedule.
4. There are frequently encountered social settings in which use of the drug is encouraged as a means of obtaining pleasure, amusement, or friendship.
5. Tolerance develops with continuous use.
6. Physiological dependence develops with continuous use.
7. There is cross-tolerance and cross-dependence with other readily available drugs that are known to have addiction liability.

In our following discussion of the extent to which benzodiazepines and other sedative–hypnotics possess each of these properties, we conclude that the threat of addiction to benzodiazepines is real but significantly less than the threat of addiction to alcohol or the older prescription sedative–hypnotics.

Property 1: Euphoria

Do benzodiazepines produce euphoria, a high, or other pleasurable feelings? The clinical opinion expressed in major medical textbooks is: perhaps, but not marked ones, at least not when taken orally by normally healthy people and not in comparison with other drugs of addiction such as opiates, alcohol, many barbiturates, meprobamate, methaqualone, amphetamine, and cocaine. Valium is probably the member of the benzodiazepine family with the greatest potential for producing euphoria. Librium is apparently almost useless as a euphoriant and, accordingly, is very seldom encountered on the illicit drug market.[13]

The comparative ineffectiveness of the benzodiazepines as pleasure drugs is attested by experiments on animals. Monkeys were trained to administer drugs to themselves through tubes that were inserted into a vein or into the stomach. By pressing a lever, the monkeys activated the delivery of a small dose of drug through the tube. Monkeys usually pressed the lever more frequently to obtain a benzodiazepine than to obtain a simple salt solution, but benzodiazepines typically motivated less bar pressing than barbiturates, alcohol, other sedative–hypnotics, codeine, and cocaine. Among the benzodiazepines, Valium motivated more bar pressing than Librium. In one experiment, a monkey that was addicted to Librium was given the choice of continuing with Librium or, by pressing another bar, obtaining a barbiturate; the monkey switched to the barbiturate.[14]

Experiments with humans suggested the same conclusion. One such experiment compared the desirability of placebo, amphetamine, and Valium. The participants, healthy college students, reported to the laboratory in the morning, three times per week for three weeks. On the first four laboratory visits, the students took the various drugs to experience their effects. Each drug was presented in a different colored capsule so that the participants could associate the effects of the drug with the appearance of the capsule. On the remaining five visits, the participants were shown two colored capsules and asked to choose the one they preferred to take. Thus, on each of five drug comparison trials, the participants judged the preferability of two drugs or drug dosages, identifying them by color. Neither the experimenter nor the participants knew which drug was in which colored capsule. The participants showed no preference between 2 milligrams of Valium and placebo. This dose of Valium was presumably so small that it was a placebo itself. They preferred placebo, however, to either 5 or 10 milligrams of Valium, and they preferred amphetamine to placebo. Apparently, these normal, presumably anxiety-free, college students positively disliked Valium.[15]

A drug choice experiment was also done with men who were in the hospital recovering from alcoholism. Every day the men were offered pills that allegedly were to help them in their recovery. They could take as many pills as they wanted, up to a maximum of 10. Some of the patients received placebo pills and others received pills containing 5 milligrams of Valium. The group given Valium and the group given placebo took approximately the same number of pills; each group averaged 1.7 pills per day. In contrast to alcohol addicts, former pill addicts, appeared to enjoy Valium. If offered

offered as much of the drug as they wanted, they escalated their dose and became readdicted even though they did not know what drug they were taking.[16]

The overall impression from these studies is that the benzodiazepines only weakly support self-medication in subjects who are healthy and who have no demonstrated propensity to overuse sedative–hypnotic pills. In fact, people who value their powers of thinking and concentration may dislike the benzodiazepines precisely because they can cause a loss of mental acuity that may linger for 24 hours or more.

In contrast, a person with chronic insomnia or anxiety might respond very differently to a benzodiazepine. For this person, the drug might bring about a wonderfully welcome relaxation that he does not know how to achieve in any other way. He might recognize Valium as a friend the first time he takes it and might resolve to take it again the next time he feels anxious or tense. One might expect, therefore, that a person with chronic anxiety or insomnia would be much more likely to develop an addiction to benzodiazepines, or any other sedative–hypnotic, than a person who becomes anxious only intermittently in response to the stresses of everyday life. This expectation was borne out in the study by Dr. Christer Allgulander in Stockholm. An unusually large fraction of the patients who had developed an addiction to prescription sedative–hypnotics suffered from long-lasting, nagging anxiety disorders.[17]

Property 2: Rapid Onset of Action

How rapidly do benzodiazepines and other sedative–hypnotics take effect? Valium and Librium begin to take effect 30 minutes to one hour after a pill is ingested. Valium acts somewhat faster than Librium. This long delay is due to the rather slow absorption of the compound from the stomach and intestine into the bloodstream.[18] The most addicting barbiturates and meprobamate are absorbed from the stomach more rapidly than are the benzodiazepines.[19] Alcohol can be effective within only minutes of drinking.[20] For most addicting drugs, the delay between ingestion and effect is much less than 30 minutes.

The reason rapid onset of action enhances a drug's addiction liability is fairly obvious. If a person takes a drug and is rewarded immediately with a desirable feeling, she will like the drug more than if she has to wait a half hour for its effect. Also, if a drug is absorbed slowly, the onset of action will be gradual rather than sudden, and she will have more difficulty appreciating the effect; there will be no "rush." If she has to wait too long, she will decide the drug is worthless. As we pointed out in Chapter 11, people with depression may quit taking tricyclic antidepressants because they lose hope of any benefit before the benefit begins.

Slow onset of action also reduces a drug's suitability for recreational use. A recreational benzodiazepine user would have to plan ahead in order to take the drug 30 minutes before he wants the effect to begin. Advance planning is a bother that most recreational users would rather avoid by using a drug whose action is almost immediate. As we have said, alcohol is one drug that acts relatively promptly. Cocaine, when snorted, is effective without significant delay. Nicotine arrives in the brain about eight seconds after inhaling tobacco smoke. Heroin, by injection, is also effective within seconds. By these standards, benzodiazepines are hopelessly slow. Their onset of action could be drastically speeded up by injecting them directly into a vein, but only users who are already abusing other drugs are likely to use benzodiazepines in this way.

Property 3: Freedom from Medical Supervision

It is obvious that using a drug on one's own, without considering the advice of a physician, presents a greater risk of addiction than using the drug only with a physician's advice. Although physicians can make mistakes, their professional training is a resource that drug users should exploit. The requirement for a physician's prescription is probably a significant barrier to sedative–hypnotic addiction.

With alcohol, of course, there is no prescription barrier, and with sedative-hypnotic pills, the barrier can be circumvented more or less easily by determined drug users. Many people can obtain a small amount of a benzodiazepine for unauthorized use by going to the medicine cabinet and taking pills that are left over from a previous illness.[21] A supply sufficient to sustain significant overuse, however, requires additional measures such as going to several different physicians and getting a separate prescription from each of them. The non-benzodiazepine sedative-hypnotic pills, such as barbiturates, methaqualone, and meprobamate, are less available as left overs and less available through multiple prescriptions, but they are rather freely available on the illicit market. The necessity of dealing with a criminal element of society, however, will deter many from unauthorized drug use.

Property 4: Social Setting

There is a greater temptation to overuse a drug that is taken among friends as an aid to companionship, pleasure, and fun than a drug taken for medical purposes only. Most people who use cocaine, marijuana, or alcohol take these drugs primarily at parties. They enjoy the drugs' pleasant effects in the company of friends who are also under the influence. The same drugs taken in a hospital setting during a pharmacology experiment would have considerably less euphoric impact.

By custom, alcohol is the sedative-hypnotic most used socially. The nonbenzodiazepine prescription sedative–hypnotic drugs, are less popular than alcohol, but they are nonetheless used socially for pleasure. These drugs are reasonably effective as euphoriants, and they are rapidly absorbed and metabolized.

Of the sedative-hypnotics, the benzodiazepines are the least desirable as party drugs. They are unwieldy because they have slow onset of action and are metabolized slowly. The return to normality may be postponed until hours after the party is over. Finally, there are no customs surrounding the use of benzodiazepines that are comparable to pouring a drink for a guest or sharing a joint with friends. In our judgement the social temptation for recreational overuse is less for the benzodiazepines than for other sedative-hypnotic pills and alcohol.

Property 5: Tolerance

Most drugs, including almost all sedative–hypnotics, produce tolerance, which means that the effect of the drug decreases if the drug is continuously present in the blood for a long time. Tolerance is caused by an increase in the body's capacity to metabolize and eliminate the drug and by the body's ability to compensate biochemically for the drug's effects. As tolerance develops for a desired drug effect, a person must increase the dose to continue experiencing the effect. The longer the drug is used and the higher the dose, the greater is the tolerance that develops. Clearly, tolerance for the desired effect increases the addiction liability of a drug because it encourages escalation of dose.

Most people are familiar with how tolerance develops from everyday experience. If you have ever smoked cigarettes, you may remember the first time you inhaled. The nicotine probably made your blood pressure drop so fast that your vision went black. You might have had to hold on to the furniture to keep your balance. After smoking a while, though, your blood pressure became so resistant to the effects of nicotine that inhaling cigarette smoke no longer even made you feel dizzy. The process is similar with alcohol tolerance. If you are not used to alcohol, you may stagger and sway after drinking a single cocktail on an empty stomach. If you are a heavy drinker, you may consume considerably more alcohol and feel almost no intoxicating effects.

Some effects of a drug are subject to faster and more pronounced tolerance than others. We already pointed out examples of this variation in previous chapters. For example, tolerance develops to the sedative (sleep-producing) actions of phenothiazines and tricyclic antidepressants but not to the antipsychotic and antidepressant effects. With alcohol, barbiturates, meprobamate, and other nonbenzodiazepine sedative–hypnotics, tolerance develops to the sedative and antianxiety actions but not to the lethal dose. Therefore, a person suffering from severe alcoholism or barbiturate addiction is caught between a severe withdrawal illness if he cuts down his drug intake and life-threatening intoxication if he increases it ever so slightly. All the while, he gets no anxiety relief from the drug because tolerance has developed for the desired effect.[22] Thus, it is plain that the usefulness of the nonbenzodiazepine sedative–hypnotics for long-term treatment of chronic anxiety is severely limited by the development of tolerance for the desired effect. We exclude the benzodiazepines from the sweeping prohibition of long-term treatment, not because we are certain that tolerance does not develop but because these drugs are so unlikely to be lethal.

Tolerance for the sedative effects of benzodiazepines develops more rapidly than tolerance for the antianxiety effects. Dr. David Margules and Dr. Larry Stein, doing research for Wyeth Laboratories, a large pharmaceutical firm, clearly demonstrated this point in animal experiments. Dr. Margules and Dr. Stein trained rats to press a bar to obtain a small amount of milk as a reward. After this behavior was well learned, the researchers introduced a tone stimulus, and while the tone was on, a mild electric shock was delivered to the rats' feet every time the bar was pressed. Milk continued to be delivered as well. As we mentioned in our discussion of the rat experiment in Chapter 15, normal rats soon learned to stop pressing the bar when the tone sounded. A benzodiazepine injection, however, caused the rats to be less impressed with the electric shock and to resume pressing the bar even when the tone was on. This release from the suppressive effect of punishment was considered to be analogous to the antianxiety effect of the benzodiazepines in humans. When the dose of benzodiazepine was increased, the sedative effect of the drug became apparent. The rats slowed down their bar pressing, even when the tone was off. This effect was analogous to the sleep-producing effect of the benzodiazepines in humans. Dr. Margules and Dr. Stein found, that if they gave rats high doses of benzodiazepine for several days, tolerance developed to the sedative effect but not to the antianxiety effect; that is, after several days of high doses, the rats resumed pressing the bar normally when the tone was off (tolerance for sedative effect) and continued right on pressing when the tone was on (no tolerance for the antianxiety effect).[23]

Understandably, experiments with such clear-cut results have not been performed with humans, but the accumulated clinical opinion is that tolerance for the sedative effects develops after a few days or, at most, a few weeks, while tolerance for the antianxiety effects develops much more slowly.[24] Of course, if the dose were sufficiently low and the use were only intermittent, significant tolerance would not develop at all for either the sedative or the antianxiety effects. Conversely, if the dose were excessively high, tolerance could probably be demonstrated even for the antianxiety effect.

In the 1960s, there seemed to be little professional concern about the possibility of tolerance for the antianxiety effects of benzodiazepines. In the discussion of benzodiazepines in the 1970 edition of Goodman and Gilman's *The Pharmacological Basis of Therapeutics*, which was the standard textbook of medical pharmacology, the problem of tolerance was not even mentioned.[25] More recently, with the advent of negative publicity in the popular press about addiction to "tranquilizers," conflicting opinions have been expressed in the medical literature. Now some authors conservatively recommend that benzodiazepines never be used continuously for more than two months.[26] In his book *Chemotherapy in Psychiatry*, published in 1977, Dr. Ross J. Baldessarini of the Harvard Medical School and the Massachusetts General Hospital stated, "The benzodiazepines, like all of the sedative-tranquilizing agents, are limited by the development of tolerance to their main or desired antianxiety effect as well as to the degree of sedation they produce. This aspect of their actions limits the length of time they are clinically useful and contributes to their abuse."[27] And "tolerance to this class of agents can encourage innocent increases in the amount of medication."[28] Dr. Baldessarini did not give any estimation of the dose and duration of use that might lead to tolerance in humans.

In contrast, Dr. Leo E. Hollister and three of his colleagues at the Stanford University Medical School belittled the problem of tolerance. They conducted an empirical study of tolerance and dose escalation associated with long-term benzodiazepine treatment (one of the few such studies in the literature using humans).[29] Dr. Hollister and his colleagues tried to find out if patients who had been taking Valium continually for an extended period tended to escalate their dose above the recommended range. To perform their experiment, they selected a group of hospital patients who had been taking Valium for a long time, interviewed the patients about their use of Valium, and measured the concentration of Valium in their blood. Unexpectedly, they had difficulty locating a sufficient number of patients who were long-term Valium users. The vast majority of the Valium users they met among hospital patients took the drug only for intermittent brief periods. However, the researchers finally located 106 patients who seemed appropriate. For the most part, these people had been taking Valium for anxiety arising from painful back difficulties. The shortest duration of Valium use was 1 month and the longest was 16 years; half of the patients had been using Valium longer than 5 years. Eighty-seven percent of the patients thought the Valium had been beneficial, suggesting that they were not tolerant to the antianxiety benefits of the drug.

The daily doses the patients claimed to take were within the normally prescribed range and did not reflect a tendency for dose escalation. People who overuse drugs, however, often try to conceal this fact. Thus, the more critical data came from blood level measurements. Thirty-five of the 106 patients had blood levels below the established therapeutic range, and 20 patients had blood levels more than twice the average therapeutic level but not outside the probable therapeutic range. (The upper limit of the therapeutic range is not well established.) Dr. Hollister's group did not believe that the observed distribution of blood levels indicated significant dose escalation because different people taking the same dose of a benzodiazepine can have widely different blood levels due to varying rates of drug metabolism.[30] In summarizing their results, Dr. Hollister and his co-workers wrote, "Even with long-term use, diazepam seemed to retain its efficacy and did not lead to any clear-cut abuse."[31]

Dr. Karl Rickels of the University of Pennsylvania Medical School reported the results of a preliminary study of the effectiveness of Valium for long-term treatment of patients who suffered from persistent, long-lasting anxiety illnesses. In this study, 100 patients took Valium for the six-month duration of the study, though some of them had been using the drug for a long time before the study began. During the course of the study, Dr. Rickels found no evidence of tolerance for the antianxiety effects.[32] Dr. Peter Tyrer, a British psychiatrist, obtained similar results when studying benzodiazepine treatment lasting four months or longer.[33]

Thus, the research literature about the development of tolerance for the antianxiety effects of benzodiazepines is inconclusive at the present time. We think it safe to say that tolerance for the anxiety-relieving effects of benzodiazepines probably does not occur with continuous use for up to six months at the recommended therapeutic dose. For this reason, the benzodiazepines are clearly superior to the barbiturates and other nonbenzodiazepine drugs. However, the benzodiazepines are not substantially different from most nonbenzodiazepine sedative–hypnotics in their production of drowsiness and sleep. Tolerance to these effects develops after a few days or, at most, after a few weeks of continuous use. Obviously, there is greater danger of dose escalation and addiction if the benzodiazepines are used to combat chronic insomnia than if they are used to combat anxiety.

Property 6: Physiological Dependence

A drug produces physiological dependence if a withdrawal illness occurs when a habitual user suddenly stops taking the drug, provided, of course, that he did not have a similar illness before he started using the drug. The symptoms depend on the kind of drug. The symptoms of opiate withdrawal, for instance, are different from the symptoms of sedative–hypnotic withdrawal. In addition, the higher the dose of the drug and the longer the drug has been continuously present in the blood, the greater the likelihood of physiological dependence and the more severe the withdrawal illness. The illness is also more severe when the drug is withdrawn suddenly—the patient goes cold turkey. If drug taking is diminished gradually over a long period, the withdrawal illness is much milder and sometimes can be circumvented entirely. There are many psychoactive drugs that do not produce significant physiological dependence—marijuana, cocaine, lithium, and phenothiazines, for example. By contrast, all of the sedative–hypnotic drugs present a risk of physiological dependence, and some are riskier than others.

Similar withdrawal symptoms occur for all the drugs in the sedative–hypnotic class, and thus a single neurological disease called the sedative–hypnotic withdrawal illness has been identified. This disease is a dramatic and serious medical condition that can be lethal. It should always be treated by a physician in a hospital. To illustrate the typical symptoms, we describe a fictional patient, Harry, who developed a tolerance to and a physiological dependence on alcohol.

Harry had been drinking more than 600 milliliters of whiskey a day for several years. Whenever Harry stopped drinking, or when he just tried to cut down, he got sick within a few hours, but his illness always disappeared as soon as he took another drink. Harry found he could also prevent his withdrawal illness by taking barbiturates or benzodiazepines, which indeed he did on several occasions when he had been trying to convince his family that he was cutting down on his drinking.

When Harry was forced to stop drinking, cold turkey, his withdrawal illness unfolded inexorably.[34] A few hours after his final drink, Harry started to get anxious, shaky, and sweaty. He felt weak and sick to his stomach. Knowing well the cause of his problem, he started to search for whiskey or any other alcoholic beverage. He begged and pleaded with family and friends, but they were disgusted with him and would not give him any alcohol. He even resorted to asking strangers for alcohol. Not obtaining any whiskey, however, Harry started to have cramps and had an episode of vomiting. Desperate and panicky, he searched for other drugs, he looked for Valium, Librium, barbiturates, or meprobamate, but he found neither drugs nor sympathizers. Harry's hands started shaking so badly that he could not lift a glass to his lips without spilling half of the water. His reflexes became supersensitive; he jumped uncontrollably at unexpected sounds or other stimuli. When he closed his eyes, Harry began to hallucinate. He even began to hallucinate with his eyes open. He saw fire burning out of control. At this time a little more than a day had passed since his last drink. Harry knew his visions were not real and that they were caused by his need for alcohol. He was not yet disoriented. He knew where he was, who he was, and what was happening to him. It was at about this time that Harry had a grand mal seizure. He lost consciousness and the muscles throughout his body rhythmically and uncontrollably flexed and writhed. If a recording machine had been attached to Harry's scalp, abnormal brain waves similar to those seen in patients who have epilepsy would probably have been recorded. If a physician were to see him at this stage, he would probably have said Harry was in a state of *acute alcoholic hallucinosis*.

If Harry had been lucky, his withdrawal illness would have started to get better at this stage. But Harry was not lucky, and his illness got worse. He started to drift in and out of consciousness. When he was conscious, he was confused, disoriented, and weak. He did not know who he was or where he was. He lost the insight that his brain was ill and began to believe that his terrible persecutory hallucinations were real. He believed he was being tormented by the most unimaginably evil persecutors—that he was burning in the fires of hell. He was terrified. It was then the third day after his last drink, and a physician would say that Harry had *tremulous delerium*. At this stage, even a large dose of alcohol or some other sedative–hypnotic would probably not have suppressed the withdrawal symptoms as it would have earlier.

During the state of tremulous delerium, Harry had a high fever; he was exhausted. His life was in danger. His heart was racing and it could have failed any time. But now Harry was lucky; his heart did not fail, and instead he began to improve over the next few days. Six days after his last drink, Harry was fine. He had never felt better. With an alcohol-free brain, he could think and speak more clearly than he had been able to in years. Harry could remember the horrible visions he had had while in tremulous delerium. They were so vivid he almost believed they had been real.

Fortunately, people who become physiologically dependent on sedative–hypnotic drugs seldom have to suffer the full course of withdrawal symptoms to the final stage of tremulous delerium. To relieve the symptoms, they are given medically supervised treatment, usually with a sedative–hypnotic such as a barbiturate or benzodiazepine. The drug immediately relieves the withdrawal symptoms if the illness has not progressed to the tremulous delerium stage. Over a few days or weeks, the dose of the drug is diminished so gradually that no withdrawal symptoms occur. Finally, no drug at all is needed; the patient is well and no longer physiologically dependent. However, loss of physiological dependence does not mean that the addiction is cured. We do not know whether a real cure is possible. According to members of Alcoholics Anonymous, Harry will always be a "recovering alcoholic."

One of the few differences between the withdrawal illness for alcohol and the withdrawal illness for prescription drugs is that, with prescription drugs, seizures are more likely during the stage of acute hallucinosis. Other minor differences relate to the rate at which the particular drug disappears from the blood. The more rapidly the drug disappears, the more severe is the withdrawal illness. Alcohol disappears from the blood more rapidly after the last dose than do most of the prescription drugs. In consequence, the illness following alcohol withdrawal develops more rapidly, is more severe at its peak, and is shorter in duration than the withdrawal illnesses of many prescription drugs.[35]

The benzodiazepines are eliminated from the blood very slowly. It takes about a day and a half for the liver and kidney to remove half of the Valium or Librium in the bloodstream. Up to two weeks may be required to eliminate the drug completely. Withdrawal symptoms typically do not start to appear until about a day and a half after the last benzodiazepine pill has been taken, and the peak of the illness may not occur until the sixth or seventh day. At its peak, the illness may reach a stage similar to acute alcoholic hallucinosis, but full tremulous delerium or death is very unlikely. Two full weeks may be required for complete recovery.[36]

Though it has been a subject of intense interest to research pharmacologists, a biochemical explanation for the development of physiological dependence is not yet known. It seems likely, however, that physiological dependence on sedative–hypnotics involves a change in the function of brain cells that allows them to compensate for the enhancement of inhibition caused by the binding of drug molecules to GABA receptor complexes. To illustrate the idea of a compensatory mechanism, we present the following speculative hypothesis. Suppose that when benzodiazepine or barbiturate molecules are present continuously for many weeks, neurons slow down their synthesis of GABA receptors and thereby reduce the number of GABA receptors in their postsynaptic membranes. This reduction in the number of GABA receptors would diminish the neural inhibition caused by GABA and compensate for the enhancement of inhibition that is caused by the drug molecules. When the drug-induced enhancement of inhibition is then suddenly terminated, the neurons would not have enough GABA receptors to provide the amount of inhibition that is needed for proper function. The insufficiency of neural inhibition would in turn cause the symptoms of the withdrawal illness. The withdrawal illness would disappear when the neurons had had time to synthesize new GABA receptors. We emphasize that this hypothesis is speculative; at present, almost nothing concrete is known about the cellular mechanisms of physiological dependence.

Although researchers have known since the benzodiazepines were introduced that prolonged high doses produce physiological dependence, they have been uncertain about whether dependence develops when benzodiazepines are taken at the lower doses recommended as therapy for anxiety and insomnia.[37] Many medical authorities have downplayed the risk of dependence associated with benzodiazepine therapy. For instance, one authority said, "In the opinion of this investigator, the current concern for protecting the American people from over-medication with the benzodiazepines, because of their alleged 'serious' addictive potential, is largely unwarranted."[38] The risk of addiction is greater than zero, however. A group of psychiatrists headed by Dr. Andrew Winokur published a report in 1981 that conclusively demonstrated a severe withdrawal illness following the sudden discontinuation of therapeutic doses of Valium in the absence of heavy use of other sedative–hypnotics.[39] The report described a young man of 26 who lived in Chicago. In the following summary of this study, we call him Eric.

Eric was referred to Dr. Winokur by a neurologist who had examined Eric to find out if a neurological problem might be responsible for the severe shaking and dizziness that he had been experiencing. These symptoms had begun at approximately the same time that Eric discontinued the Valium he had been taking— 15 milligrams per day for six years. Eric's internist had originally prescribed the Valium to help Eric with his "nervous upset stomach." The nervous stomach responded well, and Eric had been taking the medicine as prescribed ever since, never increasing or decreasing the dose. On one occasion, he stopped taking the Valium, and his nervous stomach seemed to come back. Accordingly, his doctor advised him to continue with the Valium. Finally, Eric got tired of taking medicine and decided on his own that he would reduce his dose. This act of assertiveness was followed by a flare-up of his nervous stomach, dizziness, ringing in the ears, blurred vision, and generalized shakiness. Alarmed, Eric went to the neurologist, thinking that maybe he had some menacing neurological disease that Valium had been controlling.

The neurologist found no neurological problem and, recognizing the possibility of a Valium withdrawal illness, referred Eric to Dr. Winokur's group. Dr. Winokur suggested that Eric participate in a rigorous experiment to find out if he did indeed suffer from Valium dependence or whether Valium was controlling a more ominous underlying problem. Eric agreed and entered the hospital. Dr. Winokur's plan was to terminate the Valium for several days, then restore it, then terminate it again while Eric was in the hospital and under professional observation. Every day a psychiatrist talked with Eric and recorded any apparent symptoms of anxiety, the sedative–hypnotic withdrawal illness, or any other psychiatric disturbance. The nurses on the ward, who were trained in behavioral observation, also kept detailed notes on Eric's behavior. Twice a day, at 8:00 A.M. and 8:00 P.M., a nurse took a blood sample, which was analyzed for its Valium content. The entire procedure was carried out double blind; neither Eric, the nurses, nor the doctors knew whether the pills Eric took four times a day contained Valium or an inert substance. Only the hospital pharmacist knew, and he prepared the drug and the placebo in capsules that looked identical. In fact, Eric was kept on Valium for four days, then was switched to placebo for four days, then put back on Valium for four days, and finally put back on placebo for twenty-one days.

The results were clear-cut. On the first day in the hospital, Eric was a bit nervous, as might be expected of one who has just been incarcerated in a strange place. But he was relaxed on the second, third, and fourth days. On the fifth day, the first day of placebo, Eric continued to have no problems. By the middle of the sixth day, however, Eric began to complain of anxiety, dizziness, blurred vision, ringing in the ears, constipation, and a pounding heart. An increase in anxious behavior was also apparent to the nurses and psychiatrists. The symptoms got worse on the third and fourth day of drug withdrawal. Eric became extremely anxious and irritable. He began to sweat. His hands began shaking. Soon the shakiness spread to his arms and body. He got a severe headache and could not sleep. Then he became so agitated that he could not verbalize his thoughts coherently. Eric's senses became supersensitive; he could not tolerate the sound of a clock ticking or the smell of an orange peel. At one point, he became so sensitive to touch that even the feeling of his clothes against his body was intolerable. Valium was restored on the ninth day. Thirty minutes after the first pill, Eric announced, "I feel remarkably better, never felt better." He remained normal for the next three days while taking Valium.

The second placebo period began on the thirteenth day in the hospital. Exactly as before, Eric felt fine on the first placebo day, but in the middle of the second, began to complain of anxiety. Again the symptoms got worse, and on the fourth placebo day, Eric became uncooperative and wanted to quit the experiment. The symptoms continued to be severe for eleven more days. During this time, in addition to all the symptoms that he previously had, Eric became disoriented. He could not tell where he was or what time it was. He could not find his way to the nursing station, and his hands and body shook so uncontrollably that he could not take his pills (now placebos) without help. On the sixteenth placebo day, the symptoms began to improve and by the twenty-first placebo day, he finally felt healthy again, with a normal level of anxiety. He was discharged from the hospital.

The blood tests showed that Eric began to have withdrawal symptoms when the level of Valium in the blood fell to about half the amount that was present while Eric was taking Valium. This blood level was reached in about the middle of the second placebo day. By the sixteenth placebo day, when Eric's symptoms began to improve, no detectable Valium remained in his blood.

Eric's experience shows clearly that physiological dependence can develop with long-term therapeutic doses of benzodiazepines, but it does not indicate whether dependence of this severity is common. Eric is probably unusual in that he continued taking the drug for such an extended period without significant stress, chronic illness, or compulsive involvement with alcohol and other sedative–hypnotics.

Some information on the length of time patients typically use benzodiazepines is available from studies of the prescribing practices of physicians. According to records obtained in the late 1970s from a large family-medicine clinic in Rochester, New York, prescriptions for benzodiazepines were given to a total of 835 patients over a two-year period (7 percent of all patients).[40] Most of these patients were given only a single prescription. Only 5 percent of the benzodiazepine patients (0.35 percent of all patients) were given benzodiazepine prescriptions for more than four months. The single patient who was the heaviest benzodiazepine consumer received 17 prescriptions in the two-year period and was probably taking the drug almost continuously. This study, of course, would not have detected those patients who were obtaining additional benzodiazepine prescriptions from doctors outside the clinic, and for this reason, the percentage of patients who are long-term users of benzodiazepines might be slightly underestimated. Also, this study, because it was conducted in a family practice clinic, would not have identified patients with more serious psychiatric disorders. Dr. Peter Tyrer of Southampton, England, collected data on prescriptions written by general practitioners for patients referred to a psychiatric outpatient clinic.[41] He studied 287 patients, and more than two-thirds of them had been taking benzodiazepines for more than two months prior to referral. These studies indicated that, except for psychiatric patients, very few people were given long-term treatment with benzodiazepines. Thus, patients such as Eric are probably very rare.

Dr. Karl Rickels tried to find out how frequently patients who take benzodiazepines therapeutically for more than a few months experience withdrawal symptoms when they suddenly stop taking the drug. He studied 100 patients whose Valium was suddenly withdrawn after they had used it for four months under the supervision of Dr. Rickels and his co-workers. Only 11 patients experienced any withdrawal symptoms at all. Six of these patients had mild withdrawal symptoms that they described with such comments as: "For a few days, I felt like I did when I stopped smoking," and "For a few days I felt a little tense." The remaining five had more serious symptoms, which included anxiety, insomnia, weakness, and tremors. Two of these five had been taking benzodiazepines for eight months or more before Dr. Rickels's study began, and one of them confessed to being a heavy drinker.[42] In a similar study, Dr. Tyrer reported that, after four or more months of benzodiazepine treatment, 27 percent of patients showed at least mild withdrawal symptoms when going cold turkey.[43]

Dr. Tyrer's and Dr. Rickels's observations indicated that physiological dependence arising from the therapeutic use of benzodiazepines for a few months or less is not to be feared. For patients who need long-term treatment, however, the risk is more significant. Such patients should probably have a drug holiday lasting several weeks after any two-month period of continuous benzodiazepine treatment. During the drug holiday, the patient might make use of psychotherapy to combat anxiety.

It is important to remember that physiological dependence is only one of the factors contributing to drug addiction. Even when a physiological dependence exists, there need be no residual craving for benzodiazepines after recovery from the withdrawal illness. Eric was not an addict by the definition we presented at the beginning of this chapter. Although he may have taken more Valium than was medically justified, he did not seriously harm himself in the process. He did not believe that the drug was necessary for his well-being and, had he used gradual withdrawal, he probably never would have encountered any problems.

Property 7: Cross-Tolerance and Cross-Dependence

Development of tolerance to or dependence on to one of the sedative–hypnotic drugs results in at least some degree of tolerance to or dependence on the other drugs in the sedative–hypnotic class.

For example, a heavy drinker who has developed tolerance for many of the effects of alcohol will be tolerant to Valium the first time he takes it. Accordingly, Valium and alcohol show a cross-tolerance. A person who experiences withdrawal symptoms when he abstains from alcohol can stave off the sedative–hypnotic withdrawal illness by taking a barbiturate. Therefore, barbiturates and alcohol show a cross-dependence. Because of cross-dependence, the withdrawal illness associated with any of the sedative–hypnotic drugs can be treated by prescribing a single therapeutic sedative–hypnotic, usually Valium, and then withdrawing it gradually.

The existence of cross-tolerance within the sedative–hypnotic class increases addiction liability because people frequently take two or more drugs at the same time. Alcohol and a benzodiazepine are the most common combination. The combined drug doses can cause significant tolerance and, hence, dose escalation even though the dose of each drug alone would not produce noticeable tolerance. If a woman who takes Valium regularly for anxiety relief drinks more than usual for a certain amount of time—for example, for three weeks while on a vacation cruise—she may find that she must increase her dose of Valium when she returns home and resumes her usual drinking pattern. The fact that benzodiazepines remain in the blood for several days compounds the problem.

Cross-dependence contributes to addiction because it provides a method for an addict to remain addicted. When drug abuse becomes obvious and embarrassing or when the preferred drug becomes unavailable, the user can switch to another drug to avoid the withdrawal illness. Therefore, a wife who does not want her husband to know how badly she needs to drink might substitute some Valium for her morning eye opener. A Quaalude addict, whose illicit supplier has landed in jail, might satisfy his need by switching to alcohol. Clearly, a person who wants to take more than one kind of sedative–hypnotic should be forcefully made aware that his drug habits may be leading to addiction.

Summary of Addiction Risks

Considering all seven of the drug properties relating to addiction liability, it seems clear that the benzodiazepines are the safest drugs presently available for anxiety relief. Alcohol is probably the most dangerous, and the other pills fall somewhere in between. In review, our reasons for this conclusion are as follows.

The benzodiazepines are clearly preferable to both alcohol and barbiturates with respect to five of the properties. The benzodiaze-pines produce the least euphoria; their actions take effect most slowly; the social settings in which benzodiazepines are used is not as conducive to overuse as are the settings in which alcohol and illicitly obtained drugs are used; tolerance to the anxiety-relieving effect is comparatively slight; and the withdrawal illness is less severe than the withdrawal illness associated with other popular prescription drugs and alcohol.

The benzodiazepines are preferable to alcohol but not clearly preferable to the other sedative–hypnotic pills with respect to one property: availability. Alcohol is the only sedative–hypnotic that an addict can purchase legally without a prescription.

All drugs have about equal potential for overuse with respect to the seventh property: cross-tolerance and cross-dependence.

Unfortunately, we cannot report that the addiction risk for benzodiazepines is zero, nor that it is as low as it is for a tricyclic antidepressant, a phenothiazine, or lithium. It would seem safe to say, though, that if you start taking benzodiazepines to relieve anx-iety, your chances of becoming an addict are considerably less than if you used alcohol or any of the other sedative–hypnotic pills for the same purpose.

Weighing the Benefits and Risks of Benzodiazepine Use

When we ask whether the benzodiazepines are safe enough to use, we are asking whether people can benefit from the drugs without paying too high a price—in the forms of reduced mental acuity and risk of addiction. The price will be low if the drug is taken in low doses, for durations of no more than a few months, and in the absence of significant amounts of other sedative–hypnotic drugs. The unrestricted and unsupervised use of alcohol greatly increases the likelihood of overmedication. The personality and particular situation of the patient, of course, are additional important deter-minants of risk. Therefore, a woman who lives under constant pres-sure in a pyrotechnical whirl of cocktail parties (as did Betty Ford) is clearly at higher risk than a Methodist minister in Marshall, Missouri. In light of these factors, we might advise the anxious lady of high society to seek counseling and simplify her life. For the anxious minister, we might recommend that he take Valium for a month or two and also that he discuss his problems with a sympathetic fellow minister. In any case, there are no professional psychotherapists in Marshall. No matter what the situation and personality type, the patient and the physician should remember that the side effects of the benzodiazepines rarely result just from taking prescribed doses. Problems occur when the dose is escalated, when drug use is continued for many months without a drug holiday, or when the drug is used in combination with other sedative–hypnotic drugs.

Recommendations for Use

As an aid to detecting the existence of danger in your particular situation, we offer ten recommendations for the use of benzodiazepines:

1. Do not think of benzodiazepines as cures. Their purpose is to give relief from suffering until the cause of the anxiety can be treated.

2. Do not take benzodiazepines as the only treatment for anxiety. Get appropriate medical, psychological, or pastoral help.

3. Do not take benzodiazepines without first having a psychiatric examination to make sure that your anxiety is not being caused by depression, bipolar disorder, or some other treatable mental illness.

4. Do not use benzodiazepines if you are a heavy drinker or have suffered from alcoholism or any other form of sedative–hypnotic or opiate addiction.

5. Do not use benzodiazepines for insomnia for more than three or four nights in a row. Tolerance develops rapidly for the sleep-inducing effects.

6. Do not take benzodiazepines continuously for more than two months without a drug holiday lasting several weeks.

7. Do not increase the dose of benzodiazepine beyond the recommended therapeutic range for nontolerant individuals.

8. Do not keep more than 14 daily doses of benzodiazepine on hand.

9. Do not get your benzodiazepine prescription refilled without another visit to the doctor.

10. Do not drive under the influence of benzodiazepines. Whatever you do, do not drive under the influence of benzodiazepines and alcohol.

If you take benzodiazepines and adhere to all ten recommendations, your risk of addiction will be nil. However, from time to time, most people suffer lapses of judgment and fail to adhere to reasonable precautions. In some circumstances, either the patient or physician will knowingly take a risk and forgo rigorous adherence to these recommendations. Therefore, the benzodiazepines cannot be considered perfectly safe.

The decision to use a risky treatment depends on the severity of the patient's suffering and the likelihood that the treatment will work. In Chapter 6, we advocated that schizophrenia be treated with antipsychotic drugs despite the high risk of tardive dyskinesia, a drug-induced illness that can be more permanent and debilitating than benzodiazepine addiction. Likewise, anxiety is sometimes so intense and alternative treatments so impractical that a high risk of addiction might be justified. The number of recommendations you disregard while using benzodiazepines will depend on how you and your physician evaluate the risks and benefits of benzodiazepine therapy and the availability, cost, risks, and benefits of alternative therapies.

Recommended Treatments for Anxiety Victims

We now review the symptoms of the five anxiety victims mentioned at the beginning of Chapter 15 and consider what might be appropriate treatments. For each patient, the likely benefits of benzodiazepine therapy must be balanced against its risks and against the benefits of other types of therapy. Addiction is the risk of greatest concern for benzodiazepines.

Jane Able was a freshman college student who got so anxious she lay awake at night. She vomited before her math tests. If test anxiety was her only problem, we suggest she seek help from someone who specializes in nondrug therapy for excessive situational anxiety. While learning how to cope without drugs, she could try taking a Valium pill the night before a math test. The Valium would let her sleep and in the morning, it would still be present in her blood to combat debilitating anxiety during the test. Because excessive anxiety was Jane's major problem, any loss of mental acuity she suffered in the morning probably would be more than offset by the relief from anxiety. Jane might be able to give up the Valium completely after her freshman year, when she became more adapted to college stress. Her entire experience with Valium might consist of taking only five or six pills. Because her anxiety was situational and intermittent rather than chronic, Jane did not have a high addiction liability.

Annie Hall was frightened practically out of her senses whenever she saw a spider. What should she do? Our advice to Annie is, do nothing. Being frightened of spiders is not really incapacitating if one lives in the city, as Annie did. It is fairly easy to keep the spider population down in a sixteenth-floor apartment. If Annie were really intent on therapy, benzodiazepines would probably not be the answer. These drugs are not a very effective treatment for simple phobias. In addition, they act much more slowly than spiders do. A spider would probably crawl down the drain before Valium could take effect. Therefore, if Annie were to use Valium in an attempt to counteract her spider phobia, she would have to use the drug continuously, a procedure that makes addiction a real danger. Perhaps Annie should consider behavior therapy which has some record of success in treating simple phobias.

Mrs. Angst was always anxious and occasionally was immobilized by panic. She had not gone out of the house alone for weeks because she was afraid she would become panic-stricken. She feared the shortness of breath and the heart palpitations. She also feared that a panic attack would cause her to do something embarrassing. Maybe she would become frozen with panic in a store. Then the store manager might have to call the police to take her home. But most of all, she feared the terror.

Mrs. Angst suffered from agoraphobia with panic attacks. She had a more serious problem than Jane or Annie. Her fear of fear itself was constant and incapacitating. She might benefit from treatment, and she needed all the help she could get. We would recommend that she try a combination of psychotherapy and drug therapy. Her drug therapy would probably consist of a tricyclic antidepressant for the panic attacks and a benzodiazepine for the generalized anxiety generated by years of fearing panic attacks.

Unfortunately, Mrs. Angst may be highly susceptible to addiction. Her anxiety has been ever-present for years, and the pills could become dangerously rewarding. Mrs. Angst might become obsessed with pills and come to believe that Valium was her only protection against continuous anxiety and frequent panic attacks. In spite of the risk of addiction, Mrs. Angst should probably receive therapy that includes a benzodiazepine. Some risk is justified when anxiety is truly incapacitating. The benzodiazepine must, however, be prescribed with caution. Perhaps Mrs. Angst's psychiatrist should order a blood test for sedative–hypnotics at two-month intervals to make certain that Mrs. Angst is not escalating the dose. If the treatment program is successful and tricyclic antidepressants eliminate the panic attacks, Mrs. Angst will become less anxious about going out and will be able to give up Valium.

Mr. Mann had genuine serious problems. His wife had contracted cancer; his business was in a slump; and his own health was in question. His anxiety and worry were undermining his work. Mr. Mann did not have a mental illness, but he needed help with his problems. Where should he turn? One approach we definitely do not recommend is alcohol. Excessive drinking or an alcohol addiction could only amplify his difficulties. There is a good possibility that some extra support from friends would give Mr. Mann just the relief he needed, and he was fortunate to have many friends who were willing to help. As Dr. Karl Rickels said, "Praying or talking with a friend, a clergyman or a physician is often of great help and in fact may be all that is needed by some."[44] But social support may not be quite enough, and we would recommend that Mr. Mann use Valium occasionally. Mr. Mann's addiction liability is low because his anxiety is not chronic but is caused by genuine stress that will probably decrease over time. He also has substantial social support. With the aid of a therapist who can teach him techniques for coping with his current stresses, Mr. Mann should be able to manage without Valium after a few weeks or months.

John Traurig's anxiety welled up from depression. His sense of hopeless inadequacy etched lines of worry on his face. His pangs of guilt made him wince and catch his breath. He had a lump in his throat and frequent headaches. He did not enjoy anything. John became so morbid at one point that his wife got fed up and went to a lawyer about divorce—that was John's lucky break. The lawyer sent the unhappy couple to a marriage counselor. The counselor thought John was depressed and sent him to a psychiatrist. The psychiatrist started treating John with a tricyclic antidepressant and cognitive psychotherapy. The result: John got amazingly better. His anxiety and guilt went away. He began to have fun. He started skiing again, an activity he had enjoyed so much as a kid.

John was lucky that he encountered such knowledgable advisors. The lawyer saw alternatives to divorce. The marriage counselor recognized the possibility of mental illness. The psychiatrist was not fooled by John's anxiety and saw that John had depression. Benzodiazepines would have been an incorrect treatment for John for two reasons. First, they would have been far less effective than antidepressants. Second, because his problem is chronic, John has a high risk of addiction. Fortunately, John was treated correctly with antidepressants and escaped the common mistreatments for depression: alcohol and benzodiazepines.

As you can conclude from these five cases, our advice for the management of anxiety is: be flexible. Anxiety is not a single illness and has no single best treatment. Benzodiazepines can significantly reduce the distress of many patients. We think that the risk of addiction is reasonably low for most people. Therefore, physicians and patients should not try to avoid using benzodiazepines but should use them cautiously. Caution dictates that benzodiazepines not be prescribed for patients with a history of sedative–hypnotic abuse and that patients taking benzodiazepines be reevaluated frequently for signs of drug abuse. It is a mistake to rely on the benzodiazepines as the only component of treatment. The patient should receive warm human support and psychotherapy regardless of whether he also receives benzodiazepines. A physician who prescribes benzodiazepines for anxious patients just to get them out of his office or one who provides nothing but pills merely because he is unfamiliar with other possibilities is not practicing medicine competently. Pills alone cannot solve life's problems, but when used properly, they can help.

17

The Medical Model of Mental Illness

In the preceding chapters, we tried to explain the use of drugs to treat mental illness. We emphasized their benefits, their risks, their mechanisms of action, and the conditions for their proper use. Three take-home lessons that can be gleaned from this book are that psychiatric drugs are remarkably effective in relieving the suffering of several significant mental illnesses; their side effects are manageable under the conditions prevailing for most patients; and they work by modifying the strength of synaptic transmission between brain cells.

These lessons support the medical model of mental illness, which states that psychiatric illnesses are similar in important respects to other illnesses of the body: both types of illnesses are caused by a physiological malfunction that leads to the patient's distress and disability. Like other illnesses, mental illnesses can be observed and studied through scientific research. The role of the psychiatrist is analogous to the role of the physician in general medicine. His objective is to relieve suffering, to promote good health, to prolong life, and to learn more about the causes and treatment of illnesses so that he and others can give more effective service.

According to the medical model, the major distinction between psychiatric illnesses and the illnesses treated in general medicine is simply that the important physiological events, in psychiatric illness, occur in the brain rather than in some nonneural organ. The symptoms of mental illness appear as psychological and behavioral problems rather than as problems in respiration, digestion, fertility, or other functions of peripheral organs. There are, of course, many diseases of the nervous system that are not usually treated by psychiatrists. These include brain tumors, epilepsy, Parkinson's disease, and other disorders of movement and consciousness. Psychiatry is that branch of medicine that deals with illnesses in which the patient suffers impairment in the *rational control* of behavior, thought, perception, and emotion. Rational control is preeminently a prerogative of the brain.

As we pointed out in Chapter 1, the growth in the importance of drug treatment and the increasing influence of the medical model of mental illness have been met with stiff resistance from people holding a number of opposing beliefs. Four of these beliefs, also mentioned in the first chapter, are that: (1) the drug side effects are worse than the illnesses; (2) drugs and other organic treatments are not appropriate in psychiatry because organic treatments cannot correct psychological problems; (3) psychotherapy is the appropriate treatment and that drugs replace the best treatment with a second-rate one; and (4) psychiatric drugs are not treatments for illness but are agents used by the authorities in collaboration with psychiatrists to control troublesome nonconformists. In the following sections of this chapter, we describe further these four beliefs and attempt to rebut them. We believe that the medical model is a valid and humanitarian conception of mental illness and its treatment.

Side Effects: Are the Risks Worth the Benefits?

We have already explored in detail the drugs' side effects and how they can be managed. One important additional point to be made here is that the problem of side effects is no different in psychiatry than in other branches of medicine. No medical treatment is free of risk. In selecting a treatment, the magnitude of the expected harms and the certainty of their occurrence must always be weighed against the magnitude and certainty of the desired benefits. For example, the surgical treatment of appendicitis carries several risks. First, general anesthesia deeply suppresses the activity of the nervous system; occasionally, the patient stops breathing. Second, the abdominal incision can cause bleeding, infection, or damage to vital organs. Nonetheless, because the risk of death due to the treatment is less than the risk of death due to the untreated disease, the surgical treatment is widely recognized as a humanitarian practice. By contrast, no one would suggest that general anesthesia and surgery be used to relieve stomach gas, though such a procedure might be successful. Adequate relief from this stomach distress can be obtained with procedures having risks more commensurate with the desired benefit. Analogously, the risks of tardive dyskinesia and other side effects are justified when antipsychotic drugs are used to treat schizophrenia. But such grave risks are not justified in the treatment of anxiety associated with depression, somatic illness, or marital stress even though antipsychotic drugs might successfully relieve these types of anxiety. Thus, we rebut the charge that psychotherapeutic drugs cause harms that are worse than the illnesses they cure. Some psychotherapeutic drugs may have side effects that are more harmful than some mental illnesses, but for schizophrenia, depression, bipolar disorder, and many cases of excessive anxiety, drug treatments can be matched to the illness so that the likelihood of overall benefit far exceeds the likelihood of overall harm. Continued research may bring forth new treatments that have more favorable ratios of benefits to harms than the treatments now available.

Mental Illness: Biological or Psychological?

It is common to talk about the mind as if it were different from the body. When a person exhibits a mild symptom of illness, for instance, it is not unusual for someone to ask, "Do you think his headache is real or is it just psychological?" Or someone may say, "She's not really sick, she just wants attention." Conventional wisdom suggests that pills should be given if the person is "really" sick, but if the symptom is "just" psychological, medication is inappropriate. Thus, the propriety of using pills to treat depression, mania, and schizophrenia is called into question.

This type of resistance to drug treatment springs from the denial of the central axiom of the medical model, which states that mental illnesses are the behavioral and psychological expression of conditions in the brain. In contrast to the distinction between mind and body expressed in our everyday language, there is only unity of mind and brain in the medical model of mental illness. The dualist theory that the mind and the body are independent of each other is totally rejected. According to the medical model, if the mind performs a task of reasoning, then it is the nerve cells, in their ceaseless synaptic interactions in their billions of circuits, that are reasoning. If the mind experiences depression, then the nerve cells have fallen into an abnormal physiological state. If the mind hears voices, real or imagined, it is the nerve cells in a particular pattern of firing and secretion that perform the task of auditory perception. The conclusion then follows directly that agents which change the state of activity in nerve cells will change the psychological state of the mind. The converse is also true. Agents that change the state of the mind will also change the state of corresponding brain cells.

We say that the unity of mind and brain is an axiom rather than a scientific fact because there is no fully rigorous scientific proof that *all* the experiences occurring in the human mind are *nothing but* conscious expressions of corresponding neural activity. Such proof would amount to a complete explanation of *how* the brain can generate *all* the conscious states that humans experience. Providing this explanation is a larger order than neuroscience can presently fill. No one can yet say exactly which nerve cells cause depression or how the cells interact with each other during a hallucination. Nature compels neuroscientists to be satisfied with making small inroads into the horrendously complex tangle of relationships between brain activity and mental life. Scientists are constrained to make modest statements, such as "increasing the amount of transmitter or decreasing receptor sensitivity at norepinephrine and serotonin synapses frequently causes depression to lift after about ten days of treatment." This statement is considerably less than a valid proof that all aspects of depression can be explained by the details of synaptic transmission.

Nevertheless, there is ample evidence for the general proposition that changes in the state of the mind directly correspond to changes in the amount and the pattern of neural activity in the brain. Relationships between psychological functions and brain mechanisms, in fact, can easily be the subject for a sequence of six or seven college courses. Indeed, thousands of scientists work full time trying to obtain more knowledge about mind–brain relationships, and they are experiencing a great deal of success.

The drug revolution in the treatment of mental illness is one of the best pieces of evidence for the unity of the brain and the mind. As we illustrated in this book, psychological entities such as mood (depression and mania), perception (hallucinations), and thought (incoherent speech) can be significantly influenced by molecules that change the efficacy of synaptic transmission.

Other evidence also exists. Gross physical damage to the brain, caused by a head injury, a brain tumor, or a stroke, modifies thought, mood, and perception. Various specific types of brain damage can cause a person to become blind, angry, peaceful, hungry, irresponsible, or absent-minded. Surgical disconnection of one of the cerebral hemispheres from the other leads to a condition in which the two halves of the brain engage in separate and independent trains of thought. One-half of the brain may have no knowledge of what the other half is thinking. Electrical stimulation of the living brain, as performed by surgeons during some operations for epilepsy, can evoke conscious sensations and the recollection of memories. Electroconvulsive shock treatment reliably relieves depression. A person's genetic inheritance influences his susceptibility to schizophrenia and bipolar disorder. We could continue mentioning such facts, but elaboration is unnecessary to make the point that the evidence for the unity of mind and brain is voluminous.

By contrast, there is little evidence for the dualist proposition that the mind is independent of the brain. The separation of the mind from the body is an ancient belief, still present in many cultures. In the West, dualism's most intellectually respectable proponent has been Rene Descartes, the seventeenth-century philosopher and mathematician. His arguments in support of dualism were philosophical in nature. In Descartes's time, no scientific methods for exploring the relationship between mind and brain existed; so philosophical speculation was the only method of investigation available. However, even in the realm of pure philosophy, the theory that mind and body are separate led Descartes to an unsolvable contradiction.

Descartes said that the body, including the brain, is a machine. Therefore, the body must obey the laws of physics like other machines. The parts of a machine move and function because they pull and tug on each other with physical force. The parts are made of matter; they occupy space and have weight. In contrast, Descartes continued, the mind does not act like a machine. The mind does not contain material parts, but ideas. These ideas come and go under the influence of reason and will. Reason and will have no weight and occupy no space. Therefore, reason and will cannot cause movement in a machine; they cannot push on a lever or turn a heavy wheel that occupies space.

Descartes's theory sounds very plausible until one considers how the mind acts on the machinery of the body. According to dualism, the body, being a machine, cannot respond to logic or will; only minds can do that. Hence, the mind may think beautiful and logical thoughts. It may elaborate the most elegant theories of ethics, religion, and science. It may create fantastically beautiful art. But the body will continue to behave like a nonthinking robot, completely outside the influence of ideas. Thus, the mind, for example, cannot control the machinery of speech. Further, reason and will cannot govern the words one speaks, the prayers one raises, the promises one makes, or the lover one takes. The mind cannot control the hands of the painter or musician. At this point in the extension of the theory, most people conclude that the mind and the body cannot be separate.

The difficulty with dualism is that the mind and the body are so separated that they cannot interact with each other. This "interaction problem" has never been solved within the framework of dualism. Defenders of the medical model, then, respond to the dualist criticism by asserting that dualism is almost certainly an invalid theory. The brain is the machinery of the mind. The denial of dualism is supported by the discoveries of modern neuroscience as well as by the unsolvability of the interaction problem.

Psychotherapy or Drug Therapy?

Major resistance to the drug revolution has come from the supporters of the long tradition of talk therapy in psychiatry. From the time of Freud in the early twentieth century until the late 1950s, various schools of psychotherapy totally dominated the psychiatric scene in the United States. Freud's theories of psychoanalysis held sway in American medical schools, and numerous non-Freudian psychotherapies were spawned in university graduate schools of clinical psychology. The general public acquired the expectation that psychiatrists and psychologists would provide psychotherapy to relieve mental distress. There was scarcely an inkling that mental illness could be treated with any other technique. In an environment of such undaunted beliefs, it is not surprising that the advent of drug treatments inspired some objections and defensiveness.

One objection often heard from psychotherapeutic quarters was that drug treatments would bring about only superficial relief of symptoms rather than genuine cures. A second objection was that the sedative action of the drugs would dull the patient's mental powers so much that he would be unable to participate productively in psychotherapy or in any other activity requiring intense mental effort. Third, drugs were just a cheap and easy way to paper over problems without really solving them. Really solving them, people believed, would take psychotherapy and a lot of hard work. In the following sections, we defend drug therapy against these criticisms and discuss our beliefs about the proper role of psychotherapy in the treatment of mental illness.

Drugs: A Superficial Relief of Symptoms?

Drug-oriented psychiatrists freely admit that the drugs now available for mental illnesses do not bring about cures, but only symptomatic relief. In fact, the drugs often do not even relieve all the symptoms. For example, phenothiazines fail to alleviate the symptom of flat or inappropriate affect. In addition, they often do not relieve the hallucinations—the patient may only develop sufficient insight to know that his voices are not real. Of all the drug treatments, lithium for bipolar affective disorder is probably the most impressive in restoring a state of normality to patients who are markedly incapacitated without treatment. Unfortunately, drugs never cure a mental illness in the sense that drug treatment can be discontinued without risk of relapse.

According to the medical model, however, the relief of symptoms is a genuine benefit and must not be dismissed as a trivial accomplishment. The objective of using medicine is to relieve suffering, encourage good health, and prolong life. Sometimes diseases, such as bacterial pneumonia and syphilis are cured as these goals are reached. More often, however, a cure is not available. The physician and patient must be content merely to relieve the suffering caused by the symptoms of both somatic and mental diseases. Illnesses such as cancer, rheumatoid arthritis, diabetes, atherosclerosis, the common cold, the flu, schizophrenia, and affective disorders can be treated, but not cured.

The treatment of choice is the one that relieves the most symptoms with the fewest side effects, even though the treatment is not a cure. Therefore, the use of morphine may be justified to control pain that cannot be relieved in any other way. A brace that partially restores function to a withered leg may be the best alternative for a person who suffered from polio. Toes may be amputated to arrest the spread of gangrene. For patients with schizophrenia or mania, drug treatments are unquestionably the best available alternative. Psychotherapy provides no measurable benefit, not even symptomatic relief, during episodes of schizophrenia or mania (see Chapters 6 and 14). For patients suffering depression, both drugs and psychotherapy have proven effective. The treatment of choice for these patients depends, therefore, on how each one evaluates the benefits, risks, and costs of the two forms of treatment.

Sedation: Does Sedation Impair Psychotherapy?

Those who oppose drug treatment also claim that the sedative action of psychiatric drugs impairs the patient's mental acuity so greatly that he cannot engage in psychotherapy or other pursuits requiring attention and mental effort. In other words, one of the side effects of psychiatric drugs is unacceptable. We ask, "Unacceptable in comparison to what?" In medicine, one must always compare the undesirability of drug side effects with the undesirability of the symptoms that the drug relieves and choose the lesser of two evils. If the symptoms are as debilitating as incoherence, hallucinations, manic rages, or suicide attempts, some degree of sedation is a small price to pay for relief, relief that may not be available at a lower cost.

In addition, the sedation may not be as debilitating as the opponents of drug treatment claim. First, tolerance develops for the sedative effects after a few weeks of use. If excessive sedation persists longer, there is a good chance that the drug dose is excessive and should be reduced. Second, during the initial stages of treatment for mania, schizophrenia, or agitated depression, the sedative effects may actually be desirable because the objective of treatment at this stage is to calm excessive agitation. When benzodiazepines are prescribed to reduce anxiety and encourage sleep, sedation is the desired drug effect, not an unwanted side effect.

Criticism of excessive sedation is probably most valid when directed toward drug practices in public mental hospitals. Many of the patients in these institutions are chronically ill with schizophrenia. Underfunding and understaffing make it impossible for the staff to give patients the individual attention required to adjust the drug dosage for optimal balance between desired and undesired effects. As a result, many patients are probably overdosed most of the time, accounting for the "zombielike" appearance of some of them. One must remember, however, that the flat affect of schizophrenia can produce "zombielike" behavior, and this symptom often does not respond well to drug treatment.

Drugs: An Ineffectual Substitute for Psychotherapy?

Our defense of the medical model against the criticism that drugs encourage escape from the hard work psychotherapy requires, varies according to the illness. For schizophrenia and bipolar disorder, our rebuttal is simply that known methods of psychotherapy are not effective. Therefore, drugs do not displace a psychotherapeutic solution. However, the role of psychotherapy in these illnesses can be supportive. Psychotherapy may relieve the suffering of loneliness and give the patient courage, though she may not be able to reap these benefits until some improvement has been brought about by drug therapy.

Both psychotherapy and drug therapy are effective for depression, and it is legitimate to ask which form of treatment is best. At the present, there is no compelling evidence favoring one over the other. Furthermore, psychiatrists do not know how to predict whether a particular patient will respond better to psychotherapy or drug therapy (see Chapter 11). Psychotherapy will be the treatment of choice for those patients who cannot tolerate the side effects of the antidepressant drugs. Drug therapy will be the choice of those who cannot fit psychotherapy into their schedules or who cannot afford it. However, the two forms of the treatment do not have to compete with one another. The best form of treatment for depression may be a combination of psychotherapy and drug therapy.

For the treatment of excessive anxiety, drugs should never be the only form of therapy (Chapter 16). Because of the addiction risk associated with benzodiazepines and the possible complication of alcoholism, there is a definite danger associated with a drugs-only approach. Talking with a therapist or a friend and obtaining some solutions for life's problems are indisputably helpful for relieving anxiety. Perhaps the best treatment strategy is to use benzodiazepines to control brief, intense episodes of anxiety and to use non-drug methods on a long-term basis to lower the average anxiety level and lengthen the time between acute episodes.

The Role of Psychotherapy

Personal attention to the patient is always an important component of good medical care. In a general hospital, some suffering is relieved by flowers on the nightstand, clean sheets on the bed, and gentle attentive nurses. By analogy, psychiatrists, psychologists, psychiatric nurses, and family members should try to relieve the suffering of mental patients by attending to their social needs. Sometimes this care may be hard to administer because of the patient's assaultive or negativistic behavior. Nonetheless, mental patients need a confidant, an advisor, someone who gives emotional support. Visitors, nonstressful purposive activities, and esthetically pleasant surroundings are also helpful. A psychiatrist who hands out prescriptions and dismisses patients without further personal consideration will log few therapeutic successes and retain few patients.

The medical model requires that the efficacy and safety of therapeutic techniques be adequately tested before they are released for general clinical use. This testing should be done for psychotherapeutic techniques, just as it is for drugs. Obviously a useful treatment must yield more benefit than no treatment at all. If two treatments are equally safe, the more expensive one should be used only if it is more effective. It is unethical for a therapist or physician to administer a treatment that is not known to be effective, and it is patent fraud to claim that the treatment will actually work. This practice is simple quackery.

The Food and Drug Administration (FDA) regulates drug use, but there are no regulatory laws to protect the public from ineffective psychotherapies. If a person desires, he can obtain primal screaming therapy, reasoning therapy, realism cure, decision cure, orgasm cure, rest cure, feeling therapy, nude therapy, marathon therapy, nude marathon therapy, and many others. Most of these therapies have never been tested in properly controlled studies. In some cases, the therapy is conducted by people who have not had rigorous training and the odor of a confidence racket permeates the procedure. The American Group Psychotherapy Association, a highly reputable organization, has taken the stand that many of these untested therapies may actually do more harm than good.[1] About the only protection for the prospective patient is choosing a psychotherapist who is well established and highly regarded in the mental health care community.[2]

People who favor psychotherapy are frequently critics of biological treatments, yet psychotherapy can be thought of as a biological technique that fits neatly into the medical model of mental illness. Psychotherapy produces biological effects just as a drug or electroconvulsive shock does. Through talking and personal interactions, psychotherapy causes changes in the state of the brain. Under the direction of the psychotherapist, the biological mechanisms of learning alter the strength of transmission at some synapses and alter the pattern of activity in some circuits. Whether psychotherapy changes the amount of transmitter secreted or changes the sensitivity of postsynaptic receptors is not known. Whatever the details of the mechanisms, it is certain that psychotherapy has a biological impact. Psychotherapy, when it is effective, is another way of changing synapses.

Psychiatry and Patients' Rights

The Radical Psychiatry Movement

The fourth form of resistance to drug treatment has the appearance of a civil rights movement aimed at liberating psychiatric patients from unjust coercive control by psychiatrists and their allies in the sociopolitical establishment. We call this opposition the radical psychiatry movement to emphasize its antiestablishment outlook.[3] Intellectual leaders in this movement have been Thomas Szasz in the United States, R. D. Laing and David Cooper in England, and Franco Basaglia in Italy.

The radical psychiatrists do not believe in the medical model's tenet that the patients of psychiatrists are analogous to the patients of physicians in general medicine. Rather, these critics believe that the people who seek help from psychiatrists are not medically ill and do not need medical treatment. The people are either having trouble solving problems of living or are simply deviant individuals. Proponents of radical psychiatry further state that schizophrenia and other alleged illnesses are a particular individual's response to the problems encountered in today's insane world, but these responses are not evidence of illness.

These radicals also claim that the efforts of conventional psychiatrists to relieve the symptoms of schizophrenia are not medical treatments but coercive measures to produce socially acceptable behavior from nonconforming individuals. The psychiatric treatment is not for the benefit of the patient but for the benefit of psychiatrists and the established order. The role of the conventional psychiatrist is analogous to the combined roles of the judge, the jurors, and jailors in the criminal justice system, and the role of the patient is that of the accused. The supporters of the radical movement further claim that conventional psychiatrists call themselves physicians not because they deal with medical problems or make use of medical science in their practice, but because they wish to use the prestige and authority of the medical profession as a disguise. In this way, the psychiatrists can intimidate their alleged patients and mislead the public about their true function.[4]

The radicals claim that psychiatrists, when functioning in their proper role, would be allowed to advise clients (patients) about possible solutions to problems of living much as attorneys advise clients in civil matters. The use of drugs, especially against the client's will, would be strictly forbidden because it is an illegal invasion of privacy, a violation of constitutionally protected civil rights, and a denial of the individual's autonomy. A client is a free person and his behavior, no matter how deviant, cannot be coercively controlled until he becomes so harmful to others that he runs afoul of the criminal law. Then the due process of law can be administered through the criminal justice system. The resulting criminal proceedings protect society from harm while respecting the defendant's civil rights and autonomy as required by the Constitution and the Western concept of personal liberty.[5]

These ideas of radical psychiatry first became highly publicized in the 1960s. Early in that decade, the black liberation movement reached its peak. This movement probably set an example for achieving needed social change through antiestablishment agitation. Later in the sixties, the war in Vietnam alienated the country's youth from established authority. Some young men emigrated to Canada and Sweden to avoid the draft; others openly burned their draft cards as an act of defiance. Life on university campuses was in turmoil. Classes were interrupted by bomb threats, and state governors called out the National Guard in efforts to control the students. It is hardly surprising that, in this atmosphere, a movement hostile to established psychiatry arose.

A central controversy between the proponents and critics of the medical model is the definition of illness. Conventional psychiatrists interpret the behaviors of schizophrenia as evidence of illness, but the radical psychiatrists interpret them as signs of a normal response to abnormal conditions. Thomas Szasz argued that an illness, by definition, is a condition that is caused by an anatomical defect or lesion of the body. This definition, he claimed, is one of the great discoveries of modern medical science. Therefore, schizophrenia is not an illness because there is no known anatomical lesion or physiological defect underlying it.[6]

There are two simple rebuttals to Szasz's argument, which in our minds are conclusive. First, Szasz's definition of illness is not in accord with the understanding of illness shared by the vast majority of physicians, medical researchers, and the public. One does not need to know that an anatomical lesion exists to recognize that illness exists. For example, migraine headache and epilepsy are indisputably illnesses; yet many cases of these diseases are not caused by known anatomical lesions. One knows that migraines and epilepsy are illnesses because one can easily see that the patients are both suffering and disabled. It is not necessary to identify the anatomical, physiological, or biochemical causes to realize that illness exists.

The second rebuttal to Szasz is that the present state of ignorance about the causes of schizophrenia is almost certainly not permanent. In Chapter 7, we described recent research testing the dopamine hypothesis of schizophrenia, and in Chapter 5, we presented evidence that inherited factors play a substantial role in causing schizophrenia. These data represent a great advance in the appreciation of the biology of schizophrenia beyond the level that had been achieved in 1961, the year that Szasz's *The Myth of Mental Illness* was first published. In accordance with the medical model, we believe that research will eventually uncover the precise causes of schizophrenia. Dr. Seymour Kety pointed out that the biological causes of general paresis (the psychiatric manifestations of syphilis) and pellagrous psychosis (a mental illness caused by a deficiency of the B vitamin, niacin) were not known in the nineteenth century. However, these illnesses were probably the most common reasons for psychiatric hospitalization in the 1800s. Could it be true, Kety asked, that pellagrous psychosis and general paresis were myths before their causes were understood and that they became illnesses only when medical science reached a particular stage of development?[7]

Advocates of the medical model vigorously take issue with the radical opinion that the best course for psychiatrists to follow in their battle against schizophrenia is to engage in political action to liberate patients from the bonds of drug treatment and free them from an oppressive environment. There is not a shred of evidence that such political action would relieve the suffering or restore the capacity of patients who are now being treated with drugs. As we argued in Chapter 5, evidence does not support the idea that schizophrenia would disappear under conditions of social organization different from those found in industrialized societies today. Furthermore, the incidence of schizophrenia in Europe and North America has not appreciably changed over the past one hundred years, a period of substantial change in political, economic, and social organization. By contrast, there is overwhelming evidence that modern drug treatments do relieve suffering and restore capacity. The idea that schizophrenia, bipolar disorder, and depression are illnesses has survived critical scientific scrutiny for nearly a century.[8]

In contrast to other contentions of the radical psychiatrists, the charge that conventional psychiatrists unjustly punish and control innocent nonconformists has received broader public support. Indeed, the radical psychiatry movement has probably been an important stimulus for the recent growth of judicial restraints on psychiatrists' power over their patients. Since about 1960, state and federal courts have been elaborating a body of law to ensure and clarify the civil rights of patients who are involuntarily committed to mental hospitals. Prior to 1965, there were few legal restraints on the power of a psychiatrist to commit a patient to the hospital if he thought the patient needed treatment. Before 1955, the hospital staff could order bleeding, purging, cold baths, or whirling chair therapy without the patient's consent. Recently patients have obtained judicial protections and psychiatrists have been forced to be responsive to patients' legitimate wishes.[9]

Abuse of a Patient's Rights

There have been some particularly flagrant abuses of psychiatry in the Soviet Union. Gen. Pyotr Grigorievich Grigorenko was one victim of this abuse. General Grigorenko rose to the top of the Soviet military in World War II and was highly placed in the Kremlin at the time of Stalin's death. For many years, he had been dissatisfied with the undemocratic nature of the Soviet government, but usually, he kept these thoughts to himself. Then, in 1961, during the liberalization of the regime that followed Stalin's death, General Grigorenko made some of his views public in a speech at a party meeting. He advocated democratization of the government. He criticized the exorbitant salaries and special privileges enjoyed by government officials, and he called for rotation of party leaders in office.

In that speech, Grigorenko apparently went too far because he was stripped of his duties in Moscow and sent to a much less desirable post in East Asia. There, however, he intensified his dissident activities by starting a group that distributed pamphlets urging a return to the principles of Leninism. After three months of this activity, in February 1964, the KGB arrested him on a charge of anti-Soviet agitation, a criminal charge in the Soviet Union, and sent him to prison to await trial. During this internment, the investigator in charge of his case ordered a psychiatric examination, and Grigorenko was sent to the Serbsky Institute of Forensic Psychiatry in Moscow. The Serbsky Institute is an official arm of the Ministry of Health, but some knowledgeable observers believe that it has close ties with the Ministry of Internal Affairs, which is responsible for prisons and the police.[10]

After five weeks of observation, a commission of four Serbsky psychiatrists made their report. Grigorenko, they said, suffered from a "psychological illness in the form of a paranoid development of the personality involving delusions, combined with the first signs of cerebral arteriosclerosis."[11] Further, they said that Grigorenko was not legally responsible, was incompetent to defend himself in court, and was in need of compulsory treatment. In support of this diagnosis, the commission reported that Grigorenko had symptoms of "reformist ideas, in particular for the reorganization of the state apparatus; and this was linked with ideas of over-estimation of his own personality that reached messianic proportions. He felt his experiences with emotional intensity and was unshakeably convinced of the rightness of his actions."[12]

The court accepted the Serbsky diagnosis, and in a proceeding that neither Grigorenko nor any of his relatives were allowed to attend, ordered that he be sent to a special hospital for the criminally insane. At no point during the proceeding was he allowed to consult with a lawyer or participate in the investigation. This incarceration without public trial would have violated Soviet legal codes had not the Serbsky psychiatrists diagnosed Grigorenko as mentally ill and incompetent to defend himself in court.

Grigorenko was discharged from the hospital nine months later, but he was required to make periodic contact with psychiatric clinics and was kept under constant surveillance by the KGB. This supervision, however, did not prevent him from continuing his dissident activities. He became a promoter of human rights reforms, writing letters to governmental authorities, participating in protests, and making speeches. While on a trip to Tashkent in 1969, he was arrested a second time, again diagnosed as mentally ill and incompetent to defend himself, and again sent to a prison hospital. This time he remained incarcerated for more than five years. When he finally left the hospital at the age of 67, he was in poor health due to a heart condition. In 1978, Grigorenko secured a visa to come to the United States to obtain medical treatment and visit his son. While he was in the United States, his Soviet citizenship was revoked, banishing him from his homeland.[13]

Grigorenko had never believed he was mentally ill and was keenly interested in setting the record straight. Accordingly, he approached Dr. Walter Reich, a psychiatrist at the Harvard Medical School, and requested a psychiatric evaluation. Dr. Reich was reluctant at first to assume this task. He feared that either the outcome of an honest evaluation would be embarrassing to General Grigorenko or that the general was asking him to participate in a political publicity stunt. General Grigorenko, however, gave assurances that he wanted an honest evaluation and that he was willing to take the risk that he would be diagnosed as mentally ill.[14]

With these assurances, Dr. Reich assembled a team of psychiatrists and experts in psychiatric and neurological diagnosis, including Dr. Alan Stone, Professor of Law and Psychiatry at Harvard University, Dr. Norman Geschwind, Professor of Neurology, Harvard Medical School, and Dr. Lawrence Kolb, Director of New York State Psychiatric Institute. This team exhaustively examined General Grigorenko in December of 1978. They found him to be lucid, rational, conscientious, idealistic, nonrigid, nongrandiose, intelligent, and persuadable by reason. According to diagnostic criteria that were broadly accepted in the United States, he had no diagnosable mental illness. Approximately fifty psychiatrists from the United Kingdom, West Germany, and the United States had the opportunity to examine Grigorenko's Soviet case reports. In their opinion, these reports contained no evidence of mental illness.[15]

The case of General Grigorenko was a civil liberties nightmare. It appears that a person with a long-established record of public service was diagnosed as mentally ill and involuntarily confined for over six years because he expressed ideas that were not approved by the governmental authority. The inconvenience of a public trial, at which the accused might have publicly embarrassed his accusers, was avoided, and the defendant was deprived of the right to counsel. All this action was justified by an incorrect psychiatric diagnosis and the consequent incorrect judgment that the victim was legally incompetent.

Several hundred Soviet cases suspected to be similar to General Grigorenko's came to the attention of psychiatrists in North America and Western Europe. In response, there was an attempt at the World Congress of Psychiatry held in 1977 in Honolulu to pass a resolution condemning the psychiatric misdiagnosis of political dissidents. After much political maneuvering at the congress, the resolution narrowly passed, but the Soviets claimed that the voting rules were unfairly slanted against them. They vigorously defended their diagnostic practices and vehemently denied that people accused of criminal dissident activity were being diagnosed for political rather than medical reasons. Further, the Soviet delegation said that a person was better treated and probably was released sooner if he was committed to a prison hospital than if he was sent to regular prison. Therefore, the psychiatric diagnoses had a humanitarian effect.[16]

The diagnostic theories of Dr. Andrei Snezhnevsky, a leading Soviet authority on psychiatric diagnosis, appear to hold sway at the Serbsky Institute of Forensic Psychiatry. According to Dr. Snezhnevsky, schizophrenia is an illness that can be expressed in many different degrees of severity, ranging from very mild to severely psychotic. In a mild case, the symptoms can hardly be distinguished from normal behavior (and would not be seen as symptoms of illness by psychiatrists in Western Europe and North America). Symptoms qualifying for schizophrenia include reformist tendencies, confrontation with authority, and philosophical concerns. In the Soviet Union, a patient who is diagnosed as having schizophrenia (even with only mild symptoms such as reformist tendencies) can be declared incompetent to defend himself in court and sent to the "hospital" without the benefit of a trial, a lawyer, or other legal niceties.[17]

We should not be too quick to say that such abuse never happens in the West. In certain situations in the United States, psychiatric professionals may be suspected of acting unjustly on behalf of authority. For instance, in an underfinanced state mental hospital, the overworked staff may not try to optimize the mental health of the patients. Instead, they try to minimize the work of maintaining control. Likewise, a military psychiatrist may try to preserve officers' authority over the troops rather than to restore the soldier's mental health. One of us knew a young psychiatrist who was sent to Vietnam and was assigned the job of treating shell-shocked troops. He felt he was being asked to rehabilitate the men just enough to get them back into battle.

Civil Commitment in the United States

The recent growth of United States law on the civil rights of mental patients has been focused on the rights of those who are committed to mental hospitals for treatment against their will. These are the patients who, like General Grigorenko, may be victims of illegal coercive control. Obviously, forcing a person who is charged with no crime to live in a state mental hospital is a massive curtailment of liberty, a procedure replete with possibilities for violating that person's civil rights. In general medicine, it has become an accepted principle that the physician gives treatment only with the *informed consent* of the patient. What justifications are there for departing from this principle in psychiatry?

In American law, the authority to detain a person who has not been charged with a crime derives from the states' power of *parens patriae*, the ability of the state to act as a substitute parent. According to this doctrine, the state can intervene to take care of a person who cannot take care of himself or to protect society and the person himself from dangerous acts that he might commit. "Civil commitment" is the name of the procedure that legally authorizes the forcible detention of a person under the power of *parens patriae*. Civil commitment involves a hearing before a judge so that the judge can decide whether the person should be detained.[18]

In recent years, the American courts have progressively restricted the civil commitment of mental patients to those whose potential danger to society clearly justifies their detention. The courts have been looking less and less favorably on the concept that a mental patient should be involuntarily hospitalized for his own good or for the mere convenience of others.[19] In this stance, the courts are moving toward the standard set by John Stuart Mill in his famous essay "On Liberty":

The only purpose for which power can be rightfully exercised over any member of a civilized community, against his will, is to prevent harm to others. His own good, either physical or moral, is not a sufficient warrant. He cannot rightfully be compelled to do or forbear because it will be better for him to do so, because it will make him happier, because, in the opinion of others, to do so would be wise, or even right. These are reasons for remonstrating with him, or reasoning with him, or persuading him, or entreating him, but not for compelling him, or visiting him with any evil in case he do otherwise.[20]

American judges have also been moving toward a narrow interpretation of what is meant by a patient who is "dangerous to society." A "dangerous patient" is being construed as one who is imminently likely to become so violent that he will do bodily harm to himself or others. A patient who is merely troublesome or embarrassing is not considered to be dangerous. The courts do not see as dangerous a patient who is likely to disturb the peace, damage property, or destroy her family life. Furthermore, judges are requiring that the imminent possibility of bodily harm be proven "beyond reasonable doubt." This standard of proof is very rigorous, requiring almost a 90 percent certainty that the patient will commit a violent act in the near future if she is not restrained. Data show that psychiatric patients are no more likely to commit violent acts (except for suicide) than are people in the general population. In addition, sound statistical arguments illustrate that it is completely impossible for a psychiatrist to predict with a level of certainty that is "beyond reasonable doubt" which patients will become violent. The result of these developments is that even a person's being a danger to society is no longer used much as a justification for civil commitment of mental patients.[21]

John Stuart Mill acknowledged that there are certain exceptions to the principle that the state ought not coerce an individual for his own good. One exception is when the individual is incapable of thinking for himself, incapable of being persuaded by logic, or incapable of rationally deciding on his own course of action. This exception would apply, for instance, to a young child who is being abused by her parents or to an adult who is mentally retarded and cannot take care of himself. It might also apply to mental patients who have certain types of illnesses. Thus, the issue of the patient's "competence" to think rationally may be the key issue in judging whether the patient can be legally hospitalized against his will.[22]

Sometimes the disease itself renders a person incompetent to make rational decisions. For instance, a severely depressed patient might refuse to go into the hospital because he believes he is so worthless that he does not deserve to be treated or to recover. A patient with schizophrenia may believe that the doctors are espionage agents of a foreign government who are conspiring to thwart her plans. With patients like these, it may be totally impossible to follow the advice of John Stuart Mill to remonstrate with them, reason with them, persuade them, or implore them to enter the hospital. There is excellent reason to believe that their refusal of hospitalization is not a rational choice, but a product of their illness. To allow them to exercise their right to refuse might simply prevent desperately needed care and allow them to "rot with their rights on."[23] Courts have generally recognized that when a patient, because of his illness, is not competent to make his own decision, someone other than the patient himself must make the decision.[24]

How should competence or incompetence be determined? At present, there is no single test that is generally accepted in all jurisdictions. This question is still being debated and studied. Words that are often used in an effort to define *competence to decide* are "rational," "responsible," "knowingly," "understandingly," and "capable." These are words that signify the capacity to decide an issue by applying the normal processes of thought. It is very difficult, however, to objectively evaluate whether the thought process a person uses to make a particular decision is normal or abnormal.

Alan A. Stone, a recognized scholar of legal issues in psychiatry, suggested that judges apply the following three tests of competency. First, a judge should ask whether the patient is able to give a reason for his refusal of hospitalization. If the patient cannot provide a reason, then a judgment of incompetence would be justified. Second, if the patient can give a reason, a judge must determine whether the reason is a rational one, or an irrational one caused by the patient's illness. For instance, if a patient who has been diagnosed as having schizophrenia says, "I don't want to go in because the doctors are going to transplant my brain to an android," the reason is clearly an irrational product of the illness and thus would indicate incompetence. But if the patient says truthfully, "I can't go into the hospital because 500 people are depending on me to lead a peace march next Sunday," the excuse would not be evidence for incompetence. Even though the judge might personally consider the reason to be objectionable, it is not a response caused by the illness. On the contrary, it is a reason that can be clearly understood by the other peace marchers. It is not an idiosyncratic reason that is the product of disordered thought, delusions, or hallucinations. Third, a judge should consider that those patients who will neither consent to nor refuse hospitalization have made an incompetent refusal.[25]

Stone's suggested requirement that the irrationality be a recognizable product of the illness is a particularly important one. This test would prevent abridgment of individual rights that could occur when the patient is not ill but holds an opinion that is merely unpopular or behaves in a way that is merely annoying.

Stone further suggested that four conditions in addition to incompetence should be satisfied if a patient is to be involuntarily committed. First, the patient must have a reliable diagnosis. *Reliable* means that numerous psychiatrists agree on the patient's category of illness. If psychiatrists cannot agree on the diagnosis, neither the patient nor the public can be confident that the patient is actually ill. The consequence of incarcerating people without a reliable diagnosis may be the incarceration of dissidents, which is exactly what Szasz believes happens through psychiatrists' coercive control and what did happen to General Grigorenko.

One effect of Stone's insistence on reliable diagnosis would be the restriction of civil commitment to patients whose illnesses fall into a clearly recognizable broad category, such as schizophrenia or affective disorder. Broad classifications like these are agreed upon by almost all psychiatrists. Disagreement occurs when psychiatrists try to distinguish between subtypes of depression or subtypes of schizophrenia, or when they try to diagnose mild disorders that do not justify involuntary hospitalization.

Stone's second test for justifiable commitment is that the immediate prognosis for illness portends severe distress and disability for the patient. The distress might be extreme anxiety, panic, depression, or frenzy. The rationale for this requirement is that depriving a patient of his liberty under the power of *parens patriae* should be allowed only when there is a psychiatric emergency situation in which potential exists for significant harm to the patient. If the patient is not being significantly harmed by the illness, then there is no need for the state to provide parental protection. Also, when the involuntary commitment is restricted to cases of great severity, diagnostic reliability is improved, and the chances are reduced further that the objecting patient will be incarcerated for some nonmedical reason. This test, then, along with the first test, prevents the involuntary commitment of people like General Grigorenko, who, at worst, suffer from the symptom called "reformist ideas."

The third test requires the state to show that commitment would actually benefit the patient. Thus, the hospital must have a program of treatment and/or care that is better for the patient's welfare than the conditions prevailing for the patient outside the hospital. Obviously, the state cannot legitimately exercise its power to give parental protection and commit a patient to an institution that causes his mental health to get worse. Unfortunately, the conditions inside many state hospitals are such that this third criterion would be difficult to meet. State legislatures are characteristically reluctant to appropriate funds to bring mental hospitals up to adequate standards.

The fourth and final test is designed to determine whether a reasonable person, given the circumstances of the particular patient, would reject the hospitalization. To make this decision, the judge must weigh all the benefits and harms of hospitalization. He should reject involuntary commitment if the hospital environment is a snake pit, even though the hospital could provide medication that would alleviate the psychiatric symptoms. Of course, the judge's decision must suit the particular circumstances of each case. Therefore, for a particular patient, he may ask whether involuntary commitment is better than the available alternatives. If the patient has no place to live other than the streets, the state mental hospital may be the better course. However, if the patient can be cared for by family members, the hospital may not be the better course.

The implementation of Stone's proposed tests for the legitimacy of involuntary commitment would prevent the incarceration of those who are not ill and those whose welfare would not be improved by hospitalization. Indeed, incarcerating people who are well has been viewed as a violation of the Eighth Amendment and Fourteenth Amendment to the U.S. Constitution. The Eighth Amendment says that the state shall not require excessive bail, excessive fines, or cruel and unusual punishment. Courts have ruled that forcible hospitalization without criminal charge is a form of cruel and unusual punishment referred to in the Eighth Amendment and is therefore prohibited, unless, of course, the patient has been found incompetent to refuse hospitalization or is a danger to society. The Fourteenth Amendment requires that citizens shall not be deprived of life, liberty, or property without due process of law and that all persons shall have equal protection under the laws. The incarceration of a competent person against his will without the benefit of a trial or other procedural rights associated with a criminal proceeding is a patent violation of the right of a fair trial and due process of law.[26]

The Right to Refuse Treatment

Once committed to the hospital, an involuntary patient soon encounters authority figures who want him to take drugs. Thus, another power struggle ensues. Until recently, it was customary for a psychiatrist in a state hospital to give drugs forcibly by injection if an involuntary patient refused to take them willingly. Because the patients were committed to the hospital for the purpose of treatment, psychiatrists reasoned that the patients were required to accept the treatments the hospital staff thought appropriate. This practice changed in 1975, when federal district Judge Joseph L. Tauro issued a restraining order prohibiting psychiatrists at the Boston State Hospital from giving mental patients drugs against their will, except in emergencies. The restraining order was the first step in the long adjudication of a suit brought by several involuntarily committed patients to stop the forced medication of mental patients in nonemergency situations at the Boston State Hospital. A final decision in the case was not reached until 1979. A similar case was decided by federal district Judge Stanley S. Brotman in New Jersey in 1978.[27]

In the Boston State Hospital case, the patients claimed that the drug treatments violated six constitutional amendments: their First Amendment right of free speech; their Fourth Amendment right to the inviolability of person; their Fifth Amendment and Fourteenth Amendment rights of due process; their Eighth Amendment right of freedom from cruel and unusual punishment; and a right to refuse medication implied by the Ninth Amendment, which says that the enumeration of rights in the Constitution does not deny other unmentioned rights which are retained by the people. In its own defense, the state countered that granting the patients' request would prevent effective treatment for all patients by causing pandemonium in the hospital, resignations of the staff, and reversion to the abysmal conditions that existed before the drug era. The state also claimed that court permission for drug treatment is implicit for involuntary patients because treatment is the justification for commitment to the hospital. To deny treatment, then, would convert hospitalization into simple preventive detention, which is constitutionally prohibited.[28]

Judge Tauro's final ruling was substantially in favor of the patients. He ruled that, except in emergencies, involuntary patients have the right to refuse medication, even though they have been committed for the purpose of treatment and even though the treatment may be in the patient's best interest. He quoted from an opinion written in 1914 by Justice Benjamin N. Cardozo: "Every human being of adult years and sound mind has a right to determine what shall be done with his own body."[29] In this ruling, Judge Tauro himself stated:

Whatever powers the Constitution has granted our government, involuntary mind control is not one of them, absent extraordinary circumstances. The fact that mind control takes place in a mental institution in the form of medically sound treatment for mental disease is not, in itself, an extraordinary circumstance warranting an unsanctioned intrusion on the integrity of a human being.[30]

The doctrine expressed by Justice Cardozo, that a person has the right to control his body, has long been accepted as a part of an individual's common law right to privacy, and the Supreme Court has ruled that the right to privacy is protected by the Constitution. In general medicine, it is accepted that a competent patient can refuse medical treatment, even if such a decision would certainly lead to his death. According to this doctrine, a contract is understood to exist between physician and patient. A valid contract for treatment can be formed only with the "informed consent" of the patient. Judge Tauro ruled that this form of contractual arrangement must also exist between an involuntarily hospitalized mental patient and his psychiatrist.[31]

Judge Tauro also found support for his decision in the First Amendment's guarantee of the right of free speech. He defined the antipsychotic drugs as agents that influence the process of thinking and, therefore, as constraints on the patient's ability to produce thoughts and speech. Psychiatrists express consternation at this aspect of the court opinion because, according to their values, the antipsychotic drugs do not control the mind but liberate it from the bonds of delusions, hallucinations, and incoherence.[32]

In the New Jersey case, Judge Brotman also ruled that, except in emergencies, involuntary patients could not be forced to take medication. He based his decision on the patient's rights of privacy and the Fourteenth Amendment's guarantee of due process of law.[33]

Both judges stated that drugs could be given against the patient's will in emergencies. Emergencies were defined as situations in which there was imminent danger of violent behavior leading to bodily harm to the patient himself, to other patients, or to the hospital staff. This definition was considerably narrower than state psychiatrists wanted. During the Boston State trial, the psychiatrists proposed that a psychiatric emergency should consist of suicidal gestures even when not seriously meant, property destruction, assaultiveness, extreme anxiety or panic, bizarre behavior, emotional disturbance having potential to interfere with the patient's ability to maintain daily functions, and the prospect of rapid deterioration in the patient's psychological condition. According to the court, the prevention of these nonviolent behaviors was not a sufficient reason to override a patient's desire to remain drug free. It is interesting that many of the behaviors that do not justify drug intervention, according to Judge Tauro's decision, could legitimately trigger forcible intervention by a police officer or a prison guard.[34]

Both judges also ruled that patients could be given drugs against their will if they had been found incompetent to refuse drugs. Judge Tauro specified that a patient's incompetence to refuse drugs must be established by a court and that the court must appoint a guardian to make decisions about drug use for the incompetent patient.

Judge Brotman did not require that incompetence be established by court decree. Rather, he specified that the patient's competence be determined by a consulting psychiatrist from outside the hospital. The outside consultant is to conduct an informal hearing attended by the responsible hospital psychiatrist, the patient, and a patient advocate. The function of the patient advocate is similar to that of an attorney; he is to argue the patient's case with a view toward safeguarding the patient's constitutional rights against authoritarian encroachments by hospital personnel. The patient advocate is to be a state employee, responsible not to the hospital administration, but to the Department of Human Services. Using the information developed at the hearing about the patient's competence and the nature of his illness, the consulting psychiatrist was to prescribe drug treatment or prohibit it.[35]

Legal procedures in this area are still evolving. Many years will pass before all the issues are resolved through the process of review and appeal. It is noteworthy that in 1980 the United States First Circuit Court of Appeals issued a decision that overturned Judge Tauro's requirement that treatment decisions for an incompetent patient be made by a court-appointed guardian. The appeals court gave the hospital psychiatrists more freedom to proceed according to their own judgment.[36]

The Costs of the Legalistic Approach

The resolution of conflict by rational argument in the courts is a praiseworthy custom, but it has its price. Court hearings, legal guardians, patient advocates, and outside consultants greatly increase the delay and expense of treatment. The appointment of guardians may require as many as three lawyers for each case, and these services probably cannot be afforded on a wide scale.[37] Moreover, the judicial system would not have the capacity to handle all the cases were it to erect elaborate due process safeguards for all mental patients that parallel the safeguards for persons charged with a crime. Even if the courts were to adopt relatively simple procedures, like those instituted by Judge Brotman in New Jersey, the judicial protection of patient rights is costly. Dr. Irwin Perr reported that legal procedures required by Judge Brotman's ruling added $30,000 to the cost of treatment for two drug-refusing patients in a New Jersey private hospital.[38] Most of the added expense was a consequence of the time required to obtain a court order for involuntary commitment. Waiting for the ruling delayed the onset of drug treatment and prolonged hospitalization for several months. The nonmonetary costs of the delay were also substantial. When treatment is delayed, relief of suffering is delayed.[39]

The litigious approach to patients' rights may lower the quality of care for all patients in mental hospitals. Psychiatrists may have to spend more hours consulting with lawyers and judges and fewer hours attending to patients. The uncontrolled behavior of drug-refusing but competent patients may increase the violence and tension on hospital wards. This problem may be exacerbated by the tendency of judges to commit only those patients who are prone to violence. The hospital staff may become demoralized from the difficulty of coping with drug-free patients and from the necessity of controlling patients by the use of physical restraint. Staff turnover may increase, with qualified staff leaving the public hospitals in favor of private ones, which serve only voluntary patients.[40]

Many of the negative repercussions of the patients' rights movement might be alleviated, of course, if state legislatures would appropriate funds to cover the extra work required by elaborate judicial protections. But this funding is unlikely in today's political climate. It is more likely that the public institutions will simply discharge patients who refuse treatment, even though they are not well enough to take care of themselves. Thus, the patients' rights movement provides an incentive, for releasing patients from the public mental hospitals. This particular incentive for deinstitutionalization, however, will probably save little money and relieve little suffering, for most of the discharged drug-refusing patients will immediately become patrons of charitable organizations, the public welfare system, or the criminal justice system.[41]

Protecting Patients' Rights

Mental patients require legal procedures that are sensitive to their needs as well as to their rights. Accordingly, the legislators and judges involved in developing new laws should design procedures that are rapid and inexpensive, yet still respectful of patients' rights. A suggestion often made by psychiatrists is that the court should determine a patient's competence to refuse drugs when it commits him to the hospital. This procedure has been adopted by the State of Utah. In Utah, the criterion for incompetence to refuse drugs is that the patient "lacks the ability to engage in the rational decision-making process regarding the acceptance of mental treatment, as demonstrated by evidence of inability to weigh the possible costs and benefits of the treatment."[42] The Utah law does not call for a court-appointed guardian, but leaves the treatment decisions to the responsible psychiatrist. Those favoring the Utah approach argue that guardians are not needed because existing laws against medical malpractice adequately protect involuntary patients against unethical and coercive treatment.[43]

Stone suggested that an entire treatment plan, including the proposed method of treatment and the anticipated length of hospitalization, be reviewed and approved by legal authorities at the time of commitment. If a patient being committed were found competent to refuse treatment and if he later refused to participate in the proposed treatment plan, then he would be released from the hospital. However, he would be held legally responsible for his actions. He would have all the safeguards provided by due process of law but would receive no special consideration by virtue of his mental illness. Dr. Stone's suggested procedure and the Utah procedure would protect the therapeutic environment of the hospital against threatening and disruptive patients and would reduce the legal expense of handling patients who refuse drugs. These procedures would also avoid the absurdity of committing a person to the hospital and then allowing him to refuse treatment, thus turning the hospital into an institution of purely preventive detention.[44]

Unfair power relationships between psychiatrists and their patients will never be fully prevented by judicial measures alone. The only genuine prevention is good treatment delivered by conscientious psychiatrists who respect the individuality of each patient. A psychiatrist should strive to achieve an egalitarian relationship between herself and her patients. She must be direct with her patients about the goals and effectiveness of the proposed treatment. Above all, she must avoid misleading her patients so that they think that the drugs can deliver more than is realistically possible. She must explain that the drugs relieve many symptoms of illness, but they do not necessarily cure people or solve their personal problems.[45]

Drugs are feared because they are perceived as being too powerful and giving psychiatrists too much authority. In the opinion of Judge Tauro, the drugs are a form of "involuntary mind control," a view also held by the radical psychiatrists. However, we believe this evaluation is profoundly incorrect. There is no evidence that psychiatric drugs have the power to coerce conformist behavior, except by eliminating nonconformist behaviors that are symptoms of illness, throwing food around the dining hall or undressing in public. The drugs are not useful in suppressing the proscribed nonconformities called crime. Furthermore, they do not suppress genius or nonschizophrenic eccentricity. On the contrary, when used properly for the treatment of illness, the drugs vastly increase the variety of behaviors and mental activities that the patient can perform. The drugs routinely reduce the patient's dependence on others. They restore the patient's capacity to think freely and to use his powers of thought to achieve his own objectives. If a person who wanted to reform society through revolutionary social change were to be stricken with schizophrenia or depression, he would be much more likely to overthrow the government if he took chlorpromazine or antidepressants than if he did not.

The legitimate scope of psychiatry is narrow. Only a limited number of well-defined illnesses can be treated. Psychiatry is not political activity. Diagnosing mental illness to suit political needs— as occurred with General Grigorenko—is political repression, not psychiatry. Political diagnosis is an unjustified extension of the concept of mental illness to include political dissidence. We believe that normality should be given the broadest possible range of variation. Rigorous adherence to the concept that an illness involves the patient's suffering and disability will help check the tendency for psychiatrists to treat nonill, nonconforming people as if they were ill. An objective method of diagnosis, as encouraged by the American Psychiatric Association in the *Diagnostic and Statistical Manual of Mental Disorders*, Third Edition, will open diagnostic decision making to public scrutiny and further inhibit misdiagnosis and malicious diagnosis.[46]

The Medical Model: A Summation

In this book, we explained and defended the medical model of mental illness. We believe that this model is a valid blueprint for understanding and dealing with the problem of irrational thought, perception, emotion, and behavior. According to the model, mental illnesses are biological phenomena having diverse genetic and environmental causes. They are not defects of character or lapses in morality, and they are not an occasion for casting blame. Mental illnesses are not sane responses to an insane world or sets of bad habits acquired through unfortunate learning experiences. As Wilhelm Greisinger declared in the nineteenth century, "mental diseases are brain diseases."[47] They should be treated if effective treatment is available.

Advocates of the medical model invest faith in the scientific method of inquiry. Admittedly, science is now ignorant of many important aspects of mental illness. But during the past three decades, neuroscientists have learned much about how the brain works and have developed laboratory methods for learning still more. Three important new scientific discoveries are: antipsychotic drugs block dopamine receptors, antidepressant drugs alter norepinephrine and dopamine synapses in several ways, and antianxiety drugs enhance inhibition at GABA synapses. These discoveries have produced a major advance in scientists' ability to form hypotheses about possible causes and more effective treatments of severe mental illness.

According to the medical model, it is unethical to give treatments that are not based on the best available scientific knowledge or to give treatments that are not known to be effective. Proponents of the medical model are adamantly opposed to treatment cults or allegedly therapeutic procedures that are based on little more than superstition, especially when these treatments are accompanied by promises that cannot be kept.

The role of the psychiatrist is to relieve suffering, encourage good health, and prolong life through the application of accumulated scientific knowledge. The psychiatrist has no responsibility, and should assume none, for enforcing society's norms for good and bad behavior. Instead, the psychiatrist should respect the patient and strive to enhance the value of human life.

Appendix

Selected Drugs Used to Treat Mental Illness in the United States

Generic Name	Trade Name	Usual Daily Dose (mg)
I. Drugs for Schizophrenia		
A. Phenothiazines		
Chlorpromazine	Thorazine	300–800
Triflupromazine	Vesprin	100–150
Thioridazine	Mellaril	200–600
Fluphenazine	Permitil, Prolixin	2.5–20
Perphenazine	Trilafon	8–32
Trifluoperazine	Stelazine	6–20
Loxapine	Daxolin, Loxitane	60–100
Molindone	Lindone, Moban	50–225
B. Thioxanthene		
Thiothixene	Navane	6–30
C. Butyrophenone		
Haloperidol	Haldol	6–20

Generic Name	Trade Name	Usual Daily Dose (mg)
II. Drugs for Major Depression		
A. Tricyclic Antidepressants		
Imipramine	Janimine, SK-pramine, Tofranil	100–200
Desipramine	Pertofrane, Norpramin	100–200
Amitriptyline	Amitid, Elavil, Endep	75–200
Nortriptyline	Aventyl, Pamelor	75–150
Doxepin	Sinequan, Adapin	75–150
Protriptyline	Vivactyl	15–40
Amoxapine	Asendin	200–300
B. Monamine Oxidase Inhibitors		
Isocarboxazid	Marplan	10–30
Phenelzine	Nardil	15–30
Tranylcypromine	Parnate	20–30
C. Other Antidepressants		
Maprotiline	Ludiomil	75–150
III. Drugs for Bipolar Affective Disorder		
Lithium Carbonate	Eskalith, Lithane, Lithonate, Lithotabs, Pfi-Lith	900–1500
IV. Drugs for Anxiety		
A. Benzodiazepines		
Chlordiazepoxide	Librium, SK-Lygen	15–60
Chorazepate	Tranxene	13–52
Diazepam	Valium	4–40
Lorazepam	Avitan	2–6

Generic Name	Trade Name	Usual Daily Dose (mg)
Oxazepam	Serax	30–60
Prazepam	Verstran, Centrax	20–60
B. Barbiturates		
Amobarbital	Amytal	44–150
Aprobarbital	Alurate	120–240
Butabarbital	Butisol	20–240
Pentobarbital	Nembutal	60–80
Phenobarbital	Luminal, many others	30–90
Secobarbital	Seconal	90–200
C. Other Antianxiety Drugs		
Meprobamate	Miltown, Equanil	1200–1600
Glutethimide	Doriden	125–750
Methyprylon	Noludar	150–400
Methaqualone	Quaalude, Sopor	225–300
Ethchlorvynol	Placidyl	200–600

Source: R. J. Baldessarini. "Drugs and the Treatment of Psychiatric Disorders." In A. G. Gilman, L. S. Goodman, and A. Gilman (eds.), *The Pharmacological Basis of Therapeutics* (New York: Macmillan, 1980), pp. 391–447. S. C. Harvey. "Hypnotics and Sedatives." In A. G. Gilman, L. S. Goodman, and A. Gilman (eds.), *The Pharmacological Basis of Therapeutics* (New York: Macmillan, 1980), pp. 339–375. *Physicians' Desk Reference*, 36th Edition (Oradell, N.J.: Medical Economics, 1982).

Notes

Chapter 1

1. Ayd, F. J., and Blackwell, B. (eds.). *Discoveries in Biological Psychiatry.* Philadelphia: Lippincott, 1970.
2. Berger, P. A. "Medical Treatment of Mental Illness." *Science,* 1978, 200:974–981.
3. Ibid. Berger, P. A., Hamburg, B., and Hamburg, D. "Mental Health: Progress and Problems." *Daedalus,* 1977, 106:261.
4. Szasz, T. *The Myth of Mental Illness.* Revised Edition. New York: Harper & Row, 1974.
5. Drummond, H. "Power, Madness and Poverty." *Mother Jones,* 1980, 5(1):20–25.
6. Szasz, T., *The Myth of Mental Illness,* p. 101.
7. Ibid., p. 196.
8. Kesey, K. *One Flew Over the Cuckoo's Nest.* New York: Viking Press, 1962.

Chapter 2

1. More information about nerve cells and how drugs affect them can be found in neuroscience textbooks. Among our favorites are:
   Carlson, N. R. *The Physiology of Behavior.* Boston: Allyn & Bacon, 1980.
   Cooper, J. R., Bloom, F. E., and Roth, R. H. *The Biochemical Basis of Neuropharmacology.* New York: Oxford University Press, 1978.
   Kuffler, S. W., and Nicholls, J. G. *From Neuron to Brain.* Sunderland, Mass.: Sinauer Associates, 1977.

Chapter 3

1. Spitzer, R. L., and Wilson, P. "Nosology and the Official Psychiatric Nomenclature." In H. I. Kaplan, A. M. Freedman, and B. J. Sadock (eds.), *Comprehensive Textbook of Psychiatry*, Second Edition. Baltimore: Williams & Wilkins, 1975, pp. 826–845.
   Spitzer, R. L., and Williams, J. B. W. "Classification of Mental Disorders and *DSM-III*." In H. I. Kaplan, A. M. Freedman, and B. J. Sadock (eds.), *Comprehensive Textbook of Psychiatry*, Third Edition. Baltimore: Williams & Wilkins, 1980, pp. 1035–1072.
2. Spitzer, R. L., and Wilson, P. "Nosology and Nomenclature," pp. 826–845.
3. *New York Times*, "Reagan Wounded by Gunman," 31 March 1981, p. 1.
4. *New York Times*, "Jury Finds Hinkley Not Guilty, Accepting His Defense of Insanity," 22 June 1982, p. 1.
5. Klerman, B., Endicott, J., and Spitzer, R. "Neurotic Depressions: A Systematic Analysis of Multiple Criteria and Meanings." *American Journal of Psychiatry*, 1979, 136: 57–67.
6. Kendall, R. E., et al. "Diagnostic Criteria of American and British Psychiatrists." *Archives of General Psychiatry*, 1971, 25:123–130.
   Katz, M. M., Cole, J. O., and Lowery, H. R. "Studies of Diagnostic Process: The Influence of Symptom Perception, Past Experience, and Ethnic Background on Diagnostic Decisions." *American Journal of Psychiatry*, 1969, 125:937–947.
7. Endicott, J., and Spitzer, R. L. "Use of the Research Diagnostic Criteria and Schedule for Affective Disorders and Schizophrenia to Study Affective Disorders." *American Journal of Psychiatry*, 1979, 136:52–56.
8. Spitzer, R. L., and Wilson, P. "Nosology and Nomenclature," pp. 826–845; and Spitzer, R. L., and Williams, J. B. W. "Classification of Disorders," pp. 1035–1072.
9. American Psychiatric Association. *Diagnostic and Statistical Manual of Mental Disorders*, Third Edition. Washington, D.C.: American Psychiatric Association, 1980. Spitzer, R. L., and Wilson, P. "Nosology and Nomenclature," pp. 826–845. Spitzer, R. L., Williams, J. B. W., and Skodol, A. "*DSM-III*: The Major Achievement and an Overview." *American Journal of Psychiatry*, 1980, 137:161–163.
10. Rolata, G. B. "Clues to the Cause of Senile Dementia." *Science*, 1981, 211:1032–1033.
11. Kety, S. "Disorders of the Human Brain." *Scientific American*, 1979, 241 (September):202–214. Szasz, T. "Schizophrenia: The Sacred Symbol of Psychiatry." *British Journal of Psychiatry*, 1976, 129:308–316. Spitzer, R. L., and Wilson, P. "Nosology and Nomenclature," pp. 826–845. Spitzer, R. L., and Williams, J. B. W. "Classification of Disorders," pp. 1035–1072.
12. Spitzer, R. L., and Wilson, P. "Nosology and Nomenclature," pp. 826–845.

13. Ibid.
14. Ibid. American Psychiatric Association. *DSM-III*. Spitzer, R. L., and Williams, J. B. W. "Classification of Disorders," pp. 1035–1072.
15. Spitzer, R. L., and Wilson, P. "Nosology and Nomenclature," pp. 826–845.
16. Carroll, B. J., et al. "A Specific Laboratory Test for the Diagnosis of Melancholia." *Archives of General Psychiatry*, 1981, 38:15–23.
17. Spitzer, R. L., and Wilson, P. "Nosology and Nomenclature," pp. 826–845; and Spitzer, R. L., and Williams, J. B. W. "Classification of Disorders," pp. 1035–1072.
18. American Psychiatric Association. *DSM-III*.
19. Spitzer, R. L., Williams, J. B. W., and Skodol, A. "*DSM-III:* An Overview," pp. 151–163. American Psychiatric Association. *DSM-III*. Spitzer, R. L., and Williams, J. B. W. "Classification of Disorders," pp. 1035–1072.
20. American Psychiatric Association, *Diagnostic and Statistical Manual of Mental Disorders.* Washington, D.C.: American Psychiatric Association, 1952.
21. American Psychiatric Association. *Diagnostic and Statistical Manual of Mental Disorders.* Second Edition. Washington, D.C.: American Psychiatric Association, 1968.
22. Spitzer, R. L., Williams, J. B. W., and Skodol, A. "*DSM-III:* An Overview," pp. 151–163. American Psychiatric Association. *DSM-III*, pp. 1–12. Spitzer, R. L., and Williams, J. B. W. "Classification of Disorders," pp. 1035–1072.
23. Spitzer and Wilson, "Nosology and Nomenclature," pp. 826–845; and Spitzer and Williams, "Classification of Disorders," pp. 1035–1072.
24. Spitzer, R. L., Williams, J. B. W., and Skodol, A. "*DSM-III:* An Overview," pp. 151–163. American Psychiatric Association. *DSM-III*, pp. 1–12.
25. Feighner, J. P., et al. "Psychiatric Research." *Archives of General Psychiatry*, 1972, 26:52–63.
26. American Psychiatric Association. *DSM-III*, pp. 1–12. Spitzer, R. L., and Williams, J. B. W. "Classification of Disorders," pp. 1035–1072.
27. American Psychiatric Association. *DSM-III*, pp. 1–12. Spitzer, R. L., and Williams, J. B. W. "Classification of Disorders," pp. 1035–1072.
28. Endicott, J., and Spitzer, R. L. "A Diagnostic Interview: The Schedule for Affective Disorders and Schizophrenia." *Archives of General Psychiatry*, 1978, 35:837–844. Spitzer, R. L., and Williams, J. B. W. "Classification of Disorders," pp. 1035–1072.

Chapter 4

1. The description of schizophrenia in this chapter is based on the following sources:
   Cancro, R. "Overview of Schizophrenia." In H. I. Kaplan, A. M. Freed-

man, and B. J. Sadock (eds.), *Comprehensive Textbook of Psychiatry,* Third Edition. Baltimore: Williams & Wilkins, 1980, pp. 1093–1104.

Lehmann, H. E. "Schizophrenia: Clinical Features." In H. I. Kaplan, H. M. Freedman, and B. J. Sadock (eds.), *Comprehensive Textbook of Psychiatry,* pp. 1153–1192.

Bemporad, J. R., and Pinsker, H. "Schizophrenia: The Manifest Symptomatology." In S. Arieti and E. B. Brody (eds.), *American Handbook of Psychiatry,* Second Edition. New York: Basic Books, 1974, pp. 524–550.

American Psychiatric Association. *Diagnostic and Statistical Manual of Mental Disorders.* Third Edition. Washington, D.C.: American Psychiatric Association, 1980, pp. 181–224.

2. American Psychiatric Association. *DSM-III,* pp. 188–189.
3. Lehmann, H. E., "Schizophrenia: Clinical Features," pp. 1153–1192.
4. Ibid.
5. Sheehan, S. "A Reporter at Large (Creedmoor—Part II)." *The New Yorker,* June 1, 1981, p. 74. Sheehan, S. "A Reporter at Large (Creedmoor—Part IV)." *The New Yorker,* June 15, 1981, p. 121.
6. American Psychiatric Association. *DSM-III,* p. 189.
7. Ibid.
8. Ibid., p. 190.
9. Lewis, N. D. C., and Piotrowski, Z. A. "Clinical Diagnosis of Manic Depressive Illness." In P. H. Hoch and J. Zubin (eds.), *Depression.* New York: Grune & Stratton, 1954, pp. 25–38.
10. Kendell, R. E., et al. "Diagnostic Criteria of American and British Psychiatrists." *Archives of General Psychiatry,* 1971, 25:123–130.
11. American Psychiatric Association. *DSM-III,* p. 190.
12. Lipowski, Z. J. "Organic Mental Disorders: Introduction and Review of Syndromes." In H. I. Kaplan, A. M. Freedman, and B. J. Sadock (eds.), *Comprehensive Textbook of Psychiatry,* pp. 1359–1391.
13. American Psychiatric Association. *DSM-III,* p. 190.
14. Bemporad, J. R., and Pinsker, H. "Schizophrenia: The Manifest Symptomatology," pp. 524–550. Lehmann, H. E. "Schizophrenia: Clinical Features," pp. 1153–1192.

Chapter 5

1. Luchins, D. L., Weinberger, D. R., and Wyatt, R. J. "Schizophrenia: Evidence of a Subgroup with Reversed Cerebral Asymmetry." *Archives of General Psychiatry,* 1979, 36:1309–1311.

Weinberger, D. R., et al. "Lateral Cerebral Ventricle Enlargement in Chronic Schizophrenia." *Archives of General Psychiatry,* 1979, 36:735–739.

Weinberger, D. R., et al. "Structural Abnormalities in the Cerebral Cortex of Chronic Schizophrenic Patients." *Archives of General Psychiatry,* 1979, 36: 935–939.

Andreasen, N. C., et al. "Hemispheric Asymmetries and Schizophrenia." *American Journal of Psychiatry*, 1982, 139: 427–430.

Weinberger, D. R., et al. "Computed Tomography in Schizophreniform Disorder and Other Acute Psychiatric Disorders." *Archives of General Psychiatry*, 1982, 39: 778–783.

Jernigan, T. L., et al. "Computed Tomography in Schizophrenics and Normal Volunteers. I. Fluid Volume." *Archives of General Psychiatry*, 1982, 39: 765–770.

Jernigan, T. L., et al. "Computed Tomography in Schizophrenics and Normal Volunteers. II. Cranial Asymmetry." *Archives of General Psychiatry*, 1982, 39: 771–773.

Luchins, D. J. "Computed Tomography in Schizophrenia." *Archives of General Psychiatry*, 1982, 39: 859–860.

2. Kety, S. S. "Disorders of the Human Brain." *Scientific American*, September 1979, pp. 202–214.

3. Scheinberg, I. H., and Sternlieb, I. "Wilson's Disease." In G. G. Gaull (ed.), *Biology of Brain Dysfunction*. Vol. III. New York: Plenum Press, 1975, pp. 247–264.

4. Rosenberg, L. E., and Scriver, C. R. "Disorders of Amino Acid Metabolism." In P. K. Bondy and L. E. Rosenberg (eds.), *Duncan's Diseases of the Metabolism*. Vol. I. Philadelphia: Saunders, 1975, pp. 465–644. (See especially pp. 596–605.)

5. Gardner, L. I. "Deprivation Dwarfism." *Scientific American.*, July 1972, pp. 76–82.

6. Powell, G. F., Brasel, J. A., and Blizzard, R. M. "Emotional Deprivation and Growth Retardation Stimulating Idiopathic Hypopituitarism. I. Clinical Evaluation of the Syndrome." *New England Journal of Medicine*, 1967, 276: 1271–1278.

Powell, G. F., et al. "Emotional Deprivation and Growth Retardation Simulating Idiopathic Hypopituitarism. II. Endocrinologic Evaluation of the Syndrome." *New England Journal of Medicine*, 1967, 276:1279–1283.

7. Kety, S. S. "Disorders of the Human Brain," pp. 202–214.

8. Kety, S. S. "The Biological Roots of Mental Illness; Their Ramifications Through Cerebral Metabolism, Synaptic Activity, Genetics and the Environment." In *Harvey Lectures 1975–76*. New York: Academic Press, 1978, pp. 1–22.

Kety, S. S., et al. "Mental Illness in the Biological and Adoptive Families of Adopted Individuals Who Have Become Schizophrenic: A Preliminary Report Based on Psychiatric Interviews." In R. R. Fieve, A. Rosenthal, and H. Brill (eds.), *Genetic Research in Psychiatry*. Baltimore: Johns Hopkins University Press, 1975, pp. 147–166.

9. Kendler, K. S., Gruenberg, A. M., and Strauss, J. S. "An Independent Analysis of the Copenhagen Sample of the Danish Adoption Study of Schizophrenia. III. The Relationship Between Paranoid Psychosis (Delusional Disorder) and the Schizophrenia Spectrum Disorders." *Archives of General Psychiatry*, 1981, 38: 985–987.

10. Laing, R. D. *The Politics of Experience*. New York: Ballantine, 1967, p. 115.
11. Kety, S. S. "From Rationalization to Reason." *American Journal of Psychiatry*, 1974, 131: 957–963.
12. Bleuler, M. "The Offspring of Schizophrenics." *Schizophrenia Bulletin*, 1975, 8: 93–107.
13. Fuller, J. L., and Thompson, W. R. *Foundations of Behavior Genetics*. St. Louis, Mo.: Mosby, 1978, p. 370.
14. For a review of this subject see Hirsch, S. R. "Do Parents Cause Schizophrenia?" *Trends in Neurosciences*, 1979, 2:49–52.
15. Wender, P. H., et al. "Cross Fostering, a Research Strategy for Clarifying the Role of Genetic and Experiential Factors in the Etiology of Schizophrenia." *Archives of General Psychiatry*, 1974, 30:121–128.
16. Rosenhan, D. "On Being Sane in Insane Places." *Science*, 1973, 179:250–258.
17. Murphy, J. M. "Psychiatric Labelling in Cross-Cultural Perspective." *Science*, 1976, 191:1019–1028.
18. Babigian, H. M. "Schizophrenia: Epidemiology." In H. I. Kaplan, A. M. Freedman, and B. J. Sadock (eds.), *Comprehensive Textbook of Psychiatry/III*. Baltimore: Williams & Wilkins, 1980, pp. 1113–1121. Murphy, J. M. "Psychiatric Labelling," pp. 1019–1028.
19. Goldhammer, H., and Marshall, A. W. *Psychosis and Civilization*. New York: Free Press, 1949.
20. Turner, R. J. "Social Mobility and Schizophrenia." *Journal of Health and Social Behavior*, 1968, 9:194–203.
    Hare, E. H., Price, J. S., and Slater, E. "Parental Social Class in Psychiatric Patients." *British Journal of Psychiatry*, 1972, 121:515–524.

Chapter 6

1. Swazey, J. P. *Chlorpromazine in Psychiatry*. Cambridge, Mass: M.I.T. Press, 1974.
2. Baldessarini, R. J. "Drugs and the Treatment of Psychiatric Disorders." In A. G. Gilman, L. S. Goodman, and A. Gilman (eds.), *The Pharmacological Basis of Therapeutics*. New York: Macmillan, 1980, pp. 408–411.
3. Rosenhan, D. L. "On Being Sane in Insane Places." *Science*, 1973, 179:250–258.
4. National Institutes of Health Pharmacology Service Center, Collaborative Study Group. "Phenothiazine Treatment in Acute Schizophrenia." *Archives of General Psychiatry*, 1964, 10:246–261. Hymowitz, P., and Spohn, H. "The Effects of Antipsychotic Medication on the Linguistic Ability of Schizophrenics." *Journal of Nervous and Mental Disease*, 1980, 168:287–296.
5. Swazey, J. P. *Chlorpromazine in Psychiatry*, p. 209.
6. Ibid., p. 219.

7. Vonnegut, M. *The Eden Express.* New York: Bantam, 1976.
8. Ibid., p. 164.
9. North, C., and Cardoret, R. "Diagnostic Discrepancy in Personal Accounts of Patients with Schizophrenia." *Archives of General Psychiatry*, 1981, 38:133–137.
10. Sheehan, S. "A Reporter at Large" (Creedmoor—Parts I–IV). *The New Yorker*, May 25, June 1, June 8, June 15, 1981.
11. National Institutes of Health Pharmacology Service Center, Collaborative Study Group. "Phenothiazine Treatment in Acute Schizophrenia," pp. 246–261.
12. May, P. R. A. *Treatment of Schizophrenia.* New York: Science House, 1968, pp. 151–154. May, P. R. A., and Tuma, A. H. "A Followup Study of the Results of Schizophrenia Treatment." In R. L. Spitzer and D. F. Klein (eds.), *Evaluation of Psychological Therapies.* Baltimore: Johns Hopkins University Press, 1979, pp. 256–284.
13. Davis, J. M. "Antipsychotic Drugs." In H. I. Kaplan, A. M. Freedman, and B. J. Sadock (eds.), *Comprehensive Textbook of Psychiatry/III.* Baltimore: Williams & Wilkins, 1980, pp. 2257–2289.
14. Hogarty, G. W., and Goldberg, S. C. "Drugs and Sociotherapy in the Aftercare of Schizophrenic Patients. I. One Year Relapse Rates." *Archives of General Psychiatry*, 1973, 28:54–64. Hogarty, G. W., et al. "Drug and Sociotherapy in the Aftercare of Schizophrenic Patients. II. Two Year Relapse Rates." *Archives of General Psychiatry*, 1974, 31:603–606.
15. Hogarty, G. E., et al. "Fluphenazine and Social Therapy in the Aftercare of Schizophrenic Patients." *Archives of General Psychiatry*, 1979, 36:1283–1294.
16. Hogarty, G. E., Goldberg, S. C., and Schooler, N. R. "Drug and Sociotherapy in the Aftercare of Schizophrenic Patients. III. Adjustment of Nonrelapsed Patients." *Archives of General Psychiatry*, 1964, 31:609–618.
17. Gardos, G., and Cole, J. O. "Maintenance Antipsychotic Therapy: For Whom and How Long?" In M. A. Lipton, A. DiMascio, and K. F. Killam (eds.), *Psychopharmacology: A Generation of Progress.* New York: Raven Press, 1978, pp. 1169–1178.
18. Davis, J. M. "Antipsychotic Drugs," pp. 2257–2289. Hollister, L. E. "Antipsychotic Medications and the Treatment of Schizophrenia." In J. D. Barchas et al. (eds.), *Psychopharmacology, From Theory to Practice.* New York: Oxford University Press, 1977, pp. 121–150. Baldessarini, R. J. *Chemotherapy in Psychiatry.* Cambridge, Mass.: Harvard University Press, 1977, pp. 46–48.
19. Cheung, H. K. "Schizophrenics Fully Remitted on Neuroleptics for 3–5 Years—To Stop or Continue Drugs." *British Journal of Psychiatry*, 1981, 138:490–494.
20. Lehmann, H. E. "Schizophrenia: Clinical Features." In H. I. Kaplan, A. M. Freedman, and B. J. Sadock (eds.), *Comprehensive Textbook of Psychiatry*, pp. 1153–1192. Hollister, L. E. "Antipsychotic Medications and the Treatment of Schizophrenia," pp. 121–150. Harrow, M., Grinker,

R. R., and Silvester, M. L. "Is Modern Day Schizophrenia Outcome Still Negative?" *American Journal of Psychiatry*, 1978, 135:1156–1162. Tsuang, M. T., Woolson, R. F., and Flemming, J. A. "Long-Term Outcome of Major Psychoses. I. Schizophrenia and Affective Disorders Compared with Psychiatrically Symptom-Free Surgical Conditions." *Archives of General Psychiatry*, 1979, 36:1295–1301. Bland, R. C., Parker, R. C., and Orn, H. "Prognosis in Schizophrenia: A Ten-Year Follow-Up of First Admissions." *Archives of General Psychiatry*, 1976, 33:949–954.

21. Lehmann, H. E. "Schizophrenia: Clinical Features," pp. 1153–1192.
22. Bland, R. C., Parker, R. C., and Orn, H. "Prognosis in Schizophrenia," pp. 949–954.
23. Lehmann, H. E. "Schizophrenia: Clinical Features," pp. 1153–1192.
24. Harrow, M., Grinker, R. R., and Silvester, M. L. "Is Schizophrenia Outcome Negative?" pp. 1156–1162.
25. Kesey, K. *One Flew Over the Cuckoo's Nest.* New York: Viking Press, 1962.
26. Davis, J. M. "Antipsychotic Drugs," pp. 2257–2289.
27. Ibid.
28. Vonnegut, M. *The Eden Express*, pp. 253, 272.
29. Kane, J. M., et al. "Fluphenazine vs Placebo in Patients with Remitted Acute First-Episode Schizophrenia." *Archives of General Psychiatry*, 1982, 39:70–73.
30. Jarvik, M. E. "Drugs Used in the Treatment of Psychiatric Disorders." In L. S. Goodman and A. Gilman, *The Pharmacological Basis of Therapeutics*. Fourth Edition. New York: Macmillan, 1970, p. 169.
31. Vonnegut, M. *The Eden Express*, p. 248.
32. Ibid., p. 269.
33. Carpenter, W. T., McGlashan, T. H., and Strauss, J. S. "The Treatment of Acute Schizophrenia Without Drugs: An Investigation of Some Current Assumptions." *American Journal of Psychiatry*, 1977, 134:14–20.
34. May, P. R. A. *Treatment of Schizophrenia*, pp. 151–154.
35. May, P. R. A., Tuma, A. H., and Dixon, W. J. "Schizophrenia—A Followup Study of the Results of 5 Forms of Treatment." *Archives of General Psychiatry*, 1981, 38:776–784.
36. Greenblatt, M. In foreword to May, P. R. A. *Treatment of Schizophrenia*.
37. May, P. R. A., and Simpson, G. M. "Evaluation of Treatment Methods." In H. I. Kaplan, A. M. Freedman, and B. J. Sadock (eds.), *Comprehensive Textbook of Psychiatry*, pp. 1240–1274. Feinsilver, D. B., and Gunderson, J. G. "Psychotherapy for Schizophrenics—Is It Indicated? A Review of the Relevant Literature." *Schizophrenia Bulletin*, 1972, 6:11–23.
38. Vonnegut, M. *Eden Express*, p. 249.
39. May, P. R. A. *Treatment of Schizophrenia*, pp. 231–242.
40. Hogarty, G. E., et al. "Two Year Relapse Rates," pp. 603–606.
41. Hogarty, G. E., Goldberg, S. C., and Schooler, N. R. "Adjustment of Nonrelapsed Patients," pp. 609–618.
42. Hogarty, G. E., et al. "Fluphenazine in Aftercare," pp. 1283–1294.

43. May, P. R. A. "Rational Treatment for an Irrational Disorder. What Does the Schizophrenic Patient Need?" *American Journal of Psychiatry*, 1976, 133:1008–1011.

44. Osmond, H., and Hoffer, A. "Massive Niacin Treatment in Schizophrenia: Review of a Nine-Year Study." *The Lancet*, 1962, 1:316–319.

45. Pauling, L. "On the Orthomolecular Environment of the Mind: Orthomolecular Theory." *American Journal of Psychiatry*, 1974, 131:1251–1257.

46. APA Task Force on Vitamin Therapy in Psychiatry. *Megavitamin and Orthomolecular Therapy in Psychiatry*. Washington, D.C.: American Psychiatric Association, 1973. May, P. R. A., and Simpson, G. M. "Evaluation of Treatment Methods," pp. 1240–1274.

47. Hoffer, A., and Osmond, H. *Megavitamin Therapy*. Regina, Saskatchewan: Canadian Schizophrenia Foundation, 1976, p. 14.

48. Autry, J. H., III. "Workshop on Orthomolecular Treatment of Schizophrenia: A Report." *Schizophrenia Bulletin*, 1975, 12:94–103.

49. Wittenborn, J. R., Weber, E. S. P., and Brown, M. "Niacin in the Long-Term Treatment of Schizophrenia." *Archives of General Psychiatry*, 1973, 28:308–315.

50. Wittenborn, J. R. "A Search for Responders to Niacin Supplementation." *Archives of General Psychiatry*, 1974, 31:547–552.

Chapter 7

1. Snyder, S. H., Burt, D. R., and Creese, I. "The Dopamine Receptor of Mammalian Brain: Direct Demonstration of Binding to Agonist and Antagonist Sites." In A. J. Ferendelli, B. S. McEwen, and S. H. Snyder (eds.), *Neurotransmitters, Hormones, and Receptors: Novel Approaches*. Bethesda, Md.: Society for Neuroscience, 1976, pp. 28–49. Creese, I., Burt, D. R., and Snyder, S. H. "Biochemical Actions of Neuroleptic Drugs: Focus on Dopamine Receptor." In L. L. Iversen, S. D. Iversen, and S. H. Snyder (eds.), *Handbook of Psychopharmacology*, Vol. 10. New York: Plenum Press, 1978, pp. 37–89.

2. Burt, D. R., Creese, I., and Snyder, S. H. "Dopamine Receptor Binding in the Corpus Striatum of Mammalian Brain." *Proceedings of the National Academy of Sciences*, 1975, 72:4655–4659. Seeman, P., et al. "Antipsychotic Drug Classes and Neuroleptic/Dopamine Receptors." *Nature*, 1976, 261:717–719.

3. Kebabian, J. W., Petzgold, G. L., and Greengard, P. "Dopamine-Sensitive Adenylate Cyclase in Caudate Nucleus of Rat Brain and its Similarity to the 'Dopamine Receptor.' " *Proceedings of the National Academy of Sciences*, 1972, 69:2145–2149. Clement-Cormier, Y. C., and Greengard, P. L. "Dopamine Sensitive Adenylate Cyclase in Mammalian Brain: A Possible Site of Action of Antipsychotic Drugs." *Proceedings of the National Academy of Sciences*, 1974, 71:1113–1117. Iversen, L. L. "Catecholamine-Sensitive Adenylate Cyclases in Nervous Tissue." *Journal of Neurochemistry*, 1977, 29:5–12.

4. Bunney, B. S., and Aghajanian, G. K. "Mesolimbic and Mesocortical Dopaminergic Systems: Physiology and Pharmacology." In M. A. Lipton, A. DiMascio, and K. F. Killam (eds.), *Psychopharmacology: A Generation of Progress*. New York: Raven Press, 1978, pp. 159–170.

5. Burt, D. R., Creese, I., and Snyder, S. H. "Properties of ^{3}H Haloperidol and ^{3}H Dopamine Binding Associated with Dopamine Receptors in Calf Brain Membranes." *Molecular Pharmacology*, 1976, 12:800–812. Snyder, S. H., Burt, D. R., and Creese, I. "Dopamine Receptor of Mammalian Brain," pp. 28–49. Seeman, P., et al. "Drug Classes and Receptors," pp. 717–719.

6. Snyder, S. H., Burt, D. R., and Creese, I. "Dopamine Receptor of Mammalian Brain," pp. 28–49.

7. Ibid.

8. Snyder, S. H. "Neurotransmitter and Drug Receptors in the Brain." *Biochemical Pharmacology*, 1975, 24:1371–1374.

9. Snyder, S. H. "Amphetamine Psychosis: A 'Model' Schizophrenia Mediated by Catecholamines." *American Journal of Psychiatry*, 1973, 130:60–61. Biel, J. H., and Bopp, B. A. "Amphetamines: Structure-Activity Relationships." In L. L. Iversen, S. D. Iversen, and S. H. Snyder (eds.), *Handbook of Psychopharmacology*, Vol. 11. New York: Plenum Press, 1978, pp. 1–39.

10. Angrist, B., and Sudilovsky, A. "Central Nervous System Stimulants: Historical Aspects and Clinical Effects." In L. L. Iversen, S. D. Iversen, and S. H. Snyder (eds.), *Handbook of Psychopharmacology*, Vol. 11, pp. 99–165.

11. Janowsky, D. S., et al. "Provocation of Schizophrenic Symptoms by Intravenous Injection of Methylphenidate." *Archives of General Psychiatry*, 1973, 28:185–191. Janowsky, D. S., and Davis, J. M. "Methylphenidate, Dextroamphetamine and Levamphetamine: Effects on Schizophrenic Symptoms." *Archives of General Psychiatry*, 1976, 33:304–308. Snyder, S. H., et al. "Drugs, Neurotransmitters, and Schizophrenia." *Science*, 1974, 184:1243–1253.

12. Janowsky, D. S. et al. "Provocation of Schizophrenic Symptoms," pp. 185–191.

13. Snyder, S. H., et al. "Drugs, Neurotransmitters, and Schizophrenia," pp. 1243–1253. Hollister, L. E. "Drug-Induced Psychoses and Schizophrenic Reactions: A Critical Comparison." *Annals of the New York Academy of Sciences*, 1962, 96:80–92.

14. Angrist, B., and Sudilovsky, A. "Central Nervous System Stimulants," pp. 99–165. Snyder, S. H., et al. "Drugs, Neurotransmitters, and Schizophrenia," pp. 1243–1253. Angrist, B., Lee, H. K., and Gershon, S. "The Antagonism of Amphetamine-Induced Symptomatology by a Neuroleptic." *American Journal of Psychiatry*, 1974, 131:817–819. Baldessarini, R. J. *Chemotherapy in Psychiatry*. Cambridge, Mass.: Harvard University Press, 1977, p. 124.

15. Snyder, S. H., Burt, D. R., and Creese, I. "Dopamine Receptor of Mammalian Brain," pp. 28–49.

16. Angrist, B., Sathananthan, G., and Gershon, S. "Behavioral Effects of L-Dopa in Schizophrenic Patients." *Psychopharmacologia*, 1973, 31:1–12.

17. Muller, P., and Seeman, P. "Dopaminergic Supersensitivity After Neuroleptics: Time Course and Specificity." *Psychopharmacology*, 1978, 60:1–11. Burt, D. R., Creese, I., and Snyder, S. H. "Antischizophrenic Drugs: Chronic Treatment Elevates Dopamine Receptor Binding in Brain." *Science*, 1977, 196:326–328.

18. Baldessarini, R. J., and Tarsy, D. "Dopamine and the Pathophysiology of Dyskinesias Induced by Antipsychotic Drugs." *Annual Review of Neurobiology*, 1980, 3:23–41. Creese, I., and Snyder, S. H. "Behavioral and Biochemical Properties of the Dopamine Receptor." In M. A. Lipton, A. DiMascio, and K. F. Killam (eds.), *Psychopharmacology: A Generation of Progress*, pp. 377–388.

19. Sedvall, G. "Receptor Feedback and Dopamine Turnover in the Central Nervous System." In L. L. Iversen, S. D. Iversen, and S. H. Snyder (eds.), *Handbook of Pharmacology*, Vol. 6. New York: Plenum Press, 1975, pp. 127–177. Carlsson, A. "Mechanism of Action of Neuroleptic Drugs." In M. A. Lipton, A. DiMascio, and K. F. Killam (eds.), *Psychopharmacology: A Generation of Progress*, pp. 1057–1070.

20. Gerlach, J., Thorsen, K., and Fog, R. "Extrapyramidal Reactions and Amine Metabolites in Cerebrospinal Fluid During Haloperidol and Clozapine Treatment of Schizophrenic Patients." *Psychopharmacologia*, 1975, 40:341–350.

21. Bacapoulos, N. C., et al. "Regional Sensitivity of Primate Brain Dopaminergic Neurons to Haloperidol: Alterations Following Chronic Treatment." *Brain Research*, 1978, 157:396–401.

22. Bacapoulos, N. C., et al. "Antipsychotic Drug Action in Schizophrenic Patients: Effect on Cortical Dopamine Metabolism After Long-Term Treatment." *Science*, 1979, 205:1045–1047.

23. von Praag, H. M. "The Significance of Dopamine for the Mode of Action of Neuroleptics and the Pathogenesis of Schizophrenia." *British Journal of Psychiatry*, 1977, 130:463–474.

24. Owen, F., et al. "Increased Dopamine-Receptor Sensitivity in Schizophrenia." *Lancet*, 1978, 2:223–226. Lee, T., and Seeman, P. "Elevation of Brain Neuroleptic/Dopamine Receptors in Schizophrenia." *American Journal of Psychiatry*, 1980, 137:191–197.

Chapter 8

1. Baldessarini, R. J. "Drugs and the Treatment of Psychiatric Disorders." In A. G. Gilman, L. S. Goodman, and A. Gilman (eds.), *The Pharmacological Basis of Therapeutics*. New York: Macmillan, 1980, pp. 391–447. Davis, J. M. "Antipsychotic Drugs." In H. I. Kaplan, A. M. Freedman, and B. J. Sadock (eds.), *Comprehensive Textbook of Psychiatry/III*. Baltimore: Williams & Wilkins, 1980, pp. 2257–2289.

2. Baldessarini, R. J. "Drugs and Psychiatric Disorders," pp. 391–447. Davis, J. M. "Antipsychotic Drugs," pp. 2257–2289. Berger, P. A. "Medical Treatment of Mental Illness." *Science,* 1978, 200:974–981.
3. Hollister, L. E. "Antipsychotic Medications and the Treatment of Schizophrenia." In J. D. Barchas et al. (eds.), *Psychopharmacology. From Theory to Practice.* New York: Oxford University Press, 1977, pp. 121–150.
4. Baldessarini, R. J., and Tarsy, D. "Dopamine and the Pathophysiology of Dyskinesias Induced by Antipsychotic Drugs." *Annual Review of Neuroscience,* 1980, 3:23–41. Baldessarini, R. J., and Tarsy, D. "Tardive Dyskinesia." In M. A. Lipton, A. DiMascio, and K. F. Killam (eds.), *Psychopharmacology: A Generation of Progress,* pp. 993–1004.
5. Berger, P. A. "Medical Treatment of Mental Illness," pp. 974–981. Casey, D. E. "The Differential Diagnosis of Tardive Dyskinesia." *Acta Physiologica Scandinavica,* 1981, sup. 291, 63:71–87. Smith, J. M., and Baldessarini, R. J. "Changes in Prevalence, Severity and Recovery in Tardive Dyskinesia with Age." *Archives of General Psychiatry,* 1980, 37:1368–1373. Baldessarini, R. J., and Tarsy, D. "Tardive Dyskinesia," pp. 993–1004. Kane, J. M., and Smith, J. M. "Tardive Dyskinesia." *Archives of General Psychiatry,* 1982, 39:473–482. Jeste, D. V., and Wyatt, R. J. "Changing Epidemiology of Tardive Dyskinesia: An Overview." *American Journal of Psychiatry,* 1981, 138:297–309.
6. Smith, J. M., and Baldessarini, R. J. "Changes in Tardive Dyskinesia with Age," pp. 1368–1373. May, P. R. A., and Simpson, G. M. "Schizophrenia: Overview of Treatment Methods." In H. I. Kaplan, A. M. Freedman, and B. J. Sadock (eds.), *Comprehensive Textbook of Psychiatry/III,* pp. 1192–1216. Kane, J. M., and Smith, J. M. "Tardive Dyskinesia," pp. 473–482. Jeste, D. V., and Wyatt, R. J. "Epidemiology of Tardive Dyskinesia, pp. 297–309.
7. Baldessarini, R. J., and Tarsy, D. "Dopamine and the Pathophysiology of Dyskinesias," pp. 23–41.
8. Ibid.
9. Smith, J. M., and Baldessarini, R. J. "Changes in Tardive Dyskinesia with Age," pp. 1368–1373. Geclach, J. "Prevention/Treatment of Tardive Dyskinesia." *Acta Physiologica Scandinavica,* 1981, sup. 219, 63:117–126. Baldessarini, R. J., and Tarsy, D. "Dopamine and the Pathophysiology of Dyskinesias," pp. 23–41.
10. Baldessarini, R. J., and Tarsy, D. "Dopamine and the Pathophysiology of Dyskinesias," pp. 23–41. Baldessarini, R. J., and Tarsy, D. "Tardive Dyskinesia," pp. 993–1004.
11. May, P. R. A., and Simpson, G. M. "Schizophrenia: Treatment Methods," pp. 1192–1216. Quitkin, F., et al. "Tardive Dyskinesia: Are First Signs Reversible?" *American Journal of Psychiatry,* 1977, 134:84–87.
12. Baldessarini, R. J., and Tarsy, D. "Dopamine and the Pathophysiology of Dyskinesias," pp. 23–41.
13. Quitkin, F., et al. "Tardive Dyskinesia: First Signs," pp. 84–87.
14. Meltzer, H. Y., Goode, D. J., and Fang, V. S. "The Effects of Psycho-

tropic Drugs on Endocrine Function. I. Neuroleptics, Precursors and Agonists." In M. A. Lipton, A. DiMascio, and K. F. Killam (eds.), *Psychopharmacology: A Generation of Progress.* New York: Raven Press, 1978, pp. 509–529.

15. Davis, J. M. "Antipsychotic Drugs," pp. 2257–2289.
16. Creese, I., Burt, D. R., and Snyder, S. H. "Biochemical Actions of Neuroleptic Drugs; Focus on Dopamine Receptor." In L. L. Iversen, S. D. Iversen, and S. H. Snyder (eds.), *Handbook of Psychopharmacology,* Vol. 10. New York: Plenum Press, 1978, pp. 37–89. Davis, J. M. "Antipsychotic Drugs," pp. 2257–2289.
17. Baldessarini, R. J. "Drugs and Psychiatric Disorders," pp. 391–447.
18. Davis, J. M. "Antipsychotic Drugs," pp. 2257–2289.
19. Baldessarini, R. J. "Drugs and Psychiatric Disorders," pp. 391–447.
20. Davis, J. M. "Antipsychotic Drugs," pp. 2257–2289.
21. Baldessarini, R. J. *Chemotherapy in Psychiatry.* Cambridge, Mass.: Harvard University Press, 1977, pp. 20–21. Davis, J. M. "Antipsychotic Drugs," pp. 2257–2289.
22. Baldessarini, R. J. *Chemotherapy in Psychiatry,* pp. 32–34. Hollister, L. E. "Antipsychotic Medications and Schizophrenia," pp. 121–150.
23. Sheehan, S. "A Reporter at Large (Creedmoor—Part II)," *The New Yorker,* June 1, 1981, p. 79.

Chapter 9

1. In this chapter, the description of affective disorders is based on the following sources: American Psychiatric Association. *Diagnostic and Statistical Manual of Mental Disorders,* Third Edition. Washington, D.C.: American Psychiatric Association, 1980, pp. 205–223. Nelson, J., and Charney, D. S. "The Symptoms of Major Depressive Illness." *American Journal of Psychiatry,* 1981, 138:1–13. Feighner, J. P., et al. "Diagnostic Criteria for Use in Psychiatric Research." *Archives of General Psychiatry,* 1972, 26:57–63. Klerman, G. "Affective Disorders: Overview of Affective Disorders." In H. I. Kaplan, A. M. Freedman, and B. J. Sadock (eds.), *Comprehensive Textbook of Psychiatry,* Third Edition. Baltimore: Williams & Wilkins, 1980, pp. 1305–1319. Wolpert, E. A. "Major Affective Disorders." In H. I. Kaplan, A. M. Freedman, and B. J. Sadock (eds.), *Comprehensive Textbook of Psychiatry,* pp. 1319–1331. Arieti, S. "Affective Disorders: Manic Depressive Psychosis and Psychotic Depression. Manifest Symptomatology, Psychodynamics, Sociological Factors, and Psychotherapy." In S. Arieti and E. B. Brody (eds.), *American Handbook of Psychiatry,* Second Edition. New York: Basic Books, 1974, pp. 449–490.
2. Wolpert, E. A. "Major Affective Disorders," pp. 1319–1331.
3. American Psychiatric Association. *DSM-III,* p. 217.
4. Ibid., p. 208.

5. Fieve, R. R. *Moodswing: The Third Revolution in Psychiatry.* New York: William Morrow, 1975.
6. Ibid., pp. 192–195.
7. American Psychiatric Association. *DSM-III*, p. 208.
8. Fieve, R. R. *Moodswing*, pp. 42–44. Machlis, J. *The Enjoyment of Music.* New York: Norton, 1955, pp. 103–104.
9. Bullock, A. *Hitler: A Study in Tyranny.* New York: Harper & Row, 1962.
10. Fieve, R. R. *Moodswing*, pp. 93–118.
11. Ibid., pp. 42–44.
12. American Psychiatric Association. *DSM-III*, p. 209.
13. Ibid.
14. Ibid.
15. Ibid., p. 213.
16. Ibid., pp. 213–214.
17. Ibid., p. 214.
18. Ibid.
19. Ibid.
20. Ibid., p. 215.

Chapter 10

1. Sheehan, S. "A Reporter at Large".(Creedmoor—Parts I–IV). *The New Yorker*, May 25, June 1, June 8, June 15, 1981.
2. Klerman, G. L. "Long-Term Treatment of Affective Disorders." In M. A. Lipton, A. DiMascio, and K. F. Killam (eds.), *Psychopharmacology: A Generation of Progress.* New York: Raven Press, 1978, pp. 1303–1312.
3. Klerman, G. L. "Overview of Affective Disorders." In H. I. Kaplan, A. M. Freedman, and B. J. Sadock (eds.), *Comprehensive Textbook of Psychiatry/Third Edition.* Baltimore: Williams & Wilkins, 1980, pp. 1305–1318. Walpert, E. A. "Major Affective Disorders." In H. I. Kaplan, A. M. Freedman, and B. J. Sadock (eds.), *Comprehensive Textbook of Psychiatry/Third Edition*, pp. 1319–1332. Boyd, J. H., and Weissman, M. M. "Epidemiology of Affective Disorders." *Archives of General Psychiatry*, 1981, 38:1039–1046. Weissman, M. M., Myers, J. K., and Thompson, D. "Depression and Its Treatment in a U.S. Urban Community 1975–1976." *Archives of General Psychiatry*, 1981, 38:417–421. Weissman, M. M., and Myers, J. K. "Affective Disorders in a U.S. Urban Community." *Archives of General Psychiatry*, 1978, 35:1304–1311. Ripley, H. S. "Depression and the Life Span—Epidemiology." In G. Usdin (ed.), *Depression: Clinical, Biological, and Psychological Perspectives.* New York: Brunner/Mazel, 1977, pp. 1–27.
4. Weissman, M. M., and Myers, J. K. "Affective Disorders in a U.S. Urban Community," pp. 1304–1311. Klerman, G. L. "Overview of Affective Disorders," pp. 1305–1318. Hirschfeld, R. M. A., and Cross, C. K. "Epidemiology of Affective Disorders." *American Journal of Psychiatry*, 1982, 39:35–46.
5. Weissmann, M. M., and Myers, J. K. "Affective Disorders in a U.S.

Urban Community," pp. 1304–1311. Amenson, C. S., and Lewinsohn, P. M. "An Investigation into the Observed Sex Difference in Prevalence of Unipolar Depression." *Journal of Abnormal Psychology*, 1981, 90:1–13. American Psychiatric Association. *Diagnostic and Statistical Manual of Mental Disorders*, Third Edition. Washington, D.C.: American Psychiatric Association, 1980.

6. Boyd, J. H., and Weissman, M. M. "Epidemiology of Affective Disorders," pp. 1039–1046.

7. Weissman, M. M., and Myers, J. K. "Affective Disorders in a U.S. Urban Community," pp. 1304–1311.

8. Amenson, C. S., and Lewinsohn, P. M. "Sex Difference in Prevalence of Unipolar Depression," pp. 1–13.

9. Tan, E. S. "The Presentation of Affective Symptoms in Non-Western Countries." In G. H. Burrows (ed.), *Handbook of Studies on Depression*, pp. 121–133.

10. Tsuang, M. T., Woolson, R. F., and Fleming, J. A. "Premature Deaths in Schizophrenia and Affective Disorders." *Archives of General Psychiatry*, 1980, 37:979–983.

11. Tsuang, M. T. "Suicide in Schizophrenics, Manics, Depressives, and Surgical Controls." *Archives of General Psychiatry*, 1978, 35:153–155. Guze, S. B., and Robins, E. "Suicide and Primary Affective Disorder." *British Journal of Psychiatry*, 1970, 17:437–438.

12. *Statistical Abstract of the United States*. Washington, D.C.: U.S. Department of Commerce, Bureau of the Census, 1980, p. 78.

13. Whitlock, F. A. "Depression and Suicide." In G. H. Burrows (ed.), *Handbook of Studies on Depression*. Amsterdam: Excerpta Medica, 1977, pp. 379–404.

14. Lloyd, C. "Life Events and Depressive Disorder Reviewed. I. Events as Predisposing Factors." *Archives of General Psychiatry*, 1980, 37:529–535.

15. Lloyd, C. "Life Events and Depressive Disorder Reviewed. II. Events as Precipitating Factors." *Archives of General Psychiatry*, 1980, 37:541–548.

16. Klerman, G. L. "Overview of Affective Disorders," pp. 1305–1318.

17. Grant, I., et al. "Life Events and Symptoms." *Archives of General Psychiatry*, 1982, 39:598–605.

18. Klerman, G. L. "Overview of Affective Disorders," pp. 1305–1318.

19. Kidd, K. K., and Weissman, M. M. "Why We Do Not Yet Understand the Genetics of Affective Disorders." In J. O. Cole, A. F. Schatzberg, and S. H. Frazier (eds.), *Depression: Biology, Psychodynamics, and Treatment*. New York: Plenum Press, 1978, pp. 107–122.

20. Ibid.

21. Winokur, G. "Mania and Depression: Family Studies and Genetics in Relation to Treatment." In M. A. Lipton, A. DiMascio, and K. F. Killam (eds.), *Psychopharmacology: A Generation of Progress*, pp. 1213–1222.

22. Ibid.

23. Mendlewicz, J., and Ranier, J. D. "Adoption Study Supporting Genetic Transmission in Manic-Depressive Illness." *Nature*, 1977, 268:327–329.

Chapter 11

1. Baldessarini, R. J. "Drugs and the Treatment of Psychiatric Disorders." In A. G. Gilman, L. S. Goodman, and A. Gilman (eds.), *The Pharmacological Basis of Therapeutics*. New York: Macmillan, 1980, pp. 391–447.
2. Davis, J. M. "Antidepressant Drugs." In H. I. Kaplan, A. M. Freeman, and B. J. Sadock (eds.), *Comprehensive Textbook of Psychiatry/Third Edition*. Baltimore: Williams & Wilkins, 1980, pp. 2240–2316.
3. Kessler, K. A. "Tricyclic Antidepressants: Mode of Action and Clinical Use." In M. A. Lipton, A. DiMascio, and K. F. Killam (eds.), *Psychopharmacology: A Generation of Progress*. New York: Raven Press, 1978, pp. 1289–1302. Berger, P. A. "Antidepressants and the Treatment of Depressions." In J. D. Barchas et al. (eds.), *Psychopharmacology, From Theory to Practice*. New York: Oxford University Press, 1977, pp. 174–207.
4. Hamilton, M. "Development of a Rating Scale for Primary Depressive Illness." *British Journal of Social and Clinical Psychology*, 1967, 6:278–296.
5. Morris, J. B., and Beck, A. T. "The Efficacy of Antidepressant Drugs." *Archives of General Psychiatry*, 1974, 30:667–674.
6. Kessler, K. A. "Tricyclic Antidepressants," pp. 1289–1302. Berger, P. A. "Antidepressants and Depressions," pp. 174–207.
7. Linnoila, M., et al. "Cloipramine and Doxepin in Depressive Neurosis." *Archives of General Psychiatry*, 1980, 37:1295–1299. Bielski, R. J., and Friedel, R. O. "Prediction of Tricyclic Antidepressant Response." *Archives of General Psychiatry*, 1976, 33:1479–1489. Raskin, A., et al. "Differential Response to Chlorpromazine, Imipramine and Placebo." *Archives of General Psychiatry*, 1970, 23:164–173. Goodwin, F. K., Cowdry, R. W., and Webster, M. H. "Predictors of Drug Response in Affective Disorders: Toward an Integrated Approach." In M. A. Lipton, A. DiMascio, and R. F. Killam (eds.), *Psychopharmacology: A Generation of Progress*, pp. 1277–1288.
8. Linnoila, M., et al. "Cloipramine and Doxepin," pp. 1295–1299.
9. Glass, R. M., et al. "Cognitive Dysfunction and Imipramine in Outpatient Depressives." *Archives of General Psychiatry*, 1981, 38:1048–1051.
10. Raskin, A., et al. "Differential Response," pp. 164–173. Bielski, R. J., and Friedel, R. O. "Prediction of Tricyclic Antidepressant Response," pp. 1479–1489.
11. Kantor, S. J., and Glassman, A. H. "Delusional Depression: Natural History and Response to Treatment." *British Journal of Psychiatry*, 1977, 131:351–360. Raskin, A., et al. "Differential Response," pp. 164–173.
12. Berger, P. A. "Antidepressants and Depressions," pp. 174–207.
13. Klerman, G. L. "Long-Term Treatment of Affective Disorders." In M. A. Lipton, A. DiMascio, and K. F. Killam (eds.), *Psychopharmacology:*

A Generation of Progress, pp. 1303–1312. Jann, M. W., Bitar, A. H., and Rao, A. "Lithium Prophylaxis of Tricyclic-Antidepressant-Induced Mania in Bipolar Patients." *American Journal of Psychiatry*, 1982, 139:683–684.

14. Glassman, A. H., et al. "Clinical Implications of Imipramine Plasma Levels for Depressive Illness." *Archives of General Psychiatry*, 1977, 34:197–204.

15. Ibid.

16. Coppen, A., and Peet, M. "The Long-Term Management of Patients with Affective Disorders." In E. S. Paykel and A. Coppen (eds.), *Psychopharmacology of Affective Disorders*. New York: Oxford University Press, 1979, pp. 249–256. Klerman, G. L. "Long-Term Treatment," pp. 1303–1312. Mindham, R. H. S., Howland, C., and Shepherd, M. "Continuation Therapy with Tricyclic Antidepressants in Depressive Illness." *Lancet*, 1972, 2:854–855.

17. Klerman, G. L., et al. "Treatment of Depression by Drugs and Psychotherapy." *American Journal of Psychiatry*, 1974, 131:186–191.

18. Weissman, M. M., and Klerman, G. L. "The Chronic Depressive in the Community: Unrecognized and Poorly Treated." *Comprehensive Psychiatry*, 1977, 18:523–532.

19. Ibid.

20. Bialos, D., et al. "Recurrence of Depression After Discontinuation of Long-Term Amitriptyline Treatment." *American Journal of Psychiatry*, 1982, 139:325–329.

21. Hankin, J. R., et al. "Use of General Medical Care Services by Persons with Mental Disorders." *Archives of General Psychiatry*, 1982, 39:225–231.

22. Weissman, M. M. "Psychotherapy and Its Relevance to the Pharmacotherapy of Affective Disorders: From Ideology to Evidence". In M. A. Lipton, A. DiMascio, and K. F. Killam (eds.), *Psychopharmacology: A Generation of Progress*, pp. 1313–1321.

23. Weissman, M. M., et al. "Treatment Effects on the Social Adjustment of Depressed Patients." *Archives of General Psychiatry*, 1974, 30:771–778.

24. Beck, A. T., et al. *Cognitive Therapy of Depression*. New York: Guilford Press, 1979. Kovacs, M., et al. "Depressed Outpatients Treated with Cognitive Therapy or Pharmacotherapy. *Archives of General Psychiatry*, 1981, 38:33–39.

25. Lewinsohn, P. M., Sullivan, J. M., and Grosscup, S. J. "Changing Reinforcing Events: An Approach to the Treatment of Depression." *Psychotherapy: Theory, Research and Practice*, 1980, 17:322–334.

26. Weissman, M. M., Prusoff, B. A., and DiMascio, A. "The Efficacy of Drugs and Psychotherapy in the Treatment of Acute Depressive Episodes." *American Journal of Psychiatry*, 1979, 136:555–558.

27. Covi, L., et al. "Drugs and Group Psychotherapy in Neurotic Depression." *American Journal of Psychiatry*, 1974, 131:191–198.

28. Kovacs, M., et al. "Depressed Outpatients," pp. 33–39.

29. Freedman, A. "Interaction of Drug Therapy with Marital Therapy in Depressed Patients." *Archives of General Psychiatry*, 1975, 32:619–637. Blackburn, I. M., et al. "The Efficacy of Cognitive Therapy in Depression—A Treatment Trial Using Cognitive Therapy and Pharmacotherapy, Each Alone and in Combination." *British Journal of Psychiatry*, 1981, 139:181–189. Bellack, A. S., Hersen, M., and Himmelhoch, J. "Social Skills Training Compared with Pharmacotherapy and Psychotherapy in the Treatment of Unipolar Depression." *American Journal of Psychiatry*, 1981, 138:1562–1567. Weissman, M. M., Prusoff, B. A., and DiMascio, A. "The Efficacy of Drugs and Psychotherapy," pp. 555–558.

30. DiMascio, A., et al. "Differential Symptom Reduction by Drugs and Psychotherapy in Acute Depression." *Archives of General Psychiatry*, 1979, 36:1450–1460. Weissman, M. M., et al. "Depressed Outpatients Results One Year After Treatment with Drugs and/or Interpersonal Psychotherapy." *Archives of General Psychiatry*, 1981, 38:51–55. Herceg-Baron, R., et al. "Pharmacotherapy and Psychotherapy in Acute Depressed Patients: A Study of Attrition Patterns in a Clinical Trial." *Comprehensive Psychiatry*, 1979, 20:315–325. Beck, A. T. et al. "Differential Effects of Cognitive Therapy and Pharmacotherapy on Depressive Symptoms." *Journal of Affective Disorders*, 1981, 3:221–229. Weissman, M. M., et al. "Treatment Effects on Social Adjustment," pp. 771–778.

31. Rush A. J., et al. "Differential effects of cognitive therapy and pharmacotherapy on depressive symptoms." *Journal of Affective Disorders*, 1981, 3:221-229.

32. Kovacs, M., et al. "Depressed Outpatients," pp. 33–39. Herceg-Baron, R., et al. "Pharmacotherapy and Psychotherapy in Acute Depressed Patients," pp. 315–325.

33. Prusoff, B. A., Weissman, M. M., and Klerman, G. L. "Research Diagnostic Criteria Subtypes of Depression: Their Role as Predictors of Differential Response to Psychotherapy and Drug Treatment." *Archives of General Psychiatry*, 1980, 37:796–801.

34. Blackburn, I. M., et al. "The Efficacy of Cognitive Therapy in Depression," pp. 181–189.

35. Rush, A. J., et al. "Differential Effects of Cognitive Therapy and Pharmacotherapy on Depressive Symptoms." *Journal of Affective Disorders*, pp. 221–229.

36. Brown, R. A., and Lewinsohn, P. M. "A Psychoeducational Approach to Treatment of Depression: Comparison of Group, Individual and Minimal Contact Procedures." Unpublished manuscript, University of Oregon.

37. Weissman, M. M., et al. "Depressed Outpatient Results," pp. 51–55. Kovacs, M., et al. "Depressed Outpatients," pp. 33–39.

38. Klerman, G. L., et al. "Treatment of Depression," pp. 186–191.

39. Shopsin, B. "Second Generation Antidepressants." *Journal of Clinical Psychiatry*, 1980, 41(12):45–56. Smith, R. S., Jr., and Ayd, F. J., Jr. "A Critical Appraisal of Amoxapine." *Journal of Clinical Psychiatry*, 1981,

42(6):238–242. Al-Yassiri, M. M., Ankier, S. F., and Bridges, P. K. "Tra-zodone—A New Antidepressant." *Life Sciences*, 1981, 2:449–458. Hol-lister, L. E. "Current Antidepressant Drugs: Their Clinical Use." *Drugs*, 1981, 22:129–152.

40. Kessler, K. A. "Tricyclic Antidepressants," pp. 1289–1302. Klerman, G. L. "Long-Term Treatment," pp. 1303–1312.
41. Baldessarini, R. J. "Treatment of Psychiatric Disorder," pp. 391–447.
42. Ibid.
43. Johnson, D. A. W. "Treatment Compliance in General Practice." *Acta Psychiatrica Scandinavica*, 1981, sup. 290, 63:447–453.
44. Weissman, M. M., Myers, J. K., and Thompson, D. "Depression and Its Treatment in a U.S. Urban Community 1975–1976." *Archives of General Psychiatry*, 1981, 38:417–421.
45. Barbar, J. H. "Depressive Illness in General Practice." *Acta Psychiatrica Scandinavica*, 1981, sup. 290, 63:441–446.
46. Johnson, D. A. W. "Treatment Compliance," pp. 447–453.
47. Fauman, M. A. "Tricyclic Antidepressant Prescription by General Hospital Physicians." *American Journal of Psychiatry*, 1980, 137:490–491.
48. Baldessarini, R. J. "Treatment of Psychiatric Disorders," pp. 391–447.
49. Ibid.

Chapter 12

1. Appleton, W. S., and Davis, J. M. *Practical Clinical Psychopharmacology*. Baltimore: Williams & Wilkins, 1980, pp. 117–120. Berger, P. A. "Antidepressant Medications and the Treatment of Depression." In J. D. Barchas et al. (eds.), *Psychopharmacology, From Theory to Practice*. New York: Oxford University Press, 1977, pp. 174–207. Revaris, C. L., et al. "Phenelzine and Amitriptyline in the Treatment of Depression." *Archives of General Psychiatry*, 1980, 37:1075–1080. David, J. M. "Antidepressant Drugs." In H. I. Kaplan, A. M. Freedman, and B. J. Sadock (eds.), *Comprehensive Textbook of Psychiatry/Third Edition*. Baltimore: Williams & Wilkins, 1980, pp. 2290–2316.
2. Appleton, W. S., and Davis, J. M. *Practical Clinical Psychopharmacology*, pp. 117–120. Berger, P. A. "Antidepressant Medications," pp. 174–207. Davis, J. M. "Antidepressant Drugs," pp. 2290–2316.
3. Davis, J. M. "Antidepressant Drugs," pp. 2290–2316.
4. Robinson, D. S., et al. "Clinical Psychopharmacology of Phenelzine: MAO Activity and Clinical Response." In M. A. Lipton, A. DiMascio, and K. F. Killam (eds.), *Psychopharmacology: A Generation of Progress*. New York: Raven Press, 1978, pp. 961–973. Quitkin, F., Rifkin, A., and Klein, D. F. "Monamine Oxidase Inhibitors." *Archives of General Psychiatry*, 1979, 36:749–760.
5. Davis, J. M. "Antidepressant Drugs," pp. 2290–2316.
6. Robinson, D. S., et al. "Clinical Psychopharmacology of Phenelzine," pp. 961–973. Quitkin, F., Rifkin, A., and Klein, D. F. "MAOIs," pp. 749–760.

7. Revaris, C. L., et al. "Phenelzine and Amitriptyline," pp. 1075–1080. Robinson, D. S., et al. "Clinical Psychopharmacology of Phenelzine," pp. 961–973.

8. Kesey, K. *One Flew Over the Cuckoo's Nest.* New York: Viking Press, 1962.

9. Ibid., p. 236.

10. Ibid., p. 242.

11. Weiner, R. D. "The Psychiatric Use of Electrically Induced Seizures." *American Journal of Psychiatry,* 1979, 131:1507–1517. Turek, I. S., and Hanlon, T. P. "The Effectiveness and Safety of Electroconvulsive Therapy (ECT)." *Journal of Nervous and Mental Disease,* 1977, 164:419–431.

12. Glassman, A., Kantor, S. J., and Shostak, M. "Depression, Delusions and Drug Response." *American Journal of Psychiatry,* 1975, 132:716–719. Fink, M. "Efficacy and Safety of Induced Seizures (EST) in Man." *Comprehensive Psychiatry,* 1978, 19:1–18. Avery, D., and Lubrano, A. "Depression Treated with Imipramine and ECT: The DeCarolis Study Reconsidered." *American Journal of Psychiatry,* 1979, 136:559–562.

13. Avery, D., and Lubrano, A. "Depression Treated with Imipramine and ECT," pp. 559–562.

14. Avery, D., and Winokur, G. "Mortality in Depressed Patients Treated with Electroconvulsive Therapy and Antidepressants." *Archives of General Psychiatry,* 1976, 33:1029–1037.

15. Kay, D., Fahy, T., and Garside, R. "A Seven Month Double-Blind Trial of Amitriptyline and Diazepam in ECT-Treated Patients." *British Journal of Psychiatry,* 1970, 117:667–671. Perry, P., and Tsuang, M. T. "Treatment of Unipolar Depression Following Electroconvulsive Therapy." *Journal of Affective Disorders,* 1979, 1:123–129. Coppen, A., and Peet, M. "The Long-Term Management of Patients with Affective Disorders." In E. S. Paykel and A. Coppen (eds.), *Psychopharmacology of Affective Disorders.* New York: Oxford University Press, 1979, pp. 248–256.

16. Coppen, A., et al. "Lithium Continuation Following Electroconvulsive Therapy." *British Journal of Psychiatry,* 1981, 139:284–287.

17. Wolpert, E. A. "Major Affective Disorders." In H. I. Kaplan, A. M. Freedman, and B. J. Sadock (eds.), *Comprehensive Textbook of Psychiatry, Third Edition,* pp. 1319–1331.

18. Avery, D., and Winokur, G. "Mortality in Depressed Patients," pp. 1029–1037.

19. Kalinowsky, L. B. "Convulsive Therapies." In H. I. Kaplan, A. M. Freedman, and B. J. Sadock (eds.), *Comprehensive Textbooks of Psychiatry, Third Edition,* pp. 2335–2342. Fink, M. "Efficacy and Safety of Induced Seizures," pp. 1–18.

20. Frankel, F. H. "Current Perspectives on ECT: A Discussion." *American Journal of Psychiatry,* 1977, 134:1014–1019.

21. Fink, M. "Myths of Shock Therapy." *American Journal of Psychiatry,* 1977, 134:991–996.

22. Frankel, F. H. "Current Perspectives on ECT," pp. 1014–1019.

23. Menken, M., et al. "Multiple ECT: Morphologic Effects." *American Journal of Psychiatry*, 1979, 136:456.
24. Squire, L. R. "ECT and Memory Loss." *American Journal of Psychiatry*, 1977, 134:997–1001. Squire, L. R., Slater, P. C., and Miller, P. L. "Retrograde Amnesia and Bilateral Electroconvulsive Therapy." *Archives of General Psychiatry*, 1981, 38:89–95.
25. D'Elia, G., and Raotma, H. "Is Unilateral ECT Less Effective Than Bilateral ECT?" *British Journal of Psychiatry*, 1975, 126:83–89. Davis, J. M. "Antidepressant Drugs," pp. 2290–2316. Squire, L. R. "ECT and Memory Loss," pp. 997–1001. Kalinowsky, L. B. "Convulsive Therapies," pp. 2335–2342. Fink, M. "Efficacy and Safety of Induced Seizures," pp. 1–18. Greenblatt, M. "Efficacy of ECT in Affective and Schizophrenic Illness." *American Journal of Psychiatry*, 1977, 134:1001–1005. Glassman, A., Kantor, S. J., and Shostak, M. "Depression, Delusions and Drug Response," pp. 716–719. Zung, W. W. K. "Evaluating Treatment Methods for Depressive Disorders." *American Journal of Psychiatry*, 1968, 124:40–48.

Chapter 13

1. Schildkraut, J. J. "The Catecholamine Hypothesis of Affective Disorders: A Review of the Supporting Evidence." *American Journal of Psychiatry*, 1965, 122:509–522. Bunney, W. E., Jr., and Davis, J. M. "Norepinephrine in Depressive Reactions." *Archives of General Psychiatry*, 1965, 13:483–494.
2. Baldessarini, R. J. "Drugs and the Treatment of Psychiatric Disorders." In A. G. Gilman, L. S. Goodman, and A. Gilman (eds.), *The Pharmacological Basis of Therapeutics*. New York: Macmillan, 1980, pp. 391–447.
3. Glowinski, J., and Axelrod, J. "Inhibition of Uptake of Tritiated Noradrenaline in the Intact Rat Brain by Imipramine and Structurally Related Compounds." *Nature*, 1964, 204:1318–1319.
4. Goodwin, F. K., Cowdry, R. W., and Webster, M. H. "Predictors of Drug Response in the Affective Disorders: Toward an Integrated Approach." In M. A. Lipton, A. DiMascio, and K. F. Killam (eds.), *Psychopharmacology: A Generation of Progress*. New York: Raven Press, 1978, pp. 1277–1288. Goodwin, F. K., and Potter, W. Z. "The Biology of Affective Illness: Amine Neurotransmitters and Drug Response. In J. O. Cole, A. F. Schatzberg, and F. H. Frazier (eds.), *Depression: Biology, Psychodynamics and Treatment*. New York: Plenum Press, 1978 pp. 41–73.
5. Goodwin, F. K., Cowdry, R. W., and Webster, M. H. "Predictors of Drug Response," pp. 1277–1288. Lindbrink, P., Jonsson, G., and Fuxe, K. "The Effect of Imipramine-Like Drugs and Antihistamine Drugs on Uptake Mechanisms in the Central Noradrenaline and 5-Hydroxytryptamine Neurons." *Neuropharmacology*, 1971, 10:521–536. Schildkraut, J. J. "The Catecholamine Hypothesis of Affective Disorders,"

pp. 509–522. Bunney, W. E., Jr., and Davis, J. M. "Norepinephrine in Depressive Reactions," pp. 483–494. Kessler, K. A. "Tricyclic Antidepressants: Mode of Action and Clinical Use." In M. A. Lipton, A. DiMascio, and K. F. Killam (eds.), *Psychopharmacology: A Generation of Progress*, pp. 1289–1302. Berger, P. A., and Barchas, J. D. "Biochemical Hypotheses of Affective Disorders." In J. D. Barchas, et al. (eds.), *Psychopharmacology, From Theory to Practice*. New York: Oxford University Press, 1977, pp. 151–173.

6. Schildkraut, J. J. "The Catecholamine Hypothesis of Affective Disorders," pp. 509–522. Bunney, W. E., Jr., and Davis, J. M. "Norepinephrine in Depressive Reactions," pp. 483–494.

7. Garver, D. L., and Davis, J. M. "Biogenic Amine Hypothesis of Affective Disorder." *Life Sciences*, 1979, 24:383–394.

8. Maas, J. W. "Biogenic Amines and Depression: Biochemical and Pharmacological Separation of Two Types of Depression." *Archives of General Psychiatry*, 1975, 32:1357–1361. Goodwin, F. K., Cowdry, R. W., and Webster, M. H. "Predictors of Drug Response," pp. 1277–1288.

9. Garver, D. L., and Davis, J. M. "Biogenic Amine Hypothesis," pp. 383–394. Mass, J. W. "Biogenic Amines and Depression," pp. 1357–1361. Goodwin, F. K., Cowdry, R. W., and Webster, M. H. "Predictors of Drug Response," pp. 1277–1288.

10. Hollister, L. E., Davis, K. L., and Berger, P. A. "Subtypes of Depression Based on Excretion of MHPG and Response to Nortriptyline." *Archives of General Psychiatry*, 1980, 37:1107–1110. Berger, P. Personal Communication.

11. Sulser, F., Vetulani, J., and Mobley, P. L. "Mode of Action of Antidepressant Drugs." *Biochemical Pharmacology*, 1978, 27:257–261. Rosloff, B. N., and Davis, J. M. "Effect of Iprindole on Norepinephrine Turnover and Transport." *Psychopharmacologia*, 1974, 40:53–63. Charney, D. S., Menkes, D. B., and Heninger, G. R. "Receptor Sensitivity and the Mechanism of Action of Antidepressant Treatment." *Archives of General Psychiatry*, 1981, 38:1160–1180. Berger, P. A., and Barchas, J. D. "Biochemical Hypotheses of Affective Disorders," pp. 151–173.

12. Sulser, F., Vetulani, J., and Mobley, P. L. "Action of Antidepressant Drugs," pp. 257–261. Rosloff, B. N., and Davis, J. M. "Effect of Iprindole," pp. 53–63. Charney, D. S., Menkes, D. B., and Heninger, G. R. "Receptor Sensitivity and Action of Antidepressant Treatment," pp. 1160–1180.

13. Rosenblatt, J. E., et al. "The Effect of Imipramine and Lithium on Alpha and Beta Receptors Binding in Rat Brain." *Brain Research*, 1979, 160:186–191. Sulser, F., Vetulani, J., and Mobley, P. L. "Action of Antidepressant Drugs," pp. 257–261. Charney, D. S., Menkes, D. B., and Heninger, G. R. "Receptor Sensitivity and Action of Antidepressant Treatment," pp. 1160–1180.

14. Kuffler, S. W., and Nicholls, J. B. *From Neuron to Brain*. Sunderland, Mass.: Sinauer Associates, 1976, pp. 385–390. Charney, D. S., Menkes,

D. B., and Heninger, G. R. "Sensitivity and Action of Antidepressant Treatment," pp. 1160–1180. Sulser, F., Vetulani, J., and Mobley, P. L. "Action of Antidepressant Drugs." pp. 257–261.

15. Sulser, F., Vetulani, J., and Mobley, P. L. "Action of Antidepressant Drugs," pp. 257–261. Lerer, B., Ebstein, R. P., and Belmaker, R. H. "Subsensitivity of Human Beta-Adrenergic Adenylate Cyclase After Salbutamol Treatment of Depression." *Psychopharmacology*, 1981, 75:169–172. Charney, D. S., Menkes, D. B., and Heninger, G. R. "Receptor Sensitivity and Action of Antidepressant Treatment," pp. 1160–1180.

16. Baldessarini, R. J. "Drugs and the Treatment of Psychiatric Disorders," pp. 391–447. Baldessarini, R. J. *Chemotherapy in Psychiatry.* Cambridge, Mass.: Harvard University Press, 1977, pp. 101–114. Kessler, K. A. "Tricyclic Antidepressants," pp. 1289–1302. Berger, P. A. "Antidepressant Medications and the Treatment of Depression." In J. D. Barchas et al. (eds.), *Psychopharmacology, From Theory to Practice*, pp. 174–207.

17. Racy, J., and Ward-Racy, E. A. "Tinnitus in Imipramine Therapy." *American Journal of Psychiatry*, 1980 137:854–855.

18. Hollister, L. E. "Current Antidepressant Drugs: Their Clinical Use." *Drugs*, 1981, 22:129–152. Shopsin, B. "Second Generation Antidepressants." *Journal of Clinical Psychiatry*, 1980, 41(12):45–56. Smith, R. S., Jr., and Ayd, F. J., Jr. "A Critical Appraisal of Amoxapine." *Journal of Clinical Psychiatry*, 1981, 42(6):238–242.

19. Berger, P. A. "Antidepressant Medications and Depression," pp. 174–207. Baldessarini, R. J. "Drugs and the Treatment of Psychiatric Disorders," pp. 391–447. Baldessarini, R. S. "Chemotherapy in Psychiatry," pp. 118-120.

20. Baldessarini, R. J. "Drugs and the Treatment of Psychiatric Disorders," pp. 391–447. Berger, P. A. "Antidepressant Medications and Depression," pp. 174–207. Baldessarini, R. J. "Chemotherapy in Psychiatry," p. 121.

Chapter 14

1. Krauthammer, C., and Klerman, G. L. "The Epidemiology of Mania." In B. Shopsin (ed.), *Manic Illness*. New York: Raven Press, 1979, pp. 11–28. Weissman, M. M., Myers, J. K., and Thompson, D. "Depression and Its Treatment in a U.S. Urban Community 1975–1976." *Archives of General Psychiatry*, 1981, 38:417–421.

2. American Psychiatric Association. *Diagnostic and Statistical Manual of Mental Disorders*, Third Edition. Washington, D.C.: American Psychiatric Association, 1980, p. 217.

3. Krauthammer, C., and Klerman, G. L. "The Epidemiology of Mania," pp. 11–28.

4. Mendelwicz, J., and Ranier, J. D. "Adoption Study Supporting Genetic Transmission in Manic-Depressive Illness." *Nature,* 1977, 268:327–329.

5. Krauthammer C., and Klerman, G. L. "The Epidemiology of Mania," pp. 11–28.

6. Kline, N. S. "A Narrative Account of Lithium Usage in Psychiatry." In S. Gershon and B. Shopsin (eds.), *Lithium, Its Role in Psychiatric Research and Treatment.* New York: Plenum Press, 1973, pp. 5–14. Gerbino, L., Oleshansky, M., and Gershon, M. "Clinical Use and Mode of Action of Lithium." In M. A. Lipton, A. DiMascio, and K. F. Killam (eds.), *Psychopharmacology: A Generation of Progress.* New York: Raven Press, 1978, pp. 1261–1275.

7. Kline, N. S. "Lithium Usage in Psychiatry," pp. 5–14. Baldessarini, R. J. "Drugs and the Treatment of Psychiatric Disorders." In A. G. Gilman, L. S. Goodman, and A. Gilman (eds.), *The Pharmacological Basis of Therapeutics.* New York: Macmillan, 1980, pp. 391–447.

8. Kline, N. S. "Lithium Usage in Psychiatry," pp. 5–14. Baldessarini, R. J. "Drugs and the Treatment of Psychiatric Disorders," pp. 391–447.

9. Schou, M. "Lithium as Prophylactic Agent in Unipolar Affective Illness." *Archives of General Psychiatry,* 1979, 36:849–851.

10. Bunney, W. E., Jr., et al. "A Behavioral-Biochemical Study of Lithium Treatment." *American Journal of Psychiatry,* 1969, 125:499–512.

11. Quitkin, F. M., Rifkin, A., and Klein, D. F. "Lithium in Other Psychiatric Disorders." In S. Gershon and B. Shopsin (eds.), *Lithium Research and Treatment,* pp. 295–315.

12. Goodwin, F. K., and Ebert, M. E. "Lithium in Mania: Clinical Trials and Controlled Studies." In S. Gershon and B. Shopsin (eds.), *Lithium, Research and Treatment,* pp. 237–252. Shopsin, B., Georgotas, A., and Kane, S. "Psychopharmacology of Mania." In B. Shopsin (ed.), *Manic Illness.* New York: Raven Press, 1979, pp. 177–218.

13. Mendlewicz, J., Fieve, R. R., and Stallone, F. "Relationship Between the Effectiveness of Lithium Therapy and Family History." *American Journal of Psychiatry,* 1973, 130:1011–1013.

14. Schou, M. "Prophylactic Lithium Maintenance Treatment in Recurrent Endogenous Affective Disorders." In S. Gershon and B. Shopsin (eds.), *Lithium, Research and Treatment,* pp. 269–294.

15. Gerbino, L., Oleshansky, M., and Gerson, M. "Use and Action of Lithium," pp. 1261–1275. Goodwin, F. K., and Zis, A. P. "Lithium in the Treatment of Mania." *Archives of General Psychiatry,* 1979, 36:835–844. Shopsin, B., Georgotas, A., and Kane, S. "Psychopharmacology of Mania," pp. 177–218.

16. Davis, J. M. "Overview: Maintenance Therapy in Psychiatry: II. Affective Disorders." *American Journal of Psychiatry,* 1976, 133:1–13. Stallone, F., et al. "The Use of Lithium in Affective Disorders, III: A Double-Blind Study of Prophylaxis in Bipolar Illness." *American Journal of Psychiatry,* 1973, 130:1006–1010.

17. Reifman, A., and Wyatt, R. J. "Lithium: A Brake in the Rising Cost of Mental Illness." *Archives of General Psychiatry,* 1980, 37:385–388.

18. Fieve, R. R. *Moodswing*. New York: Bantam Books, 1978.
19. Ibid., pp. 47–53.
20. Gerbino, L., Oleshansky, M., and Gershon, M. "Use and Action of Lithium", pp. 1261–1275. Fieve, R. R., Platman, S. R., and Plutchik, R. R. "The Use of Lithium in Affective Disorders: I. Acute Endogenous Depression." *American Journal of Psychiatry*, 1968, 125:487–491. Fieve, R. R. "Overview of Therapeutic and Prophylactic Trials with Lithium in Psychiatric Patients." In S. Gershon and B. Shopsin (eds.), *Lithium, Research and Treatment*, pp. 317–350.
21. Shopsin, B., Georgotas, A., and Kane, S. "Psychopharmacology of Mania," pp. 177–218. Bunney, W. E., Jr. "Psychopharmacology of the Switch Process in Affective Illness." In M. A. Lipton, A. DiMascio, and K. F. Killam (eds.), *Psychopharmacology: A Generation of Progress*, pp. 1249–1259. Jann, M. W., Bitar, A. H., and Rao, A. "Lithium Prophylaxis of Tricyclic-Antidepressant-Induced Mania in Bipolar Patients." *American Journal of Psychiatry*, 1982, 139:683–684.
22. Schou, M. "Lithium as Prophylactic Agent," pp. 849–851.
23. Klerman, G. L. "Long-Term Treatment of Affective Disorders." In M. A. Lipton, A. DiMascio, and K. F. Killam (eds.), *Psychopharmacology: A Generation of Progress*, pp. 1303–1311.
24. Sack, R. L., and De Fraites, E. "Lithium and the Treatment of Mania." In J. D. Barchas et al. (eds.), *Psychopharmacology, From Theory to Practice*. New York: Oxford University Press, 1977, pp. 208–225. Sheard, M. H. "The Biological Effects of Lithium." *Trends in Neuroscience*, 1980, 3:85–86. Gerbino, L., Oleshansky, M., and Gershon, M. "Use and Action of Lithium," pp. 1261–1275.
25. Belmaker, R. H. "Receptors, Adenylate Cyclase, Depression and Lithium." *Biological Psychiatry*, 1981, 16:333–350. Ebstein, R. P., Hermoni, M., and Belmaker, R. H. "The Effect of Lithium on Noradrenaline-Induced Cyclic AMP Accumulation in Rat Brain: Inhibition After Chronic Treatment and Absence of Supersensitivity." *Journal of Pharmacology and Experimental Therapeutics*, 1980, 213:161–167. Reches, A., Ebstein, R. P., and Belmaker, R. H. "Differential Effect of Lithium on Noradrenaline and Dopamine-Sensitive Accumulation of Cyclic AMP in Guinea Pig Brain." *Psychopharmacology*, 1978, 58:213–216.
26. Sack, R. L., and De Fraites, E. "Lithium and Mania," pp. 208–225.
27. Pert, A., et al. "Long-Term Treatment with Lithium Prevents the Development of Dopamine Receptor Supersensitivity." *Science*, 1978, 201:171–173. Rosenblatt, J. E., et al. "The Effect of Imipramine and Lithium on Alpha and Beta Receptor Binding in Rat Brain." *Brain Research*, 1979, 160:186–191. Hermoni, M., et al. "Chronic Lithium Prevents Reserpine-Induced Supersensitivity of Adenylate Cyclase." *Journal of Pharmacy and Pharmacology*, 1980, 32:510–511. Zohar, J., et al. "Lithium Does Not Prevent Agonist-Induced Subsensitivity of Human Adenylate Cyclase." *Biological Psychiatry*, 1982, 17:343–350.
28. Post, R. M., et al. "Cerebrospinal Fluid Norepinephrine in Affective Illness." *American Journal of Psychiatry*, 1978, 135:907–912.

29. Shopsin B., and Gershon, S. "Pharmacology-Toxicology of the Lithium Ion." In S. Gershon and B. Shopsin (eds.), *Lithium, Research and Treatment*, pp. 107–146. Walpert, E. A. "Major Affective Disorders." In H. I. Kaplan, A. M. Freedman, and B. J. Sadock (eds.), *Comprehensive Textbook of Psychiatry, Third Edition.* Baltimore: Williams & Wilkins, 1980, pp. 1319–1331. Fieve, R. R. "Lithium Therapy." In H. I. Kaplan, A. M. Freedman, and B. J. Sadock (eds.), *Comprehensive Textbook of Psychiatry, Third Edition.* pp. 2348–2352.

30. Fieve, R. R. "Lithium Therapy," pp. 2348–2352.

31. Sack, R. L., and De Fraites, E. "Lithium and Mania," pp. 208–225.

32. Shopsin, B., and Gershon, S. "Pharmacology–Toxicology of the Lithium Ion," pp. 107–146.

33. Ibid. Baldessarini, R. J. "Drugs and the Treatment of Psychiatric Disorders," pp. 391–447. Fieve, R. R. "Lithium Therapy," pp. 2348–2352.

34. Baldessarini, R. J. "Drugs and the Treatment of Psychiatric Disorders," pp. 391–447. Jenner, E. A. "Lithium and the Question of Kidney Damage." *Archives of General Psychiatry*, 1979, 36:888–890.

35. Jenner, E. A. "Lithium and Kidney Damage," pp. 888–890. Ramsey, T. A., and Cox, M. "Lithium and the Kidney: A Review." *American Journal of Psychiatry*, 1982, 139:443–449.

36. Ibid.

37. Ramsey, T. A., and Cox, M. "Lithium and the Kidney," pp. 443–449.

Chapter 15

1. Sharpless, S. "Hypnotics and Sedatives, I. The Barbiturates." In L. S. Goodman and A. Gilman (eds.), *The Pharmacological Basis of Therapeutics*, Third Edition. New York: Macmillan, 1965, pp. 105–128.

2. Allgulander, C. "Dependence on Sedative and Hypnotic Drugs, a Comparative Clinical and Social Study." *Acta Psychiatrica Scandinavica*, 1978, Sup. 270.

3. Baldessarini, R. J. "Drugs and the Treatment of Psychiatric Disorders." In A. G. Gilman, L. S. Goodman, and A. Gilman (eds.), *The Pharmacological Basis of Therapeutics.* Sixth Edition. New York: Macmillan, 1980, p. 436.

4. Ibid. Allgulander, C. "Dependence on Drugs," p. 13. *Physicians' Desk Reference*, Thirtieth Edition. Oradell, N.J.: Medical Economics, 1976.

5. Allgulander, C. "Dependence on Drugs," p. 13. Osol, A., Robertson, P., and Altschule, M. D. *The United States Dispensatory and Physicians Pharmacology.* Philadelphia: Lippencott, 1967.

6. Allgulander, C. "Dependence on Drugs," p. 13.

7. Harvey, S. C. "Hypnotics and Sedatives." In A. G. Gilman, L. S. Goodman, and A. Gilman (eds.), *The Pharmacological Basis of Therapeutics*, Sixth Edition, pp. 339–375. Jaffe, J. H. "Drug Addiction and Drug Abuse." In A. G. Gilman, L. S. Goodman, and A. Gilman (eds.), *The Pharmacological Basis of Therapeutics*, Sixth Edition, pp. 535–584.

8. Allgulander, C. "Dependence on Drugs," p. 13.

9. Harvey, S. C. "Hypnotics and Sedatives," pp. 339–375. Baldessarini, R. J. "Drugs and Psychiatric Disorders," p. 436.

10. Rickels, K. "Use of Antianxiety Agents in Anxious Outpatients." *Psychopharmacology*, 1978, 58:1–17.

11. Harvey, S. C. "Hypnotics and Sedatives," pp. 339–375. Baldessarini, R. J. "Drugs and Psychiatric Disorders," p. 436.

12. Balter, M. B., Levine, J., and Manheimer, D. I. "Cross National Study of the Extent of Antianxiety/Sedative Drug Use." *New England Journal of Medicine*, 1974, 290:769–774. Greenblatt, D. J., Shader, R. I., and Koch-Wesser J. "Psychotropic Drug Use in the Boston Area." *Archives of General Psychiatry*, 1975, 32:518–521. Hasday, J. D., and Karch, F. E. "Benzodiazepine Prescribing in a Family Medicine Center." *Journal of the American Medical Association*, 1981, 246:1321–1325. Parry, H. J., et al. "National Patterns of Psychotherapeutic Drug Use." *Archives of General Psychiatry*, 1973, 28:769–783.

13. Greenblatt, D. J., and Shader, R. I. "Pharmacotherapy of Anxiety with Benzodiazepines and Beta-Adrenergic Blockers." In A. Lipton, A. DiMascio, and K. F. Killam (eds.), *Psychopharmacology: A Generation of Progress*. New York: Raven Press, 1978, pp. 1381–1390.

14. Ibid.

15. Parry, H. J., et al. "National Patterns of Drug Use," pp. 769–783.

16. Balter, M. B., Levine, J., and Manheimer, D. I. "Study of Antianxiety/Sedative Drug Use," pp. 769–774.

17. Allgulander, C. "Dependence on Drugs." p. 13. Greenblatt, D. J., and Shader, R. I. "Dependence, Tolerance and Addiction to Benzodiazepines: Clinical and Pharmacokinetic Considerations." *Drug Metabolism Reviews*, 1978, 8:13–28.

18. Katz, R. L. "Drug Therapy: Sedatives and Tranquilizers." *New England Journal of Medicine*, 1972, 286:757–760. Rickels, K. "Benzodiazepines: Clinical Use Patterns." In S. I. Szara and J. P. Ludford (eds.), *Benzodiazepines: A Review of Research Results*. NIDA Research Monograph 33. Washington, D.C.: Department of Health and Human Services, 1980, pp. 43–60.

19. Rickels, K. "Use of Antianxiety Agents," pp. 1–17.

20. Reinhold, R. "Tranquilizer Prescriptions Drop Sharply; So Does Reported Incidence of Abuse." *New York Times*, 9 September 1980, p. C1. Rickels, K. "Benzodiazepines: Clinical Use Patterns," pp. 43–60.

21. Greenblatt, D. J., and Shader, R. I. "Dependence, Tolerance and Addiction," pp. 13–28. Marks, J. *The Benzodiazepines: Use, Overuse, Misuse, Abuse*. Baltimore: University Park Press, 1978. Rickels, K. "Benzodiazepines: Clinical Use Patterns," pp. 43–60. Greenblatt, D. J., and Shader, R. I. *Benzodiazepines and Clinical Practice*. New York: Raven Press, 1974, p. 61.

22. Baldessarini, R. J. *Chemotherapy in Psychiatry*. Cambridge, Mass.: Harvard University Press, 1977, p. 135. Davis, J. M. "Minor Tranquilizers, Sedatives, and Hypnotics." In H. I. Kaplan, A. M. Freedman, and B. J. Sadock (eds.), *Comprehensive Textbook of Psychiatry*, Third Edition.

Baltimore: Williams & Wilkins, 1980, pp. 2316–2333. Hasday, J. D., and Karsh, F. E. "Benzodiazepine Prescribing in a Family Medicine Center," pp. 1321–1325. Parry, H. J., et al. "National Patterns of Drug Use," pp. 769–783. Rickels, K. "Use of Antianxiety Agents," pp. 1–17.

23. American Psychiatric Association. *Diagnostic and Statistical Manual of Mental Disorders*, Third Edition. Washington, D.C.: American Psychiatric Association, 1980, pp. 225–233. Greenblatt, D. J., and Shader, R. I. *Benzodiazepines and Clinical Practice*, p. 63. Rickels, K. "Use of Antianxiety Agents," pp. 1–17. Nemiah, J. C. "Anxiety State. In H. I. Kaplan, A. M. Freedman, and B. J. Sadock (eds.), *Comprehensive Textbook of Psychiatry*, pp. 1483–1493. Baldessarini, R. J. "Drugs and Psychiatric Disorders," p. 436.

24. Baldessarini, R. J. "Drugs and Psychiatric Disorders," p. 441. Greenblatt, D. J., and Shader, R. I. *Benzodiazepines and Clinical Practice*, p. 63. Nemiah, J. C. "Anxiety State." pp. 1483–1493. Rickels, K. "Use of Antianxiety Agents," pp. 1–17.

25. Schatzberg, A. F., and Cole J. O. "Benzodiazepines in Depressive Disorders." *Archives of General Psychiatry*, 1978, 35:1359–1365. Rickels, K. "Use of Antianxiety Agents," pp. 1–17.

26. American Psychiatric Association. *DSM-III*, pp. 225–239.

27. Baldessarini, R. J. *Chemotherapy in Psychiatry*, p. 136. Rickels, K. "Use of Antianxiety Agents," pp. 1–17. Rickels, K. "Benzodiazepines: Clinical Use Patterns," pp. 43–60.

28. Rickels, K. "Benzodiazepines: Clinical Use Patterns," pp. 43–60. Rickels, K. "Use of Antianxiety Agents," pp. 1–17.

29. Baldessarini, R. J. "Drugs and Psychiatric Disorders," p. 436. American Psychiatric Association. *DSM-III*, pp. 225–239.

30. Appleton, W. S., and Davis, J. M. *Practical Clinical Psychopharmacology*. Baltimore: Williams & Wilkins, 1980, pp. 144–148. Klein, D. F., Zitrin, C. M., and Woerner, M. "Antidepressants, Anxiety, Panic and Phobia." In A. Lipton, A. DiMascio, and K. F. Killam (eds.), *Psychopharmacology: A Generation of Progress*, pp. 1401–1410.

31. Greenblatt, D. J., and Shader, R. I. *Benzodiazepines and Clinical Practice*, pp. 43–59. Iversen, S. D., and Iversen, L. L. *Behavioral Pharmacology*, Second Edition. New York: Oxford University Press, 1981, pp. 236–246.

32. Hesbacher, P. T., et al. "Setting, Patient, and Doctor Effects on Drug Response in Neurotic Patients: I. Differential Attrition, Dosage Deviation, and Side Reaction Responses to Treatment." *Psychopharmacologia*, 1970, 18:180–208. Hesbacher, P. T., et al. "Setting, Patient, and Doctor Effects on Drug Response in Neurotic Patients: II. Differential Improvement." *Psychopharmacologia*, 1970, 18:209–226.

33. Davis, J. M. "Tranquilizers, Sedatives, and Hypnotics," pp. 2316–2333. Greenblatt, D. J., and Shader, R. I. *Benzodiazepines and Clinical Practice*, pp. 61–101. Greenblatt, D. J., and Shader, R. I. "Pharmacotherapy of Anxiety," pp. 1381–1390.

34. Cooper, J. R., Bloom, F. E., and Roth, R. H. *The Biochemical Basis of Neuropharmacology*, Third Edition. New York: Oxford University Press,

1978, pp. 223–247. Kuffler, S. W., and Nicholls, J. G. *From Neuron to Brain*. Sunderland, Mass.: Sinauer, 1977, pp. 219–236.

35. Olsen, R. W. "Drug Interactions at the GABA Receptor-Ionophore Complex." *Annual Review of Pharmacological Toxicology*, 1982, 22:245–277. Tallman, J. F., Skolnik, P., and Gallagher, D. W. "Receptors for the Age of Anxiety: Pharmacology of the Benzodiazepines." *Science*, 1980, 207:274–281.

36. Gavish, M., and Snyder, S. H. "Benzodiazepine Recognition Sites on GABA Receptors." *Nature*, 1980, 287:651–652. Kuhar, M. "The Benzodiazepine Receptor: Anatomical Aspects." In S. I. Szara and J. P. Ludford (eds.), *Benzodiazepines: A Review of Research Results*, pp. 12–24. Macdonald, R., and Barker, J. L. "Benzodiazepines Specifically Modulate GABA-Mediated Postsynaptic Inhibition in Cultured Mammalian Neurons." *Nature*, 1978, 271:563–564. Olsen, R. W. "Drug Interactions at the GABA Receptor-Ionosphere Complex," pp. 245–277. Stratten, W. P., and Barnes, C. D. "Diazepam and Presynaptic Inhibition." *Neuropharmacology*, 1971, 10:685–696. Tallman, J. F., Skolnik, P., and Gallagher, D. W. "Receptors for the Age of Anxiety," pp. 274–281.

37. Ho, I. R., and Harris, R. A. "Mechanism of Action of Barbiturates." *Annual Review of Pharmacology*, 1981, 21:83–111. Huang, L.-Y.M., and Barker, J. L. "Pentobarbital: Stereospecific Action of (+) and (−) Isomers Revealed on Cultured Mammalian Neurons." *Science*, 1980, 207:195–197. Leeb-Lundberg, F., Snowman, A., and Olsen, R. W. "Barbiturate Receptor Sites Are Coupled to BZ Receptors." *Proceedings of the National Academy of Sciences (US)*, 1980, 77:7468–7472. Nicoll, R. "Selective Actions of Barbiturates on Synaptic Transmission." In A. Lipton, A. DiMascio, and K. F. Killam (eds.), *Psychopharmacology: A Generation of Progress*, pp. 1337–1348. Nicoll, R. "Pentobarbital: Action on Frog Motoneurons." *Brain Research*, 1975, 96:119–123. Olsen, R. W. "Drug Interactions at the GABA Receptor-Ionophore Complex," pp. 245–277. Ticku, M. K. "Interaction of Depressant, Convulsant and Anticonvulsant Barbiturates with the [^{3}H]diazepam Binding Site of the Benzodiazepine-GABA-Receptor Complex." *Biochemical Pharmacology*, 1981, 30:1573–1579.

38. Baldessarini, R. J. "Drugs and Psychiatric Disorders," p. 436. Davis, J. M. "Tranquilizers, Sedatives, and Hypnotics," pp. 2316–2333. Greenblatt, D., and Shader, R. I. *Benzodiazepines and Clinical Practice*, pp. 231–261. Harvey, S. C. "Hypnotics and Sedatives," pp. 339–375.

39. Baldessarini, R. J. "Drugs and Psychiatric Disorders." pp. 391–447. Davis, J. M. "Tranquilizers, Sedatives, and Hypnotics," pp. 2316–2333. Greenblatt, D., and Shader, R. I. *Benzodiazepines and Clinical Practice*, pp. 61–101.

40. Greenblatt, D., and Shader, R. I. *Benzodiazepines and Clinical Practice*, pp. 83, 84.

41. Salzman, C., et al. "Chlordiazepoxide-Induced Hostility in a Small Group Setting." *Archives of General Psychiatry*, 1974, 31:401–405.

42. Greenblatt, D., and Shader, R. I. *Benzodiazepines and Clinical Practice*,

pp. 231–235, 250–252. Harvey, S. C. "Hypnotics and Sedatives," pp. 339–375. *Physicians' Desk Reference,* Thirtieth Edition, pp. 543, 571–572, 1173, 1324, 1549–1550.
43. Davis, J. M. "Tranquilizers, Sedatives, and Hypnotics," pp. 2316–2333.
44. Ho, I. R., and Harris, R. A. "Action of Barbiturates," pp. 83–111.
45. Ritchie, M. J. "The Aliphatic Alcohols." In A. G. Gilman, L. S. Goodman, and A. Gilman (eds.), *The Pharmacological Basis of Therapeutics,* pp. 376–390.
46. Department of Health, Education and Welfare. *Alcohol and Health: Second Report to the U.S. Congress.* Washington, D.C.: DHEW Publication, 1974, (ADM) 75-212, pp. 79–92. Ritchie, M. J. "The Aliphatic Alcohols," pp. 376–390.
47. Harvey, S. C. "Hypnotics and Sedatives," pp. 339–375.
48. Baldessarini, R. J. "Drugs and Psychiatric Disorders," p. 441. Greenblatt, D., and Shader, R. I. *Benzodiazepines and Clinical Practice,* pp. 231–261. Harvey, S. C. "Hypnotics and Sedatives," pp. 339–375.

Chapter 16

1. Hubbell, J. G. "Danger! Prescription Drug Abuse." *Readers' Digest,* April 1980, pp. 100–104. Hughes, R., and Brewin, R. *The Tranquilizing of America.* New York: Harcourt Brace Jovanovich, 1979.
2. Szara, S. I. Introduction in S. I. Szara and J. P. Ludford (eds.), *Benzodiazepines: A Review of Research Results.* NIDA Research Monograph 33. Washington, D.C.: Department of Health and Human Services, 1980, pp. 1–3.
3. Brecher, E. M. *Licit and Illicit Drugs.* Boston: Little Brown, 1972, pp. 414–418.
4. Jaffe, J. "Drug Addiction and Drug Abuse." In A. G. Gilman, L. S. Goodman, and A. Gilman (eds.), *The Pharmacological Basis of Therapeutics,* Sixth Edition. New York: Macmillan, 1980, pp. 535–584.
5. American Psychiatric Association. *Diagnostic and Statistical Manual of Mental Disorders,* Third Edition. Washington, D.C.: American Psychiatric Association: 1980, p. 168. Department of Health, Education and Welfare. *Alcohol and Health: First Special Report to the U.S. Congress.* New York: Scribner's 1973, p. xv. Department of Health, Education and Welfare. *Alcohol and Health: Second Special Report to the U.S. Congress.* Washington, D.C.: DHEW Publication No. (ADM) 75-212, 1974, p. 20. Department of Health Education and Welfare. *Alcohol and Health: Third Special Report to the U.S. Congress.* Washington, D.C.: DHEW Publication ADM 78-569, 1978, p. 8. Hoffmann, F. G. *A Handbook on Drug and Alcohol Abuse: The Biomedical Aspects.* New York: Oxford University Press, 1975, p. 98. Mello, N. K., and Mendelson, J. H. "Alcohol and Human Behavior." *Handbook of Psychopharmacology,* 1978, 12:235–317.
6. Department of Health, Education and Welfare. *Third Special Report,* p. 12.

7. American Psychiatric Association. *DSM-III*, p. 168. Department of Health, Education and Welfare. *Third Special Report*, pp. 8, 12. Mello, N. K., and Mendelson, J. H. "Alcohol and Human Behavior," pp. 235–317.
8. Miller, F. "Back from Drugs: The Triumph of Johnny Cash." *Readers' Digest*, September 1970, pp. 85–89. Hubbell, J. G. "Danger! Prescription Drug Abuse," pp. 100–104.
9. Ford, B., with Chase, C. *The Times of My Life*. New York: Harper & Row, 1978.
10. Gordon, B. *I'm Dancing as Fast as I Can*. New York: Harper & Row, 1979.
11. Winokur, A., et al. "Withdrawal Reaction from Long-Term, Low Dosage Administration of Diazepam: A Double-Blind, Placebo-Controlled Study." *Archives of General Psychiatry*, 1980, 37:101–105. Hollister, L. E., Motzenbecker, F. P., and Dagan, R. O. "Withdrawal Reactions to Chlordiazepoxide (Librium)." *Psychopharmacologia*, 1961, 2:63–68.
12. Allgulander, C. "Dependence on Sedative and Hypnotic Drugs: A Comparative Clinical and Social Study." *Acta Psychiatrica Scandinavica*, sup. 270, 1978.
13. Baldessarini, R. J. *Chemotherapy in Psychiatry*. Cambridge, Mass.: Harvard University Press, 1977, p. 138. Baldessarini, R. J. "Drugs and the Treatment of Psychiatric Disorders." In A. G. Gilman, L. S. Goodman, and A. Gilman (eds.), *The Pharmacological Basis of Therapeutics*, Sixth Edition, pp. 391–447. Harvey, S. C. "Hypnotics and Sedatives." In A. G. Gilman, L. S. Goodman, and A. Gilman (eds.), *The Pharmacological Basis of Therapeutics*, Sixth Edition, pp. 339–375. Jaffe, J. "Drug Addiction and Abuse," pp. 535–584. Jarvik, M. E. "Drugs Used in the Treatment of Psychiatric Disorders." In L. S. Goodman, and A. Gilman (eds.), *The Pharmacological Basis of Therapeutics*, Third Edition. New York: Macmillan, 1965, pp. 159–214. Rickels, K. "Benzodiazepines: Clinical Use Patterns." In S. I. Szara, and J. P. Ludford (eds.), *Benzodiazepines: A Review*, pp. 43–63.
14. Griffiths, R. R., and Ator, N. A. "Benzodiazepine Self-Administration in Animals and Humans: A Comprehensive Review." In S. I. Szara, and J. P. Ludford (eds.), *Benzodiazepines: A Review*, pp. 22–36.
15. Ibid.
16. Ibid.
17. Allgulander, C. "Dependence on Sedative and Hypnotic Drugs." Baldessarini, R. J. "Drugs and Psychiatric Disorders," pp. 391–347. American Psychiatric Association. *DSM-III*, pp. 225–239.
18. Baldessarini, R. J. "Drugs and Psychiatric Disorders," pp. 391–447. Harvey, S. C. "Hypnotics and Sedatives," pp. 339–375.
19. Sharpless, S. "Hypnotics and Sedatives. I: The Barbiturates." In L. S. Goodman and A. Gilman (eds.), *The Pharmacological Basis of Therapeutics*, Third Edition, pp. 105–128. Jarvik, M. E. "Drugs Used in Treatment," pp. 159–214.
20. Ritchie, J. M. "The Aliphatic Alcohols." In L. S. Goodman and A. Gil-

man (eds.), *The Pharmacological Basis of Therapeutics*, Third Edition, pp. 143–158.

21. Davis, J. M. "Minor Tranquilizers." In H. I. Kaplan, A. M. Freedman, and B. J. Sadock (eds.), *Comprehensive Textbook of Psychiatry*, Third Edition. Baltimore: Williams & Wilkins, 1980, pp. 2316–2333. Jaffe, J. "Drug Addiction and Abuse," pp. 535–584.

22. Jaffe, J. "Drug Addiction and Abuse," pp. 538, 550.

23. Margules, D., and Stein, L. "Increase of 'Antianxiety' Activity and Tolerance of Behavioral Depression During Chronic Administration of Oxazepam." *Psychopharmacology*, 1968, 13:74–80.

24. Baldessarini, R. J. *Chemotherapy in Psychiatry*, p. 22. Davis, J. M. "Minor Tranquilizers," pp. 2316–2333. Greenblatt, D. J., and Shader, R. I. "Dependence, Tolerance and Addiction to Benzodiazepines: Clinical and Pharmacokinetic Considerations." *Drug Metabolism Reviews*, 1978, 8:13–28. Rickels, K. "Use of Antianxiety Agents in Anxious Outpatients." *Psychopharmacology*, 1978, 58:1–17.

25. Jarvik, M. E. "Drugs Used in the Treatment of Psychiatric Disorders." In L. S. Goodman and A. Gilman (eds.), *The Pharmacological Basis of Therapeutics*, Fourth Edition. New York: Macmillan, 1970, pp. 151–203.

26. Baldessarini, R. J. "Drugs and Psychiatric Disorders," pp. 391–447.

27. Baldessarini, R. J. *Chemotherapy in Psychiatry*, p. 133.

28. Ibid., p. 144.

29. Hollister, L. E., et al. "Long-Term Use of Diazepam." *Journal of the American Medical Association*, 1981, 246:1568–1570.

30. Greenblatt, D. J., and Shader, R. I. *Benzodiazepines in Clinical Practice*. New York: Raven Press, 1974, p. 24. Gottschalk, L. A. "Pharmacokinetics of the Minor Tranquilizers and Clinical Response." In M. A. Lipton, A. DiMascio, and K. F. Killam (eds.), *Psychopharmacology: A Generation of Progress*. New York: Raven Press, 1978, pp. 975–985.

31. Hollister, L. E., et al. "Use of Diazepam," pp. 1568–1570.

32. Rickels, K. "Benzodiazepines: Clinical Use Patterns," pp. 43–63.

33. Tyrer, P. "Dependence on Benzodiazepines." *British Journal of Psychiatry*, 1980, 137:576–577.

34. Based on symptoms given by Jaffe, J. "Drug Addiction and Abuse," pp. 535–584.

35. Ibid.

36. Ibid. Baldessarini, R. J. *Chemotherapy in Psychiatry*, p. 133. Pevnick, J. S., Jasinski, D. R., and Haertzen, C. A. "Abrupt Withdrawal from Therapeutically Administered Diazepam." *Archives of General Psychiatry*, 1978, 35:995–998. Winokur, A., et al. "Withdrawal Reaction from Diazepam," pp. 101–105.

37. Hollister, L. E., Motzenbecker, F. P., and Dagan, R. O. "Withdrawal Reactions to Chlordiazepoxide (Librium)," pp. 63–68.

38. Rickels, K. "Use of Antianxiety Agents," pp. 1–17.

39. Winokur, A., et al. "Withdrawal Reaction from Diazepam," pp. 101–105.

40. Hasday, J. D., and Karch, F. E. "Benzodiazepine Prescribing in a Family Medicine Center." *Journal of the American Medical Association*, 1981, 246:1321–1325.
41. Tyrer, P. "Drug Treatment of Psychiatric Patients in General Practice." *British Medical Journal, 1978*, (October 7): 1008–1010.
42. Rickels, K. "Benzodiazepines: Clinical Use Patterns," pp. 43–63.
43. Tyrer, P. "Dependence on Benzodiazepines," pp. 576–577.
44. Rickels, K. "Use of Antianxiety Agents," pp. 1–17.

Chapter 17

1. Leo, J. "Danger Is Found in Some Remedies." *New York Times*, 9 February 1969, p. 92.
2. Karasu, T. B. "The Ethics of Psychotherapy." *American Journal of Psychiatry*, 1980, 137:1502–1515. Frances, A., and Clarkin, J. F. "No Treatment as the Prescription of Choice." *Archives of General Psychiatry*, 1981, 38:542–545. Leo, J. "Danger in Some Remedies," p. 92.
3. Roth, M. "Psychiatry and Its Critics." *Canadian Psychiatric Association Journal*, 1972, 17:343–350. Talbot, J. A. "Radical Psychiatry: An Appreciation of the Issues." *American Journal of Psychiatry*, 1972, 131:121–128.
4. Szasz, T. *The Myth of Mental Illness*, Revised Edition. New York: Harper & Row, 1974. Laing, R. D. *The Politics of Experience*. New York: Ballantine, 1967. Cerrolaza, M. "The Nebulous Scope of Current Psychiatry." *Comprehensive Psychiatry*, 1973, 14:299–309.
5. Roth, M. "Psychiatry and Its Critics," pp. 343–350. Cerrolaza, M. "Nebulous Scope of Psychiatry," pp. 299–309. Szasz, T. *The Myth of Mental Illness*. Laing, R. D. *Politics of Experience*.
6. Szasz, T. *The Myth of Mental Illness*, Revised Edition. New York: Harper & Row, 1974. Szasz, T. "Schizophrenia: The Sacred Symbol of Psychiatry." *British Journal of Psychiatry, 1976*, 129:308–316.
7. Kety, S. "From Rationalization to Reason." *American Journal of Psychiatry*, 1974, 131:957–963. Kety, S. "Disorders of the Human Brain." *Scientific American*, September 1979, 241:202–214. Ford, M. "The Psychiatrist's Double Bind: The Right to Refuse Medication." *American Journal of Psychiatry*, 1980, 137:332–339. Moore, M. S. "Some Myths About 'Mental Illness.'" *Archives of General Psychiatry*, 1975, 32:1483–1497.
8. Cerrolaza, M. "Nebulous Scope of Psychiatry," pp. 299–309. Kety, S. "From Rationalization to Reason," pp. 957–963.
9. Applebaum, P. "Can Mental Patients Say No to Drugs?" *New York Times Magazine*, 21 March 1982, 46:51–59. Stone, A. A. "Recent Mental Health Litigation: A Critical Perspective." *American Journal of Psychiatry*, 1977, 134:273–279. Stone, A. A. "Mental Health and the Law: A System in Transition." Washington, D.C.: National Institute of Mental Health, Center for Studies of Crime and Delinquency, DHEW Publication No. (ADM) 75-176, pp. 1–4.

10. Bloch, S., and Reddaway, P. *Psychiatric Terror: How Soviet Psychiatry Is Used to Suppress Dissent.* New York: Basic Books, 1977, p. 61.
11. Ibid., p. 107.
12. Ibid.
13. Ibid., pp. 105–127. Reich, W. "The Case of General Grigorenko: A Psychiatric Reexamination of a Soviet Dissident." *Psychiatry*, 1980, 43:303–323.
14. Reich, W. "The Case of General Grigorenko," pp. 303–323.
15. Ibid. Bloch, S., and Reddaway, P. *Psychiatric Terror*, pp. 115–116.
16. Bloch, S., and Reddaway, P. *Psychiatric Terror*, pp. 350–398. Reich, W. "Soviet Psychiatry on Trial. *Commentary*, 1978, 65:40–48.
17. Reich, W. "Soviet Psychiatry on Trial," pp. 40–48. Reich, W. "The Spectrum Concept of Schizophrenia: Problems for Diagnostic Practice." *Archives of General Psychiatry*, 1975, 32:489–498.
18. Stone, A. A. "The Right to Refuse Treatment: Why Psychiatrists Should and Can Make It Work." *Archives of General Psychiatry*, 1981, 38:358–362. Ford, M. "The Psychiatrist's Double Bind," pp. 332–339.
19. Bloch, S., and Reddaway, P. *Psychiatric Terror*, p. 45. Stone, A. A. "The Right to Refuse," pp. 358–362.
20. Mill, J. S. "On Liberty." In J. M. Robson (ed.), *Collected Works of John Stuart Mill*, Volume XVIII, Toronto: University of Toronto Press, 1977, pp. 223–224.
21. Ford, M. "The Psychiatrist's Double Bind," pp. 332–339. Stone, A. A. "Mental Health and the Law," pp. 25–42, 56.
22. Reiser, S. J. "Refusing Treatment for Mental Illness: Historical and Ethical Dimensions." *American Journal of Psychiatry*, 1980, 137:329–331. Stone, A. A. "Mental Health and the Law," pp. 25–42, 56. Reich, W. "Soviet Psychiatry on Trial," pp. 40–48. Meisel, A., Roth, L. H., and Lidz, C. W. "Toward a Model of the Legal Doctrine of Informed Consent." *American Journal of Psychiatry*, 1977, 134:285–289.
23. Gutheil, T. G., Shapiro, R., and St. Clair, L. "Legal Guardianship in Drug Refusal: An Illusory Solution." *American Journal of Psychiatry*, 1980, 137:347–352.
24. Applebaum, P. S., Mirkin, S. A., and Bateman, A. L. "Empirical Assessment of Competency to Consent to Psychiatric Hospitalization." *American Journal of Psychiatry*, 1981, 138:1170–1176. Applebaum, P. S., and Gutheil, T. G. "Drug Refusals: A Study of Psychiatric Inpatients." *American Journal of Psychiatry*, 1980, 137:347–352. Owens, H. "When Is a Voluntary Commitment Really Voluntary?" *American Journal of Orthopsychiatry*, 1977, 47:104–110. Perr, I. "Effect of the Rennie Decision on Private Hospitalization in New Jersey: Two Case Reports." *American Journal of Psychiatry*, 1981, 138:774–778. Applebaum, P. "Can Mental Patients Say No to Drugs?" pp. 51–59. Stone, A. A. "Mental Health and the Law," pp. 25–42, 56. Stone, A. A. "The Right to Refuse," pp. 358–362.
25. Stone, A. A. "Mental Health and the Law," pp. 25–42, 56. Ford, M. "The Psychiatrist's Double Bind," pp. 332–339.

26. Stone, A. A. "Mental Health and the Law," pp. 88–89.
27. Ford, M. "The Psychiatrist's Double Bind," pp. 332–339. Schultz, S. "The Boston State Hospital Case: A Conflict of Civil Liberties and True Liberalism." *American Journal of Psychiatry*, 1982, 139:183–188. Applebaum, P. "Can Mental Patients Say No to Drugs?" pp. 51–59. Curran, W. J. "The Management of Psychiatric Patients: Courts, Patients' Representatives, and the Refusal of Treatment." *New England Journal of Medicine*, 1980, 302:1297–1299. Applebaum, P. S., and Gutheil, T. G. "The Boston State Hospital Case: 'Involuntary Mind Control,' the Constitution, and the 'Right to Rot.'" *American Journal of Psychiatry*, 1980, 137:720–723.
28. Ford, M. "The Psychiatrist's Double Bind," pp. 332–339. Applebaum, P. "Can Mental Patients Say No to Drugs?" pp. 51–59. Applebaum, P. S., and Gutheil, T. G. "The Boston State Hospital Case," pp. 720–723. Meisel, A., Roth, L. H., and Lidz, C. W. "Legal Doctrine of Informed Consent," pp. 285–289.
29. Applebaum, P. "Can Mental Patients Say No to Drugs?" pp. 51–59. Meisel, A., Roth, L. H., and Lidz, C. W. "Legal Doctrine of Informed Consent," pp. 285–289.
30. Ford, M. "The Psychiatrist's Double Bind," pp. 332–339. Gutheil, T. G. "In Search of True Freedom: Drug Refusal, Involuntary Medication, and 'Rotting with Your Rights on.'" *American Journal of Psychiatry*, 1980, 137:327–328. Lebegue, B., and Clark, L. D. "Incompetence to Refuse Treatment: A Necessary Condition for Civil Commitment." *American Journal of Psychiatry*, 1981, 138:1075–1077.
31. Ford, M. "The Psychiatrist's Double Bind," pp. 332–339. Applebaum, P. S., and Gutheil, T. G. "The Boston State Hospital Case," pp. 720–723. Stone, A. A. "The Right to Refuse," pp. 358–362.
32. Gutheil, T. G. "In Search of Freedom," pp. 327–328. Ford, M. "The Psychiatrist's Double Bind," pp. 332–339. Applebaum, P. S., and Gutheil, T. G. "The Boston State Hospital Case," pp. 720–723. Stone, A. A. "The Right to Refuse," pp. 358–362.
33. Stone, A. A. "The Right to Refuse," pp. 358–362.
34. Ibid.
35. Ibid. Applebaum, P. "Can Mental Patients Say No to Drugs?" pp. 51–59. Curran, W. J. "Management of Psychiatric Patients," pp. 1297–1299. Applebaum, P. S., and Gutheil, T. G. "The Boston State Hospital Case," pp. 720–723.
36. Stone, A. A. "The Right to Refuse," pp. 358–362.
37. Gutheil, T. G., Shapiro, R., and St. Clair, L. "Legal Guardianship," pp. 347–352.
38. Perr, I. "Effect of the Rennie Decision," pp. 774–778.
39. Ibid. Ford, M. "The Psychiatrist's Double Bind," pp. 332–339. Stone, A. A. "Overview: The Right to Treatment." *American Journal of Psychiatry*, 1975, 132:1125–1134. Applebaum, P. "Can Mental Patients Say No to Drugs?" pp. 51–59. Applebaum, P. S., and Gutheil, T. G. "The Boston State Hospital Case," pp. 720–723. Schultz, S. "The Bos-

ton State Hospital Case," pp. 183–188. Gutheil, T. G., Shapiro, R., and St. Clair, L. "Legal Guardianship," pp. 347–352. Stone, A. A. "Recent Mental Health Litigation," 1975, pp. 273–279.

40. Ford, M. "The Psychiatrist's Double Bind," pp. 332–339. Gutheil, T. G., Shapiro, R., and St. Clair, L. "Legal Guardianship," pp. 347–352. Stone, A. A. "Recent Mental Health Litigation," 1975, pp. 273–279. Schultz, S. "The Boston State Hospital Case," pp. 183–188.

41. Stone, A. A. "Overview: Right to Treatment," pp. 1125–1134. Ford, M. "The Psychiatrist's Double Bind," pp. 332–339. Stone, A. A. "Recent Mental Health Litigation," pp. 273–279. Whitmer, G. E. "From Hospitals to Jails: The Fate of California's Deinstitutionalized Mentally Ill." *American Journal of Orthopsychiatry*, 1980, 50:65–75. Bonovitz, J. C., and Bonovitz, J. S. "Diversion of the Mentally Ill into the Criminal Justice System." *American Journal of Psychiatry*, 1981, 138:973–976.

42. Stone, A. A. "The Right to Refuse," pp. 358–362. Lebegue, B., and Clark, L. D. "Incompetence to Refuse Treatment," pp. 1075–1077.

43. Lebegue, B., and Clark, L. D. "Incompetence to Refuse Treatment," pp. 1075–1077. Applebaum, P. S., and Gutheil, T. G. "The Boston State Hospital Case," pp. 720–723.

44. Stone, A. A. "The Right to Refuse," pp. 358–362. Stone, A. A. "Mental Health and the Law," pp. 88–89.

45. Stone, A. A. "The Right to Refuse," pp. 358–362. Stone, A. A. "Mental Health and the Law," pp. 88–89. Karasu, T. B. "Ethics of Psychotherapy," pp. 1502–1515. Wooton, B. "Psychiatry, Ethics, and the Criminal Law." *British Journal of Psychiatry*, 1980, 136:525–532.

46. American Psychiatric Association. *Diagnostic and Statistical Manual of Mental Disorders*, Third Edition. Washington, D.C.: American Psychiatric Association, 1980. Roth, M. "Psychiatry and Its Critics," pp. 343–350.

47. Spitzer, R. L., and Wilson, P. "Nosology and the Official Psychiatric Nomenclature." In H. I. Kaplan, A. M. Freedman, and B. J. Sadock (eds.), *Comprehensive Textbook of Psychiatry*, Second Edition. Baltimore: Williams & Wilkins, 1980, pp. 826–845.

Index